# MRI Registry Review

# MRI Registry Review

## Tech to Tech Questions and Answers

Stephen J. Powers
*South Coast Hospital Group*
*Fall River, MA, USA*

WILEY Blackwell

This edition first published 2021
© 2021 John Wiley & Sons Ltd

The right of Stephen J. Powers to be identified as the author of this work has been asserted in accordance with law.

*Registered Offices*
John Wiley & Sons, Inc., 111 River Street, Hoboken, NJ 07030, USA
John Wiley & Sons Ltd, The Atrium, Southern Gate, Chichester, West Sussex, PO19 8SQ, UK

*Editorial Office*
9600 Garsington Road, Oxford, OX4 2DQ, UK

For details of our global editorial offices, customer services, and more information about Wiley products visit us at www.wiley.com.

Wiley also publishes its books in a variety of electronic formats and by print-on-demand. Some content that appears in standard print versions of this book may not be available in other formats.

*Library of Congress Cataloging-in-Publication Data*

Names: Powers, Stephen J. (Senior MRI technologist), author. | Powers,
    Stephen J. (Senior MRI technologist) MRI physics.
Title: MRI registry review : tech to tech questions and answers / Stephen
    J. Powers.
Description: First edition. | Hoboken, NJ : Wiley-Blackwell, [2021] |
    Includes index.
Identifiers: LCCN 2021007232 (print) | LCCN 2021007233 (ebook) | ISBN
    9781119757931 (paperback) | ISBN 9781119757948 (adobe pdf) | ISBN
    9781119757955 (epub)
Subjects: MESH: Magnetic Resonance Imaging | Patient Care | Problems and
    Exercises
Classification: LCC RC386.6.M34  (print) | LCC RC386.6.M34  (ebook) | NLM
    WN 18.2  | DDC 616.07/548–dc23
LC record available at https://lccn.loc.gov/2021007232
LC ebook record available at https://lccn.loc.gov/2021007233

Cover Design: Wiley
Cover Image: Courtesy of Stephen Powers

Set in 11.5/13.5pts STIX Two Text by SPi Global, Pondicherry, India
Printed and bound by CPI Group (UK) Ltd, Croydon, CR0 4YY

C9781119757931_071021

# Contents

About the Author . . . . . . . . . . . . . . . . . . . . . . . . . . . . . . . . . . . . . .vii

Acknowledgments and Advice . . . . . . . . . . . . . . . . . . . . . . . . . viii

**1** Patient Interactions and Management. . . . . . . . . . . . . . . . . . . . .1

    Below are artist renditions of the anatomical position: . . . . . . . . . . . . . . . .31

    Section 1 Patient Interactions and Management Answers. . . . . . . . . . . . . .31

    Enlarged Pictures . . . . . . . . . . . . . . . . . . . . . . . . . . . . . . . . . . . . . . . .43

**2** Parameters, Image Formation, Data Acquisition . . . . . . . . . . . . . . .45

    Section 2: Parameters, Image Formation, Data Acquisition: Answers . . . . . .93

    Section 2 Question 41–54. . . . . . . . . . . . . . . . . . . . . . . . . . . . . . . . . .96

    Section 2: Enlarged Illustrations . . . . . . . . . . . . . . . . . . . . . . . . . . . . .107

    Section 2 Questions 41–54. . . . . . . . . . . . . . . . . . . . . . . . . . . . . . . . .108

    Chapter 2: Parameters, Image Formation, Data Acquisition . . . . . . . . . . .109

**3** Pulse Sequences and MRI Math. . . . . . . . . . . . . . . . . . . . . . . . .113

    Use the factors listed below for Questions 200–203 . . . . . . . . . . . . . . . . .154

    Section 3 MR Pulse Sequences and MR Math Answers. . . . . . . . . . . . . . .177

**4** Procedures . . . . . . . . . . . . . . . . . . . . . . . . . . . . . . . . . . . . . . . .192

    Image Artifacts . . . . . . . . . . . . . . . . . . . . . . . . . . . . . . . . . . . . . . . .275

    Remember, Choose the Answer Most Correct . . . . . . . . . . . . . . . . . . . . .275

    Artifacts. . . . . . . . . . . . . . . . . . . . . . . . . . . . . . . . . . . . . . . . . . . . .293

    Miscellaneous Questions: . . . . . . . . . . . . . . . . . . . . . . . . . . . . . . . . .297

        Helpful Anatomy: The Basil Ganglia . . . . . . . . . . . . . . . . . . . . . . .307

        Helpful Anatomy: T2 Axials of Basil Ganglia . . . . . . . . . . . . . . . . . .308

        Helpful Anatomy: T1 Sagittal of Brain Stem. . . . . . . . . . . . . . . . . . .308

        Other Helpful Anatomy: The Brachial Plexus. . . . . . . . . . . . . . . . . . .309

    The Boney Pelvis . . . . . . . . . . . . . . . . . . . . . . . . . . . . . . . . . . . . . . .310

    The Cranial Nerves: O O O T T A F A G V A H. . . . . . . . . . . . . . . . . . . . .311

Cranial Nerve: Study . . . . . . . . . . . . . . . . . . . . . . . . . . . . . . . . . . . . . . . . .312

T1 and T2 Contrast Differences in the Brain . . . . . . . . . . . . . . . . . . . . . . .312

Answers . . . . . . . . . . . . . . . . . . . . . . . . . . . . . . . . . . . . . . . . . . . . . . . . . .313

MRI Math . . . . . . . . . . . . . . . . . . . . . . . . . . . . . . . . . . . . . . . . . . . . . . .339

Glossary . . . . . . . . . . . . . . . . . . . . . . . . . . . . . . . . . . . . . . . . . . . . . . . .350

Index . . . . . . . . . . . . . . . . . . . . . . . . . . . . . . . . . . . . . . . . . . . . . . . . . . .375

# About the Author

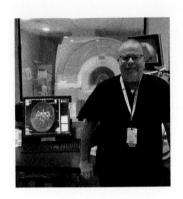

Stephen J. Powers B.S.R.T. (R), (CT), (MR)

- Author of MRI Physics: Tech to Tech Explanations.
- Received Associate Degree: Radiologic Technology, Northeastern University, Boston, MA, 1981, and Bachelor of Science: Health and Social Sciences, Roger Williams University, Bristol, RI, 1996.
- Course Instructor: MR Physics, Cross-Sectional Anatomy and Pathology for the MR Certificate Program at Massasoit Community College, Brockton, MA, 1999–2014.
- Clinical MR Instructor for Mass. College of Pharmacy, 2010–2014.
- Former MR Applications Specialist: GE Health Care.
- Presently Staff MR Technologist for Southcoast Hospital Group.
- Married with two sons and living in Southeastern Massachusetts, USA.

# Acknowledgments and Advice

This one's for you Mom.

Again I have to say Thank you to my wonderful wife Suzanne for her patience and understanding while I wrote a Registry Review on the heels of MR Physics book.

Next, thank you to **Alicia Webb R.T.R.(MR)** my friend, and colleague for her artistic talents in drawing all the illustrations in this text book. You were a great help in drawing the different illustrations that are hard to find, image, or otherwise display. Thanks Allie!!

Rachelle (Pebbles), Thanks for my inside cover Picture. **You're my favorite!!**

I also need to thank my past and present coworkers as well as my many former students for encouraging me to write this Registry Review book.

It only seemed natural that I should put together a registry review on the heels *MRI Physics: Tech to Tech Explanations*. While the advanced registry asks questions in no particular order, I have sectioned my questions by topic in a similar order to my physics book. I hope this mirroring will assist you in working on your weaknesses and not your strengths. For example, if you're weak on pulse sequences or MRI Math, I want to have all those kinds of questions grouped together and to be able to easily find further answers and explanations in the corresponding chapters in *MRI Physics: Tech to Tech Explanations*. The various sections will state the corresponding chapter(s) in *MRI Physics: Tech to Tech Explanations* hopefully making your studying easier.

I wish you good luck and good fortune in your career as an MRI Technologist. Radiology has been very good to me. I hope it is as good to you and then some. Remember, **failing to prepare is prepping to fail.**

Peace,

Steve

# Some Test-Taking Advice

I'd like to offer some suggestions, words of advice, and some FYI's on how to give yourself the best chance to successfully pass the exam.

Sitting for this exam is a big and important next step in your imaging career. Stress will be the word of the day, week, month, or even year while you prep. Chill, it's not that bad.

- **My first advice is: Scan baby Scan.** You learn a lot by doing. You know more than you think you do. You really do. Review anatomy while you scan. Look for artifacts. Studying while you scan is not just looking at questions during a sequence.
- **Practice answering questions.** Take time a few times a week to answer some questions. Correct them, the ones you got wrong, research the correct answer. This works on your weakness not your strengths.
- Try this: Answer 30 questions in 25 minutes. Train to work under some pressure. Not a lot, just some. Navy Seals train under pressure, we're not Navy seals.
- Here is a technique I've learned over the years. Explain a concept or topic to somebody. When you verbalize something, you also learn. It makes things make sense. Things start to make more sense when you talk it out. Albert Einstein is credited with saying: "You don't really understand something unless you can explain it to your Grandmother." I love that saying, try it and see if it helps.

Now for Test Day

- Don't schedule an appointment time for too early in the morning, if you oversleep, get stuck in traffic, and run late you'll be even more stressed. It's difficult to focus when stressed, you'll make bad choices.
- Be 30 minutes early! You may lose your right to sit for the test if you are late.
- Get a good night sleep the night before.
- **Don't stay up late cramming for the test**, you'll end up getting confused, frustrated, even more stressed and worse yet, less confident.
- Have a good breakfast. Don't be hungry. The brain works on sugar.
- *Raise your hand to ask bathroom breaks! Not more than 10 minutes long.*
- You will be photographed, and Palm printed.
- *Have two valid forms of I.D.: Driver's license, Passport, or ARRT card.*
- You can't bring anything in with you. Not even your pocketbook. They'll give you a locker. Dress in layers as testing locations vary in temperature.
- You'll need a calculator. One will be issued to you or use the one on the PC desktop.

- There is an 18-minute tutorial about the test. *You also need to acknowledge a Non-Disclosure agreement within two minutes after the tutorial.*
- *Then use the dry erase board!!!*
- On the dry erase board, jot notes/formulas or mnemonics before you start.
- You have 3.5 hours (210 minutes) to do 220 questions. That math is 1:00 minute per question. That may not sound like much but it really is. Many questions you'll find easy and answer quickly giving more time as you go.
- Also don't be in a rush to leave. Give yourself at least 5+ hours for the whole thing so you don't have to rush. Answers made in haste well. . ..
- Others questions will need some thought, so, DON'T DWELL ON A QUESTION FOR A LONG TIME. You must answer it, mark it as a go back, and continue. You can't move on to question 22 until you answer question 21.
- **Practice answering questions at home**!!! Practice, Practice, Practice!!

Eliminating Possible Answers

- 20 of the 220 are pilot questions which don't count for or against you. You don't know which ones they are.
- There are four answers given for each question. 1 or 2 will probably be out-right wrong. Eliminate as many as possible to make the right choice.
- Look for answers that are ridiculous. If they're too high/low or just plain can't be correct, they're probably wrong. Res Ipsa Loquitur applies.
- Look for grammatical clues. If the grammar doesn't make sense on a fill in the blank or has a wrong syntax, it's **probably** not the correct answer.
- Let one question answer another. One question may ask what the Gyromagnetic Ratio of Hydrogen is, while another one may have previously stated it while asking another question.
- **MR Terminology should be generic (not vendor specific).** They may make a cross vendor terminology chart available to you. It's not fair to ask questions using Hitachi terms if you have only scanned on GE or Siemens.
- Don't get crazy trying to know every little aspect or detail of every concept involved in MRI. You are not working on your PhD. The test is designed to test your general knowledge in MRI, anatomy, and patient care.
- As for the previous statement, the exam is looking to see if you know basic anatomy, landmarks, and the consequences of your actions when changing scan parameters. For example, what happens to SNR if you decrease the FOV? or, if you increase the TR, what happens to the T1 weighting?
- When you are done with the exam, you'll get a preliminary score. This is not your final official score. You'll get that in about three weeks.

- *Raise your hand when you're done*. You can't just get up and leave. You need to be re-palm printed before being dismissed.

The next page has a chart taken directly from the ARRT website which shows you the breakdown.

Visit the ARRT website for complete information:

WWW.ARRT.ORG

What to Know
- You may ask what do I need to know? I could say, "Know-it-All," but that's a ridiculous answer and not possible. Key on the major topics.
- The next page has a breakdown of each Category and Subcategory. Note where the concentration of the questions is heaviest: **Image Production and Procedures**.
- **Patient Care and Safety**: Includes Medical-Legal, terminology. and Ethics.
- **Image Production**: Know the consequences of your actions.
- **Procedures**: Know your Anatomy.

# ARRT Advanced MRI Exam Breakdown Displayed Below

| Content category | Number of scored questions |
|---|---|
| Patient care | 18 |
| *Patient Interactions and Management (18)* | |
| Safety | 20 |
| *MRI Screening and Safety (20)* | |
| Image Production | 105 |
| *Physical Principles of Image Formation (39)* | |
| *Sequence Parameters and Options (36)* | |
| *Data Acquisition, Processing, and Storage (30)* | |
| Procedures | 57 |
| *Neurological (25)* | |
| *Body (15)* | |
| *Musculoskeletal (17)* | |
| Total | 200 |

What's the Time Breakdown?
- The Tutorial = 18 minutes, and 2 minutes for the Non-disclosure agreement. 20 minutes total.
- A maximum of 3.5 hours to answer questions.
- Finally, 10 minutes for a post exam survey. Max. total time of four hours to complete exam.

| MRI | | | |
|---|---|---|---|
| Scored Items | 200 | NDA Time (in min.) | 2 |
| Pilot Items | 20 | Test Time (in hours) | 3.5 |
| Total Items | 220 | Survey Time (in min.) | 10 |
| Tutorial Time (in min.) | 18 | Total Time (in hours) | 4.0 |

Those charts, like I said, on the previous page are snapshots taken directly from the ARRT website. I'm betting you have seen them already. I show them as a reminder so you don't have to look them up again.

- For additional/more complete info go to WWW.ARRT.ORG
  What about if I've already taken the Advanced Certification exam and have to renew your certification?
  Then you are looking for CQR (Continuous Qualifications Requirement) information.
- Go to WWW.ARRT.ORG/CQR

*Here's the skinny on the CQR.*
- You have to take the SSA every 10 years for Credential earned **after 1 January 2011**.
- You need to complete CQR every 10 years for each eligible discipline. You have three years to complete the process. The ARRT notifies you when your window opens.
- Take the Structured Self-Assessment (SSA). **It is not a Pass/Fail test. There is no Fail.** You'll get CEU's assigned to you to improve on deficiencies based on your score. This system makes you work on your weakness and not your strengths. That's a good thing.
- Yes, most of those assigned CEU's apply to your Biennium.

# Cross-Vendor Terminology: Page 1

I include these Cross-Vendor Terminology lists only for your reference while studying. Don't try to memorize/learn every single term.

| General Electric | Siemens | Sequence/Term | Philips | Hitachi | Toshiba |
|---|---|---|---|---|---|
| SPIN ECHO | SPIN ECHO | Spin Echo | SPIN ECHO | SPIN ECHO | SPIN ECHO |
| GRE | GRE | Gradient Recalled Echo | FAST FIELD ECHO | FIELD ECHO | GE |
| SPGR | FLASH | Spoiled Gradient Echo | T1-FFE | RF SPOILED, SARGE, RSSG | FAST FE |
| GRASS | FISP | Coherent Gradient Echo | FFE | REPHASED SARGE | SSPF |
| SSFP | PSIF | Steady State Precession | T2-FFE | Time Reversed SARGE | None |
| FIESTA | True FISP | True FISP | BALANCE FE | Balanced SARGE, BASG | True SSFP |
| FIESTA-C | CISS | True FISP/Dual Excitation | None | Phase Balanced SARGE | None |
| None | DESS | Dual Echo Steady State | None | None | None |
| MERGE | MEDIC | Combined Multi Echo Gradient Echo | M-FFE | NONE | NONE |
| 3D FGRE, 3D FAST SPGR | MP-RAGE | Ultrafast 3D Gradient Echo | 3D-TFE | MP-RAGE | 3DFAST-FE |
| FAST GRE, FAST SPGR | TURBO FLASH | Ultrafast Gradient Echo | TFE | RGE | FAST FE |
| LAVA | VIBE | 3D Interpolated Gradient Echo | THRIVE | TIGRE | NONE |
| eDWI | REVEAL | Body Diffusion Weighted | DWIBS | NONE | VISION |

| General Electric | Siemens | Sequence/Term | Philips | Hitachi | Toshiba |
| --- | --- | --- | --- | --- | --- |
| SWAN | SWI | Susceptibility Weighting | VENOUS BOLD | NONE | NONE |
| TRICKS | TWIST | Dynamic MRA w/manipulated k-Space | 4D-TRAK | NONE | NONE |
| VIBRANT | VIEWS | High Res. Breast imaging | BLISS | NONE | RADIANCE |
| INHANCE INFLOW IR | NATIVE TRUE FISP | Non Contrast Angio True FISP | TRANCE | VASC FSE | FBI, CIA |
| CARTIGRAM | MAP IT | Parametric T2 Mapping | NONE | NONE | NONE |
| IR, MPIR, | IR, TIR | Inversion Recovery | IR | IR | IR |
| STIR | STIR | Short TI | STIR | STIR | IR |
| FLAIR | TURBO FLAIR | Long TI | FLAIR | FLAIR | FASTFLAIR |
| FSE | TSE | Fast Spin Echo | TSE | FSE | FSE |
| SSFSE | HASTE | Single Shot Fast Spin Echo | SS-TSE | SSFSE | FASE |
| FR-FSE | RESTORE | Fast Spin Echo with Crusher pulse | DRIVE | DE-FSE | T2 PUL FSE |
| NONE | HYPERECHO | Hyper Echo | NONE | NONE | NONE |
| CUBE | SPACE | 3D FSE | VISTA | NONE | NONE |
| ETL | TURBO FACTOR | Number of Echoes | TURBO FACTOR | SHOT FACTOR | ETL |
| ECHO SPACING | ECHO SPACING | Time between echoes | ECHO SPACING | INTER ECHO TIME (ITE) | ECHO SPACING |
| EPI | EPI | Echo Planar | EPI | EPI | EPI |
| ADC | ADC | Apparent Diffusion Coefficient Map | ADC | ADC MAP | ADC |

# Cross Vendor Terminology Page 2

| General Electric | Siemens | | Philips | Hitachi | Tosiba |
|---|---|---|---|---|---|
| FIBERTRACK | DTI FIBER TRACK | DTI Tractography or Tractography | FIBERTRACK | NONE | NONE |
| NONE | TURBO GSE | Turbo Gradient Spine echo | GRASE | NONE | NONE |
| PROPELLER | BLADE | MOTION CORRECTION | MULIVANE | RADAR | JET |
| BODY PROPELLER | BLADE | | NONE | NONE | NONE |
| ASSET | m-SENSE | PARALLEL IMAGING | SENSE | RAPID | SPEEDER |
| ARC | GRAPPA | | NONE | NONE | NONE |
| 2D/3D CSI | NONE | BRAIN SPECTRO | NONE | NONE | NONE |
| PROSE | 3D CSI | PROSTATE | NONE | NONE | NONE |
| BREASE | GRACE | BREAST | NONE | NONE | NONE |
| FLOURO TRIGGER/ SMART PREP | CARE BOLUS | CONTRAST BOLUS TIMING | BOLUS TRACK | FLUTE | VISUAL PREP |
| | | SCANNING PARAMETERS | | | |
| SPACING | DIST. FACTOR (% OF SLICE THICK) | DISTANCE BETWEEN SLICES | GAP | INTERVAL | GAP |
| PARTIAL FOV | RECTANGULAR FOV | RECTANGULAR FOV | RECTANGULAR FOV | RECTANGULAR FOV | RECTANGULAR FOV |
| REC. B/W (in kHz) | BANDWIDTH (Hz/pixel) | BANDWIDTH | FAT/WATER SHIFT/PIXEL | BANDWIDTH | BANDWIDTH |
| VARIABLE B/W | OPTIMIZED B/W | ADJUSTIBLE BANDWIDTH | OPTIMIZED B/W | VARIABLE B/W | MATCHED B/W |

| General Electric | Siemens | Philips | Hitachi | Tosiba |
|---|---|---|---|---|
| NPW | PHASE OVERSAMPLING | OVERSAMPLING/ANTI ALIASING | FOLD OVER SUPPRESSION | ANTI WRAP | PHASE WRAP SUPPRESSION |
| FRACTIONAL NEX | HALF NEX | PARTIAL K SPACE FILLING | HALF SCAN | HALF SCAN | AFI |
| PARTIAL ECHO | ASYMETRIC ECHO | PARTIAL ECHO | PARTIAL ECHO | HALF ECHO | |
| FLOW COMP | GMN (GRADIENT MOTION NULLING) | FLOW RELATED MOTION CORRECTION | FLAG/FLOW COMP | GR | FC |
| RAMP PULSE | TONE | VARIABLE RF PULSE | TONE | SSP | ISCE |
| MTC | MTC/MTS | MAGNETIZATION TRANSFER | MTC | MTC | SORS-STC |
| FAT-SAT | FAT SAT | CHEMICAL PREP PULSE | SPIR | FAT SAT | MSOFT |
| WATER EXCITATION | WATER EXCITATION | WATER EXCITATION | PROSET | WATER EXCITATION | PASTA |
| IDEAL | DIXON | DIXON TECHNIQUE | NONE | FATSEP | NONE |
| SAT PULSE | PRESAT | SPATIAL PREP PULSES | REST | PRE SAT | PRE SAT |
| CONCATINATED SAT | TRAVELING SAT | MOVING SATURATION PULSE | TRAVEL REST | SEQUENTIAL PRE SAT | BFAST |
| PURE | NORMALIZE | MULTI CHANNEL COIL SIG. CORRECTION | CLEAR | NATURAL | NONE |
| ELLIPTICAL CENTRIC | ELLIPTICAL SCANNING | CENTRAL K-SPACE FILL (FOR MRA) | CENTRA | PEAKS | DRKS |

# 1 Patient Interactions and Management

This section will concentrate on the many aspects of Patient Care including: patient monitoring, safety, and some legal/ethical aspects of taking care of a patient. There are/will be approximately 30 questions on the subject of patient care. The breakdown is listed below.

- Ethics + Legal ≈ 4
- Screening/Safety ≈ 11
- Patient assessment/Monitoring ≈ 6
- Communication skills ≈ 5
- Infection control ≈ 4 (a.k.a. aseptic technique)

Answers will be provided at the end of each section. There will be some discussions/explanations as to the how's/why's/what's for select questions. Also, I will point out/explain why some of the choices were not the correct answer. This is another way of learning. Remember, it's ok to fail here at home so you don't fail at the testing site.

1. Informed consent consists of all the following except?

|   |   |   |
|---|---|---|
| A. | Age and ability to understand statements | ☐ |
| B. | Right to stop and refuse further imaging treatment | ☐ |
| C. | Alternate imaging methods | ☐ |
| D. | Patients have all rights to bring suit | ☐ |

*MRI Registry Review: Tech to Tech Questions and Answers*, First Edition. Stephen J. Powers.
© 2021 John Wiley & Sons Ltd. Published 2021 by John Wiley & Sons Ltd.

**2.** What is the FDA safe Gauss line limit?

> **A.** 0.5 Gauss ☐
> **B.** 5 Gauss ☐
> **C.** 50 Gauss ☐
> **D.** 5 T ☐

**3.** A systolic blood pressure of below 100 is a sign of?

> **A.** Hypertension ☐
> **B.** Hyperglycemia ☐
> **C.** Cardiac arrest ☐
> **D.** Hypotension ☐

**4.** What is libel?

> **A.** Chance for a mistake ☐
> **B.** A true statement made to purposely defame a person's reputation ☐
> **C.** A false statement made to purposely defame a person's reputation ☐
> **D.** A new kind of oral contrast ☐

**5.** Res Ipsa Loquitur means "It speaks for itself". It implies that:

> **A.** There was a breach in duty harm resulting ☐
> **B.** The results are in question ☐
> **C.** A principle that the occurrence of an accident implies that negligence caused the incident ☐
> **D.** A and C ☐

**6.** What are the signs of cardiac arrest?

> **A.** No pulse ☐
> **B.** Cyanosis ☐
> **C.** Patient is unresponsive ☐
> **D.** All the above ☐

**7.** What are the contraindications for administering gadolinium?

| | |
|---|---|
| **A.** There are none | ☐ |
| **B.** C.O.P.D | ☐ |
| **C.** Renal impairment | ☐ |
| **D.** Allergy to iodine | ☐ |

**8.** What condition requires the patient to wear a mask?

| | |
|---|---|
| **A.** There are none | ☐ |
| **B.** C.O.P.D | ☐ |
| **C.** Tuberculosis | ☐ |
| **D.** Pneumonia | ☐ |

**9.** A patient on contact precautions requires technologists to wear?

| | |
|---|---|
| **A.** HazMat suits | ☐ |
| **B.** Gown, gloves, and mask | ☐ |
| **C.** Gown and gloves | ☐ |
| **D.** Eye protection | ☐ |

**10.** True or False: All patients require at least visual and verbal monitoring.

**11.** What is the preferred method to R/O metallic foreign body?

| | |
|---|---|
| **A.** Hi resolution CT | ☐ |
| **B.** P/A and lateral X-ray views of the orbits | ☐ |
| **C.** Panorex views of the orbits | ☐ |
| **D.** Visual exam by the radiologist | ☐ |

**12.** What is the accepted practice for administering gadolinium to a nursing mother?

| | |
|---|---|
| **A.** Gadolinium is not excreted thru breast milk | ☐ |
| **B.** Pump and dump for the next 24 hours | ☐ |
| **C.** Don't give them gadolinium | ☐ |
| **D.** All the above | ☐ |

**13.** What instrument is used to take a patient blood pressure?

| A. Laryngoscope | ☐ |
| B. Pulse Ox | ☐ |
| C. Sphygmomanometer | ☐ |
| D. Osteotome | ☐ |

**14.** What is a potential effect is emesis?

| A. Hives | ☐ |
| B. Hypertension | ☐ |
| C. Jaundice | ☐ |
| D. Dehydration | ☐ |

**15.** A patient on respiratory precautions requires technologists to wear?

| A. HazMat suits | ☐ |
| B. Gown, gloves, and mask | ☐ |
| C. Gown and gloves | ☐ |
| D. Eye protection | ☐ |

**16.** The localization light can possibly cause eye damage. True or False?

**17.** Why does the I.V. bag need to be above the heart at all times?

| A. Avoid infection | ☐ |
| B. Avoid blood back flow | ☐ |
| C. Avoid air bubbles | ☐ |
| D. B and C | ☐ |

**18.** Which is not a concern during a quench?

| A. Combustion | ☐ |
| B. Frost bite | ☐ |
| C. Room pressure increases | ☐ |
| D. Asphyxiation | ☐ |

**19.** Who needs to be monitored?

A. Only sedated patients ☐
B. The elderly ☐
C. Pediatric ☐
D. All patients ☐

**20.** RF irradiation is expressed as SAR. SAR is measured in:

A. kilowatts/min ☐
B. W/g ☐
C. W/kg ☐
D. What's/kg ☐

**21.** A patient with high BUN and creatinine values may have what condition?

A. Renal infection ☐
B. Renal artery stenosis ☐
C. Renal insufficiency ☐
D. Renal cysts ☐

**22.** True or False: Gadolinium will not cross a non-intact BBB.

**23.** Several factors influence the patient's ability to dissipate heat including all but:

A. Ambient room temperature ☐
B. Coil type ☐
C. Altitude ☐
D. RF amplitude ☐

**24.** Which sequence has the highest amount of time-varying magnetic fields?

A. Gradient recalled ☐
B. Spin echo ☐
C. Fast spin echo ☐
D. Echo planar ☐

**25.** Which sequence has the highest amount of RF applied to the patient?

| | |
|---|---|
| **A.** Turbo spin echo | ☐ |
| **B.** Gradient echo | ☐ |
| **C.** Spin echo | ☐ |
| **D.** MRA | ☐ |

**26.** Individuals with pacemakers should remain outside the _____ fringe field line?

| | |
|---|---|
| **A.** 5.0 Gauss | ☐ |
| **B.** 50 Gauss | ☐ |
| **C.** 2.0 Gauss | ☐ |
| **D.** 0.5 Gauss | ☐ |

**27.** FDA limits for heating due to RF is limited to:

| | |
|---|---|
| **A.** 0.5 °C in normal mode | ☐ |
| **B.** 1.0 °C in first mode | ☐ |
| **C.** 1.5 °C in either mode | ☐ |
| **D.** A and B | ☐ |

**28.** True or False: Resistive magnets should be quenched if a heavy object is drawn into it.

**29.** The attractive force that a ferrous object will see 5 feet from the bore depends on:

| | |
|---|---|
| **A.** Size of the object | ☐ |
| **B.** Field strength | ☐ |
| **C.** Metallic properties of object | ☐ |
| **D.** All the above | ☐ |

**30.** 5 Gauss is also known as:

| | |
|---|---|
| **A.** 0.5 mT | ☐ |
| **B.** 5 mT | ☐ |
| **C.** They don't convert | ☐ |
| **D.** 0.05 mT | ☐ |

**31.** True or False: Objects closest to isocenter are more likely to heat from RF exposure.

**32.** Who obtains informed consent?

|  |  |
|---|---|
| **A.** R.N | ☐ |
| **B.** R.T.R | ☐ |
| **C.** M.D. or D.O. | ☐ |
| **D.** Unit Secretary | ☐ |

**33.** Why do sedated patient need to be N.P.O.?

|  |  |
|---|---|
| **A.** Diabetes | ☐ |
| **B.** Risk of vomiting | ☐ |
| **C.** Airway managing | ☐ |
| **D.** B and C | ☐ |

**34.** Common signs and symptoms of an allergic reaction are:

|  |  |
|---|---|
| **A.** Emesis | ☐ |
| **B.** Dyspnea | ☐ |
| **C.** Urticaria | ☐ |
| **D.** All the above | ☐ |

**35.** True or False: When imaging for a Wilms tumor, you would be scanning a child's abdomen.

**36.** What is the noise level (dB) limit inside of the bore?

|  |  |
|---|---|
| **A.** 14.0 dB | ☐ |
| **B.** There is none | ☐ |
| **C.** 100 dB | ☐ |
| **D.** 140 dB | ☐ |

**37.** True or False: Objects away from isocenter see the highest amount of magnetic field change during a sequence.

**38.** Photo phosphenes can be induced during an MRI by _____.

**39.** In the event of a quench, the scan room should be evacuated to avoid

_____.

|  |  |
|---|---|
| **A.** RF burns | ☐ |
| **B.** Hearing loss | ☐ |
| **C.** Frost bite and asphyxiation | ☐ |
| **D.** B and C | ☐ |

**40.** A slight increase in body temperature is a common occurrence when exposed to _____.

| | |
|---|---|
| **A.** The static magnetic field | ☐ |
| **B.** Gradients | ☐ |
| **C.** RF | ☐ |
| **D.** All the above | ☐ |

**41.** The amount of RF deposited into the body is depends on _____.

| | |
|---|---|
| **A.** Strength of the RF field | ☐ |
| **B.** TE | ☐ |
| **C.** Flip angle | ☐ |
| **D.** A and C | ☐ |

**42.** DTPA, a chelating agent, is used to _____.

| | |
|---|---|
| **A.** Prevent rapid excretion by the kidneys | ☐ |
| **B.** Allow permeability through the BBB | ☐ |
| **C.** Decrease toxicity of gadolinium | ☐ |
| **D.** All the above | ☐ |

**43.** Extra caution when giving gadolinium is advised in cases of:

| | |
|---|---|
| **A.** Decreased renal function | ☐ |
| **B.** Known allergy to gadolinium | ☐ |
| **C.** History of sickle cell anemia | ☐ |
| **D.** All of these | ☐ |

**44.** Normal enhancing structures outside of the BBB include all but the _____.

| | |
|---|---|
| **A.** Dural sinuses | ☐ |
| **B.** Pituitary stalk and gland | ☐ |
| **C.** Basal ganglia | ☐ |
| **D.** Choroid plexus | ☐ |

**45.** _____ is the most common cryogen used to maintain superconductivity.

- **A.** Oxygen ☐
- **B.** Hydrogen ☐
- **C.** Helium ☐
- **D.** Nitrogen ☐

**46.** At isocenter, the unit of magnetic strength is measured in _____ while outside of the scanner it is measured in _____.

- **A.** Gauss, Watts ☐
- **B.** Gauss, Tesla ☐
- **C.** Tesla, Gauss ☐
- **D.** Watts, MHz ☐

**47.** True or False: A tympanoplasty is a contraindication for the patient to have an MRI.

**48.** The SAR limits are:

- **A.** 4 W/kg Body and 3 W/kg Head ☐
- **B.** 3 W/kg Body and 4 W/kg Head ☐
- **C.** 4 kW/kg Body and 3 kW/kg Head ☐
- **D.** 40 W/kg Body and 30 W/kg Head ☐

**49.** Sudden and rapid loss of superconductivity due to the release of cryogens describes a _____.

- **A.** Quatrain ☐
- **B.** Quadrilateral ☐
- **C.** Quadrant ☐
- **D.** Quench ☐

**50.** How often should imaging coils be inspected for safety?

- **A.** Monthly ☐
- **B.** Quarterly ☐
- **C.** Annually ☐
- **D.** Every time you use them ☐

**51.** Copper lining in the walls, windows, floor, and door designed to keep RF out of the scan room is called the _____?

|   |   |
|---|---|
| **A.** Shielding | ☐ |
| **B.** Faraday cage | ☐ |
| **C.** Faraday induction | ☐ |
| **D.** Passive shielding | ☐ |

**52.** Two typical sites to check a pulse is the _____ and the _____.

|   |   |
|---|---|
| **A.** Wrist and Carotids | ☐ |
| **B.** Femoral and Pedal | ☐ |
| **C.** Temporal and Wrist | ☐ |
| **D.** with a B/P cuff and Doppler | ☐ |

**53.** The hematocrit is an indicator of what?

|   |   |
|---|---|
| **A.** Volume of red blood cells | ☐ |
| **B.** Hemoglobin level | ☐ |
| **C.** Sickle cell anemia | ☐ |
| **D.** Liver function | ☐ |

**54.** What anatomical area would you image for bowel and bladder dysfunction?

|   |   |
|---|---|
| **A.** Brachial plexus | ☐ |
| **B.** Thoraco-lumbar junction | ☐ |
| **C.** Sacral plexus | ☐ |
| **D.** Cerebral pontine angle | ☐ |

**55.** When imaging, what part of the patient's EKG trace can increase/elevate?

|   |   |
|---|---|
| **A.** P wave | ☐ |
| **B.** T wave | ☐ |
| **C.** Q wave | ☐ |
| **D.** QRS complex | ☐ |

**56.** What condition is the result of decreased blood supply to bone?

A. Septic necrosis ☐
B. Hemangioma ☐
C. Avascular necrosis ☐
D. Hemangioma ☐

**57.** Islet cells are found in which organ?

A. Kidney ☐
B. Pancreas ☐
C. Liver ☐
D. Conus medullaris ☐

**58.** What part of the femur is most often affected by avascular necrosis?

A. Femoral head ☐
B. Lesser trochanter ☐
C. Surgical neck ☐
D. Mid shaft ☐

**59.** What imaging plane best demonstrates the Achilles tendon?

A. Axial ☐
B. Coronal ☐
C. Sagittal ☐

**60.** The prostate is located where in relation to the bladder?

A. Anterior and superior ☐
B. Inferior and anterior ☐
C. Inferior and posterior ☐
D. Superior and posterior ☐

**61.** What sequence is most sensitive to M.S. plaques?

A. GRE ☐
B. FSE/TSE ☐
C. T2 FLAIR ☐
D. T1 FLAIR ☐

**62.** What blood vessel has the greatest pressure?

A. Aortic arch ☐
B. Pulmonary veins ☐
C. Renal arteries ☐
D. Coronary artery ☐

**63.** T wave elevation during an MRI is an example of _____.

A. Patient anxiety ☐
B. Magneto-hemodynamic effect ☐
C. Equipment failure ☐
D. Loose skin contacts ☐

**64.** The sciatic nerve originates from the _____?

A. Sacral plexus ☐
B. L2/3 ☐
C. Upper thigh ☐
D. Medulla oblongata ☐

**65.** What is the first branch off the abdominal aorta?

A. Renal ☐
B. Celiac ☐
C. Superior mesenteric ☐
D. Inferior mesenteric ☐

**66.** Fringe magnetic fields are controlled/limited by _____.

A. Passive and active shimming ☐
B. Passive and active shielding ☐
C. Faraday cage ☐
D. Cryostat ☐

**67.** What structure in the brain is responsible for CSF production?

A. The ventricles ☐
B. Corpus collosum ☐
C. Arachnoid mater ☐
D. Choroid plexus ☐

**68.** The nerve affected by carpal tunnel syndrome is the _____?

| | |
|---|---|
| **A.** Median | ☐ |
| **B.** Carpal | ☐ |
| **C.** Ulna | ☐ |
| **D.** Brachialis longus | ☐ |

**69.** The pituitary stalk is also known as the _____.

| | |
|---|---|
| **A.** Infrundibulum | ☐ |
| **B.** Infundibulum | ☐ |
| **C.** Peduncle | ☐ |
| **D.** Falx cerebri | ☐ |

**70.** The venous drainage of the liver in through what major vessel?

| | |
|---|---|
| **A.** Portal vein | ☐ |
| **B.** IVC | ☐ |
| **C.** Hepatic veins | ☐ |
| **D.** Superior mesenteric vein | ☐ |

**71.** What is the first branch major branch off the aortic arch?

| | |
|---|---|
| **A.** Brachiocephalic | ☐ |
| **B.** Left common carotid | ☐ |
| **C.** Subclavian | ☐ |
| **D.** Tertiary | ☐ |

**72.** True or False: There are two ligamentum teres in the body. One each in the liver and hip.

**73.** _____ is the mechanism used by the kidneys for filtration.

| | |
|---|---|
| **A.** Glomus | ☐ |
| **B.** Osmosis | ☐ |
| **C.** Reverse osmosis | ☐ |
| **D.** Glomular | ☐ |

**74.** Serum creatinine is a blood test used to monitor the function of the _____?

| | |
|---|---|
| **A.** Liver | ☐ |
| **B.** Spleen | ☐ |
| **C.** Adrenals | ☐ |
| **D.** Kidneys | ☐ |

**75.** The ACL is best seen in the _____ plane?

|  |  |
|---|---|
| **A.** Axial | ☐ |
| **B.** Sagittal | ☐ |
| **C.** Coronal | ☐ |

**76.** What heart chamber is the most anterior?

|  |  |
|---|---|
| **A.** Right ventricle | ☐ |
| **B.** Left ventricle | ☐ |
| **C.** Left atrium | ☐ |
| **D.** Right atrium | ☐ |

**77.** What heart chamber is the most posterior?

|  |  |
|---|---|
| **A.** Right ventricle | ☐ |
| **B.** Left ventricle | ☐ |
| **C.** Left atrium | ☐ |
| **D.** Right atrium | ☐ |

**78.** In the pediatric brain, the best sequence to show gray/white matter differentiation is?

|  |  |
|---|---|
| **A.** FSE | ☐ |
| **B.** GRE | ☐ |
| **C.** T2 FLAIR | ☐ |
| **D.** STIR | ☐ |

**79.** What plane is useful for visualizing scoliosis in the spine?

|  |  |
|---|---|
| **A.** Axial | ☐ |
| **B.** Sagittal | ☐ |
| **C.** Oblique | ☐ |
| **D.** Coronal | ☐ |

**80.** Imaging for suspected Arnold Chiari, you should concentrate on the?

|  |  |
|---|---|
| **A.** Ventricles | ☐ |
| **B.** Frontal lobe | ☐ |
| **C.** Temporal lobe | ☐ |
| **D.** Cerebellum | ☐ |

**81.** A patient's hematocrit is a measure of _____?

| | |
|---|---|
| **A.** Volume % of RBC's | ☐ |
| **B.** Platelets | ☐ |
| **C.** White blood cells | ☐ |
| **D.** Hemoglobin | ☐ |

**82.** An infectious process will cause an increased _____ count.

| | |
|---|---|
| **A.** RBC's | ☐ |
| **B.** Platelets | ☐ |
| **C.** White blood cells | ☐ |
| **D.** Hemoglobin | ☐ |

**83.** What nerve roots typically make up the lumbar plexus?

| | |
|---|---|
| **A.** L-3 to 5 | ☐ |
| **B.** L 1 to 5 | ☐ |
| **C.** L1-4 | ☐ |
| **D.** L 3-S1 | ☐ |

**84.** Dyspnea is used to describe.

| | |
|---|---|
| **A.** Difficulty urinating | ☐ |
| **B.** Unable to swallow | ☐ |
| **C.** Difficulty breathing | ☐ |
| **D.** Unable to smell | ☐ |

**85.** Difficulty swallowing is known as:

| | |
|---|---|
| **A.** Dysphagia | ☐ |
| **B.** Disnuclear | ☐ |
| **C.** Dysarthria | ☐ |
| **D.** Decarbonate | ☐ |

**86.** Inability to speak is known as:

| | |
|---|---|
| **A.** Aphagia | ☐ |
| **B.** Disassociation | ☐ |
| **C.** Dysarthria | ☐ |
| **D.** Disarticulate | ☐ |

**87.** The vertebral arteries originate from the _____?

    **A.** Aorta ☐
    **B.** Carotids ☐
    **C.** Subclavian's ☐
    **D.** Jugular's ☐

**88.** A tangled collection of blood vessels is called a _____.

    **A.** Hematoma ☐
    **B.** Hemangioma ☐
    **C.** Hemorrhoid ☐
    **D.** Hyoid ☐

**89.** What nerve is affected by Bell's palsy?

    **A.** 5th ☐
    **B.** 6th ☐
    **C.** 7th ☐
    **D.** 8th ☐

**90.** Of the 12 cranial nerves, which 2 have the largest diameter?

    **A.** Olfactory and optic ☐
    **B.** Optic and trigeminal ☐
    **C.** Olfactory and trigeminal ☐
    **D.** Trigeminal and acoustic ☐

**91.** Imaging a patient for "Anosmia," you would concentrate on the _____.

    **A.** First cranial nerve ☐
    **B.** Mandible ☐
    **C.** Fifth cranial nerve ☐
    **D.** Soft tissue neck ☐

**92.** In a patient having bowel and bladder dysfunction, you should image the?

    **A.** Brachial plexus ☐
    **B.** Brain ☐
    **C.** Thoraco-lumbar region ☐
    **D.** Soft tissue neck ☐

**93.** What are the three layers of Meninges?

| | |
|---|---|
| **A.** Cortex, medulla, and pia | ☐ |
| **B.** Pia, dura, and arachnoid | ☐ |
| **C.** Pia, dura, and scleral | ☐ |
| **D.** Plea, dura, and subarachnoid | ☐ |

**94.** Of the three meninges, the inner most is _____ and the outer most is the _____.

| | |
|---|---|
| **A.** Dura and pia | ☐ |
| **B.** Arachnoid and dura | ☐ |
| **C.** Pia and arachnoid | ☐ |
| **D.** Pia and dura | ☐ |

**95.** What is the sequence of choice for suspected hemorrhage in the brain?

| | |
|---|---|
| **A.** T1 | ☐ |
| **B.** GRE | ☐ |
| **C.** STIR | ☐ |
| **D.** FSE | ☐ |

**96.** What nerve is affected by chronic long-term hiccups?

| | |
|---|---|
| **A.** Abducens | ☐ |
| **B.** Glossal-pharyngeal | ☐ |
| **C.** Hippocampal | ☐ |
| **D.** Vagus | ☐ |

**97.** If a patient is having a vasovagal/syncopal episode, they may demonstrate signs of?

| | |
|---|---|
| **A.** Rapid heart rate | ☐ |
| **B.** Low B/P | ☐ |
| **C.** Diaphoresis | ☐ |
| **D.** All of these | ☐ |

**98.** Syncope is commonly known as:

| | |
|---|---|
| **A.** Grand mal seizure | ☐ |
| **B.** Tinnitus | ☐ |
| **C.** Fainting | ☐ |
| **D.** Palsy | ☐ |

**99.** Common causes of syncope are?

A. Hypovolemia ☐
B. Low blood sugar ☐
C. Hypotension ☐
D. All of these ☐

**100.** Which arteries carry de-oxygenated blood?

A. Carotids ☐
B. Coronary ☐
C. Pulmonary ☐
D. SVC ☐

**101.** An Erythrocyte is a _____.

A. WBC ☐
B. RBC ☐
C. Stem cell ☐
D. Platelet ☐

**102.** Another name for hives is _____.

A. Acne ☐
B. Urticaria ☐
C. Dermatitis ☐
D. Rash ☐

**103.** A "Patent" airway means it is _____.

A. Absent ☐
B. Closed ☐
C. Open ☐
D. Constricted ☐

**104.** True or False: Oxygen is considered a medication and requires an MD order.

A. True ☐
B. False ☐

**105.** The patient is left semi-prone, with right leg bent up for support, the face is pointed downward slightly to decrease the risk of aspiration. This is called the _____ position.

| | |
|---|---|
| **A.** Trendelenburg | ☐ |
| **B.** L.A.O | ☐ |
| **C.** Recovery or Sims | ☐ |
| **D.** Left lateral recumbent | ☐ |

**106.** Discussing a patient's medical history with someone whom has no right to know it is not only a HIPPA violation but also _____.

| | |
|---|---|
| **A.** Libel | ☐ |
| **B.** Perjury | ☐ |
| **C.** An invasion of privacy | ☐ |
| **D.** Assault | ☐ |

**107.** COPD is also known as _____.

| | |
|---|---|
| **A.** Asthma | ☐ |
| **B.** Apnea | ☐ |
| **C.** Emphysema | ☐ |
| **D.** Stridor | ☐ |

**108.** A leukocyte is a _____.

| | |
|---|---|
| **A.** WBC | ☐ |
| **B.** RBC | ☐ |
| **C.** Stem cell | ☐ |
| **D.** Platelet | ☐ |

**109.** There are _____ safety zones in or around an MRI suite.

| | |
|---|---|
| **A.** 1 | ☐ |
| **B.** 2 | ☐ |
| **C.** 3 | ☐ |
| **D.** 4 | ☐ |

**110.** Zone 1 is open to the general public. True or False?

| | |
|---|---|
| **A.** True | ☐ |
| **B.** False | ☐ |

**111.** The standard of care to rule out intraocular metallic foreign body is _____.

| | |
|---|---|
| **A.** PA (Waters) view and lateral of the orbits | ☐ |
| **B.** CT scan | ☐ |
| **C.** Tomogram of the orbit | ☐ |
| **D.** MRI of the orbit | ☐ |

**112.** There are three categories that describe an implants status as to being scanned:

| | |
|---|---|
| **A.** MR safe | ☐ |
| **B.** MR conditional | ☐ |
| **C.** MR unsafe | ☐ |
| **D.** All of these | ☐ |

**113.** MR safe means:

| | |
|---|---|
| **A.** Can always be scanned at any field strength | ☐ |
| **B.** Can scan with low SAR factors | ☐ |
| **C.** Can always be scanned with no restrictions | ☐ |
| **D.** A, B, or C | ☐ |

**114.** MR conditional means:

| | |
|---|---|
| **A.** Can be scanned only at 1.5T | ☐ |
| **B.** Might be scanned with manufacture's specific conditions | ☐ |
| **C.** Can brought into the scan room with no restrictions | ☐ |
| **D.** All of these | ☐ |

**115.** MR unsafe means:

| | |
|---|---|
| **A.** Can be scanned only at 0.5T | ☐ |
| **B.** Can scan at 1.0T with low SAR factors | ☐ |
| **C.** Can never be scanned or brought into the scan room at any field strength | ☐ |
| **D.** All of these | ☐ |

**116.** The FDA limit for clinical scanning of patients is _____ T.

|   |   |
|---|---|
| **A.** 3 | ☐ |
| **B.** 4 | ☐ |
| **C.** 7 | ☐ |
| **D.** 5 | ☐ |

**117.** Doubling the flip angle from 90° to 180° will _____ times the RF deposition.

|   |   |
|---|---|
| **A.** 2 | ☐ |
| **B.** 4 | ☐ |
| **C.** 6 | ☐ |
| **D.** 8 | ☐ |

**118.** Hypoglycemia is a condition where the patient's _____ is _____:

|   |   |
|---|---|
| **A.** BUN, high | ☐ |
| **B.** Creatine, low | ☐ |
| **C.** Blood sugar, high | ☐ |
| **D.** Blood sugar, low | ☐ |

**119.** Which veins carry oxygenated blood?

|   |   |
|---|---|
| **A.** Carotids | ☐ |
| **B.** Coronary | ☐ |
| **C.** Pulmonary | ☐ |
| **D.** SVC | ☐ |

**120.** The eGFR is a representation of how well the patient's kidneys are working. In general, an eGFR of >90 is considered normal or well-functioning kidneys. True or False?

**121.** The eGFR is calculated using different factors including: Age, Serum creatinine, Gender and _____.

|   |   |
|---|---|
| **A.** BUN | ☐ |
| **B.** Race | ☐ |
| **C.** Weight | ☐ |
| **D.** Fasting blood sugar | ☐ |

**122.** A nosocomial infection is one that _____.

| | |
|---|---|
| **A.** Originates from a sinus infection | ☐ |
| **B.** Started at home | ☐ |
| **C.** Was not present prior to entering the hospital | ☐ |
| **D.** None of these | ☐ |

**123.** There are three ways to transmit infection that include droplet, contact, and _____.

| | |
|---|---|
| **A.** Airborne | ☐ |
| **B.** Nosocomial | ☐ |
| **C.** Mucosal | ☐ |
| **D.** Oral | ☐ |

**124.** Your first step in performing any imaging procedure is to _____.

| | |
|---|---|
| **A.** Verify the medical history | ☐ |
| **B.** Check for allergies | ☐ |
| **C.** Double-check the physicians order | ☐ |
| **D.** Establish the patients I.D. with at least two identifiers | ☐ |

**125.** Beneficence or Benefactor means:

| | |
|---|---|
| **A.** An act of mercy, caring, charity, or kindness | ☐ |
| **B.** Giving to a charity | ☐ |
| **C.** Lack of caring | ☐ |
| **D.** Strong connotation of doing no good | ☐ |

**126.** Nonmaleficence means:

| | |
|---|---|
| **A.** To do no more harm | ☐ |
| **B.** To reach a beneficial outcome | ☐ |
| **C.** Being paid well for a job well done | ☐ |
| **D.** A and B | ☐ |

**127.** Insulin is used to regulate a patient's blood sugar levels. If too much insulin is administered, a condition called _____ may result.

| | |
|---|---|
| **A.** Hypogastrosis | ☐ |
| **B.** Hyperglycemia | ☐ |
| **C.** Hypoglycemia | ☐ |
| **D.** Pancreatitis | ☐ |

**128.** Signs or symptoms of an anaphylactic reaction usually include

> **A.** Dilated pupils, tachycardia, low B/P ☐
> **B.** Pt is pale, hives, diff swallowing, nausea ☐
> **C.** Headache, nausea, diff swallowing ☐
> **D.** Pt. is restless, itchy, and complains of being tired ☐

**129.** The condition of lack of oxygen to the brain is called _____.

> **A.** Hypo viremia ☐
> **B.** Hypo-glioma ☐
> **C.** Hypoxia ☐
> **D.** Hypovolemia ☐

**130.** Indwelling urinary foley catheters should be kept where?

> **A.** Above the patient's head ☐
> **B.** At table level ☐
> **C.** Below table level ☐
> **D.** Wherever ☐

**131.** In an unresponsive/unconscious patient, the _____ is a primary concern.

> **A.** Pulse rate ☐
> **B.** Patient IV ☐
> **C.** B/P ☐
> **D.** Airway ☐

**132.** Bradycardia means?

> **A.** Fast heart rate ☐
> **B.** Slow heart rate ☐
> **C.** Irregular heart beat ☐
> **D.** Bleeding disorder ☐

**133.** In the event of a medical emergency in the scan room, your first step would be _____.

> **A.** Start chest compressions ☐
> **B.** Administer 2l of $O_2$ via nasal cannula ☐
> **C.** Open the airway ☐
> **D.** Remove the patient from the scan room before intervention ☐

**134.** If a patient is "Febrile," it means that they are:

A. Hungry ☐
B. Feverish ☐
C. Thirsty ☐
D. Afraid ☐

**135.** The likelihood of peripheral nerve stimulation decreases as field strength increases.

A. True ☐
B. False ☐

**136.** Peripheral nerve stimulation usually happens at the end's extremities away from isocenter.

A. True ☐
B. False ☐

**137.** Peripheral nerve stimulation usually happens with sequences that are RF intense.

A. True ☐
B. False ☐

**138.** Peripheral nerve stimulation is painful and causes long-lasting medical conditions.

A. True ☐
B. False ☐

**139.** Peripheral nerve stimulation stops when the sequence ends.

A. True ☐
B. False ☐

**140.** An MRCP is typically done to diagnose what?

A. Poly cystic kidneys ☐
B. Hepatitis ☐
C. Renal calculi ☐
D. Gall stones ☐

**141.** Aseptic technique should always be used for _____.

| | |
|---|---|
| **A.** Inserting rectal prostate probe | ☐ |
| **B.** Starting an IV | ☐ |
| **C.** Placing patient on the MR table | ☐ |
| **D.** Applying a surface coil | ☐ |

**142.** What view or plane is best for the supraspinatus muscle and tendon _____?

| | |
|---|---|
| **A.** Axial | ☐ |
| **B.** Coronal | ☐ |
| **C.** Sagittal | ☐ |
| **D.** Oblique coronal | ☐ |

**143.** Bacteria, viruses, and prions are _____.

| | |
|---|---|
| **A.** Blood cells | ☐ |
| **B.** Pathogens | ☐ |
| **C.** Contagious | ☐ |
| **D.** B and C | ☐ |

**144.** What kind of shock is caused by heavy blood loss _____?

| | |
|---|---|
| **A.** Hemolytic | ☐ |
| **B.** Hypovolemic | ☐ |
| **C.** Hypotension | ☐ |
| **D.** Hypoglycemic | ☐ |

**145.** Lateral means?

| | |
|---|---|
| **A.** Something is off to the side | ☐ |
| **B.** In the middle of the body | ☐ |
| **C.** Tossing the football behind you | ☐ |
| **D.** In front of | ☐ |

**146.** Medial means?

| | |
|---|---|
| **A.** Something is off to the side | ☐ |
| **B.** In the middle of the body | ☐ |
| **C.** Tossing the football behind you | ☐ |
| **D.** In front of | ☐ |

**147.** Inferior means?

A. Something is off to the side ☐
B. In the middle of the body ☐
C. Tossing the football behind you ☐
D. Below another ☐

**148.** Anterior means?

A. Something is below another ☐
B. In front of another ☐
C. Tossing the football behind you ☐
D. Behind ☐

**149.** Superior aspect means?

A. Something is off to the side ☐
B. In the middle of the body ☐
C. Above another ☐
D. Below ☐

**150.** Posterior aspect means?

A. Off to the side ☐
B. In the middle of the body ☐
C. Behind something else ☐
D. Below something else ☐

**151.** Which of the cranial nerves are the largest?

A. 1st and 3rd ☐
B. 1st and 5th ☐
C. 1st and 2nd ☐
D. 2nd and 3rd ☐

**152.** Going to the radiologists for clarification of an order or protocol revision is an example of:

A. Practicing avoidance ☐
B. Respondeat superior ☐
C. Carpe diem ☐
D. Semper fidelis ☐

**153.** Gadolinium will not cross a non-intact blood brain barrier.

| | |
|---|---|
| **A.** True | ☐ |
| **B.** False | ☐ |

**154.** Normal intracranial tissues that enhance with the administration of gadolinium include the pituitary, nasal mucosa turbinates, choroid plexus, dural sinuses, meninges and the _____.

| | |
|---|---|
| **A.** Infundibulum | ☐ |
| **B.** Optic nerves | ☐ |
| **C.** Frontal lobe | ☐ |
| **D.** Corpus callosum | ☐ |

**155.** What is a Bolus?

| | |
|---|---|
| **A.** A soft round mass | ☐ |
| **B.** A round mass of medication or medical substance | ☐ |
| **C.** What IV contrast is stored in | ☐ |
| **D.** A and B | ☐ |

**156.** In the event of a cardiac arrest in the magnet, your steps would be what?

| | |
|---|---|
| **A.** Start CRP instantly | ☐ |
| **B.** Remove patient from room, call a code, and start CPR | ☐ |
| **C.** Remove patient from room, close the door, call a code, start CPR, have somebody monitor the door to keep everybody out of the scan room | ☐ |
| **D.** Run the code from inside the room to keep maximize patient privacy | ☐ |

**157.** What is the definition of "ectomy"?

| | |
|---|---|
| **A.** An excision of an organ or body part | ☐ |
| **B.** Suturing two parts together | ☐ |
| **C.** An incision in order to drain | ☐ |
| **D.** Implantation of a structure | ☐ |

**158.** What is the definition of "ostomy"?

| | |
|---|---|
| **A.** An excision or artificial opening in an organ or body part | ☐ |
| **B.** Suturing two parts together | ☐ |
| **C.** An incision in order to drain | ☐ |
| **D.** Implantation of a structure | ☐ |

**159.** What is the definition of atrophy?

A. To enlarge ☐
B. To shrink ☐
C. To dry out as in dehydrate ☐
D. To become saturated ☐

**160.** What is the definition of hypertrophy?

A. To enlarge ☐
B. To shrink ☐
C. To dry out as in dehydrate ☐
D. To become saturated ☐

**161.** What is the definition of desiccate?

A. To enlarge ☐
B. To shrink ☐
C. To dry out as in dehydrate ☐
D. To become saturated ☐

**162.** What is the definition of "aberrant" mean?

A. To bend ☐
B. To narrow ☐
C. To deviate from the normal course ☐
D. To twist onto itself ☐

**163.** If a patient has had a nephrectomy, it means that they have had?

A. The uterus removed ☐
B. An ovary removed ☐
C. A kidney removed ☐
D. Part of the colon removed ☐

**164.** If a patient has had an oophorectomy, it means that they have had?

A. The uterus removed ☐
B. An ovary removed ☐
C. A kidney removed ☐
D. Part of the colon removed ☐

**165.** Popliteal refers to what location in the body?

    **A.** Above the uterus ☐
    **B.** under the tongue ☐
    **C.** below the kidney ☐
    **D.** behind the knee ☐

**166.** If a patient has had a laminectomy, it means that they have had?

    **A.** The uterus removed ☐
    **B.** an ovary removed ☐
    **C.** A kidney removed ☐
    **D.** Part of the vertebra removed ☐

**167.** The meaning of the term "Hypo" is?

    **A.** Above the normal level ☐
    **B.** Below the normal level ☐
    **C.** At a normal level ☐
    **D.** Empty ☐

**168.** "Itis" means?

    **A.** Inside another ☐
    **B.** Infected or enflamed ☐
    **C.** A lack of blood supply ☐
    **D.** Clotted with blood ☐

**169.** If a patient is in the "right lateral recumbent position," they are how?

    **A.** Lying down on their right-side ☐
    **B.** Lying down on their correct side ☐
    **C.** Semi-reclined on their right-side ☐
    **D.** Trendelenburg ☐

**170.** Adverse allergic reactions are always a concern when administering IV gadolinium for a study. This concern is heightened when the patient has what two conditions?

    **A.** Anemia ☐
    **B.** Asthma ☐
    **C.** Hypoglycemia ☐
    **D.** Prior allergic respiratory reactions ☐
    **E.** B and D ☐

**171.** Stenosis refers to what?

| | |
|---|---|
| **A.** A widening | ☐ |
| **B.** A narrowing | ☐ |
| **C.** The beginning of something | ☐ |
| **D.** The end of something | ☐ |

**172.** Tortuosity means what?

| | |
|---|---|
| **A.** Twisted/turning | ☐ |
| **B.** Straight | ☐ |
| **C.** Narrowed | ☐ |
| **D.** Deflated | ☐ |

**173.** Truncated means what?

| | |
|---|---|
| **A.** Twisted/turning | ☐ |
| **B.** Terminated | ☐ |
| **C.** Cut-off | ☐ |
| **D.** B or C | ☐ |

**174.** Coarctation means?

| | |
|---|---|
| **A.** Twisted/turning | ☐ |
| **B.** A split or division | ☐ |
| **C.** Narrowing | ☐ |
| **D.** Dilation | ☐ |

**175.** A stricture means?

| | |
|---|---|
| **A.** Twisted/turning | ☐ |
| **B.** A split or division | ☐ |
| **C.** Narrowing | ☐ |
| **D.** Dilation | ☐ |

**176.** The prefixes "BI," "Di", and "TRI" mean?

| | |
|---|---|
| **A.** 1,2,3 | ☐ |
| **B.** 2,3,4 | ☐ |
| **C.** 1,1,3 | ☐ |
| **D.** 2,2,3 | ☐ |

# Below are artist renditions of the anatomical position:

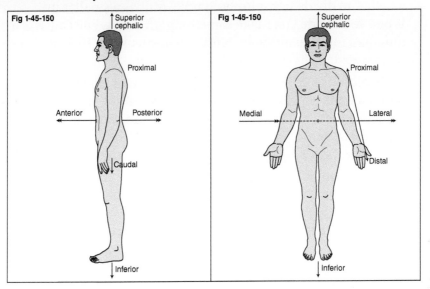

A conversion magnetic for strengths.

| Gauss | To mT | G ÷ by 10 = mT | mT ÷ by 1000 = Tesla |
|---|---|---|---|
| 1 G | 1.G ÷ 10 = | 0.1 mT | 0.0001 T |
| 5 G | 5.G ÷ 10 = | 0.5 mT | 0.0005 T |
| 10000 G | 10000.G ÷ 10 = | 1000 mT | 1 T |

G to mT; ÷ by 10 or move decimal point 1 place left. mT to T; ÷ by 1000 or move decimal point 3 places to left

| mTesla | To Gauss | mT × 10 = G |
|---|---|---|
| 0.1 mT | 0.1 × 10 = | 1 G |
| 0.5 mT | 0.5 × 10 = | 5 G |

mT to G; multiply by 10 or move decimal point 1 place

# Section 1 Patient Interactions and Management Answers

1. **D.** Informed consent does not include the patient's right to have legal counsel.
2. **B.** Everybody knows the 5. Gauss line, but if asked it in Milli-tesla, it is 0.5 mT. To convert G to mT, divide by 10, so move the decimal point

over to the left 1 place. $5.0 \div 10 = 0.5\,mT$. Conversely, mT to G you multiply by 10, so move the decimal point 1 place to the right. 750. $mT = 7500\,G$. (750. X 10. = 7500.). So how am I supposed to remember whether to divide or multiply. Simple: Milli is a smaller unit, so *divide*. When you divide you make something smaller, while Gauss is a bigger unit than milli, so *multiply*. Milli also means 1000. $1000\,ms = 1\,second$. *See conversion chart given before this section.*

3. **D.** A patient's B/P is stated as systolic over diastolic. An easy to remember, it is: **The D is down S/D**. When the heart contracts, it is called systole. The higher the systolic pressure, the more blood the heart is pumping out.

4. **C.** According to Dictionary.com, libel is often confused with liable. Libel is defamation by written or printed words, pictures, or any form about another in order to call their character into question. Liable is a legal responsibility. Technologists are legally responsible for caring for our patients and accurately document to medical record.

5. **D.** Again according to Dictionary.com, the rule that an injury is due to the defendant's negligence when that which caused it was under his or her control and the injury would not have happened had proper management been observed.

6. All the above.

7. **A.** There are no contraindications for administering gadolinium, only relative ones.

8. **C.** Tuberculosis (TB) patients wearing a mask as a form of reverse precautions.

9. **C.**

10. True.

11. **B.**

12. **B.** Department policies vary on this topic. This is the sort of question where you need to see what the answers, you are given to make a best guess. Err on the side of safety for the baby and you should be good.

13. **C.** A Sphygmomanometer is the device used to check a patient's blood pressure.

14. **D.**

15. **B.**

16. **True.** In today's scanners, localization lights are lasers and the scanner will usually have warning placards advising not let the patient stare into the light.

17. **D.** Non-infusion IV's are gravity fed and need to be kept above the heart to avoid blood back flow and possibility air bubbles getting into the bloodstream.

18. **A.** Gaseous helium is not combustible. Hydrogen is.

19. **D.** All patients need at least visual and verbal monitoring.

20. **C.** W/kg (Watts per Kilogram) is the FDA term used for SAR.

21. **D.** BUN and creatinine both relate to how well the kidneys are functioning.

22. **False.** I hate double negative questions. Stop for a second. The question is telling you that the BBB is broken. So gado **will** pass through into tumor/infection.

23. **C.** Altitude has no bearing on the patient's ability to dissipate heat.

24. **D.** EPI sequences have multiple "Base" beginnings like SE, GRE, or IR, but all end with a series of gradient reversal; each reversal causes an echo.

25. **A.** Of the four sequences listed, the FSE/TSE sequence has the most amount of RF pulses by virtue of its ETL.

26. **A.** It is a long-standing practice that pacemakers need to be kept out side of the 5 Gauss line.

27. **D.** FDA guidelines that that scanning in normal mode, the body temp is allowed to raise by $0.5\,°C$ and in first level raise by $1.0\,°C$.

28. **False.** Resistive magnets have no cryogens so cannot be quenched. Just shut off.

29. **D.** All of the above.

30. **A.** $0.5\,m/T$ is a conversion from Gauss. See Answer number 2 for more on conversions.

31. **True.** Isocenter is where all the RF is concentrated while further out from isocenter is where the gradient fields have the most interval change.

32. **C.** The only person whom can obtain an informed consent is an M.D./D.O. From the A.M.A. website: "The process of informed consent occurs when communication between a patient and physician results in the patient's authorization or agreement to undergo a specific medical intervention."

33. **D.** The risk of aspiration is a very real concern for patients that have been received either conscious sedation or general anesthesia.

34. **D.** Vomiting = Emesis, Dyspnea = Difficulty breathing and Urticaria = Hives.

35. **True.** This is a common question in multiple registry exams. A Wilms tumor is a renal tumor seen in children.

36. **D.** The noise limit is 140 dB. According to Dr. Shellock's safety website: Peak unweighted sound pressure level greater than 140-dB. In the United Kingdom, guidelines issued by the Department of Health recommend hearing protection be worn by staff exposed to an average of 85-dB over an 8-hour day. Modern MR scanners are capable of producing noise

levels from 126 to 131 dB on a linear scale, recommending the use of both earplugs and headphones for ear protection relative to the use of 3-T MR systems when certain pulse sequences are used.

37. **True.** The highest/greatest amount of magnetic field change happens at the far ends of the gradients when they are applied. The gradients all "pivot" at isocenter just like a playground "See-Saw." This is why areas away from isocenter are where PNS is felt.

38. **C.** Even though the highest amount of gradient change occurs away from isocenter, the rods and cones in the retina can be made to react to the gradient field and cause "flashes" to be seen by the patient.

39. **C.** The scan room temperature will drop when/if the cryogen escapes into the scan room. Also, gaseous helium is lighter than room air, so it will rise to the ceiling looking like a fog. It will displace room air downwardly. As the quench continues, it will displace all the room air making asphyxiation a real possibility.

40. **C.** RF will heat the patient. The RF wavelength used in MRI is very close to that of microwaves in the electromagnetic spectrum. Heating of tissue begins at the surface and gradually extends deeper into the tissues.

41. **D.** The strength or amplitude of the RF as well as the flip angle affect the amount of "SAR" the patient is exposed to. The flip angle contributes to SAR as it comes from the duration or length of time the RF ($B_1$) field is applied for.

42. **C.** Gadolinium is a rare earth metal and is therefore toxic to the human body. A chelating agent binds with the gadolinium atomic structure rendering it nontoxic as long as the chemical bonds between the two are intact.

43. **D.** Obviously a known allergy to any substance is a concern. Impaired renal function can cause the contrast agent to remain in the body long enough for the chemical bonds between Gad and the chelating agent to breakdown allowing for trace amounts of free gadolinium in the body. There is a slightly higher chance for the patient to have an allergic reaction to gadolinium when they have sickle cell anemia. *Another name for sickle cell anemia is hemolytic anemia.*

44. **C.** There are a number of structures in the brain/skull that will enhance normally when gadolinium contrast is administered. Those being the Nasal mucosa, Pituitary gland and stalk, Choroid plexus, Optic nerves, and Dural venous sinuses. The Basal ganglion are inside the BBB and will not enhance with an intact BBB.

45. **C.** Hydrogen and oxygen are both fire hazards, so less than ideal. Helium is the most common cryogen used. **Of note**: Older MR systems used to have "Dual Cryostats." This means that there were two vessels that held cryogens. One of helium and a second one with nitrogen.

46. **C.** Tesla is the denomination for the field strength at isocenter. 1.5 or 3 T. Away from isocenter as the field strength drops to less than 1 T, the term used to denote magnetic strength is in Gauss.

47. **False.** A tympanoplasty is a very common surgical procedure to repair the ear drum.

48. **A.** 4 W/kg Body and 3 W/kg Head. This a very common question in MR Registry Exams. You need to know these limits.

49. **D.** A quench is a sudden and rapid release of the cryogen. It quickly converts from a liquid to a gas. The conversion of liquid to gas is approximately 720-1 meaning 1 l of liquid becomes 720 l of gas.

50. **D.** Coils should, in reality, be inspected for the integrity of wire insulation every time you use them.

51. **B.** The Faraday cage is designed to keep our RF in and others out. It is the equivalent to the lead lining in an X-ray room.

52. **A.** The radial artery in the wrist and the carotid are two very common and easy places to feel for and count the patient's pulse rate.

53. **A.** The hematocrit is an indicator of the volume of red blood cells.

54. **B.** The thoraco-lumbar junction should be imaged with T2 axials when symptoms include loss of bowel and bladder control.

55. **B.** It is not uncommon for the T wave to elevate during a sequence.

56. **C.** Avascular ("A" meaning: non, no, or without), so avascular (without vasculature) and thus cell death (necrosis). Be careful with answer A, Septic necrosis. Septic = infection.

57. **B.** Islet cells are found in the pancreas. The pancreas has clusters of cells (Islets) which produce various hormones. There are different types of cells in an Islet, some of which produce glucagon which raises glucose levels or insulin to lower blood sugar by allowing cells to absorb glucose.

58. **A.** The most common site of avascular necrosis is the femoral head.

59. **C.** The plane of choice for imaging the Achilles is sagittal as the tendon runs S/I attaching at the calcaneus and running up and into the calf or gastrocnemius muscle.

60. **B.** The prostate is inferior to and slightly anterior to the urinary bladder.

61. **C.** The most sensitive sequence we have for MS is T2 FLAIR. Prior to the advent of FLAIR imaging, proton density was the sequence/weighting of choice.

62. **A.** The aortic arch has the highest pressure of all the blood vessels.

63. **B.** T wave elevation on an EKG is an example of the magneto-hemo-dynamic effect.

64. **A.** The sciatic nerve originates from the sacral plexus. See Section 4, Useful Anatomy for more information.

65. **B.** The celiac is the first branch off the abdominal aorta. As an FYI, the three branches off the celiac are: Hepatic, Splenic, and Left gastric. The second branch off the AA is the superior mesenteric artery or SMA.

66. **A.** The fringe magnetic field is controlled or constrained by the Passive and Active shielding systems. Be careful of the words Passive and Active. There are two systems in a scanner with Passive and Active attached to them. Slow down, read the whole question. Figure out what is being asked and look at your answer choices.

67. **D.** The choroid plexus makes CSF. All ventricles have choroid plexus.

68. **A.** The median nerve in carpal tunnel is being compressed by the flexor retinaculum.

69. **B.** The stalk of the pituitary is also known as the infundibulum. Infundibulum means funnel-shaped tube or cavity. The infundibulum connects the posterior pituitary gland to the hypothalamus. Some cells in the infundibulum are neurons that also have endocrine-type properties. It is not just a "Cherry Stem" that attaches the pituitary gland to the brain.

70. **C.**

71. **A.** The 1st branch is the brachiocephalic or innominate artery. An easy way to remember the names of the "Great Vessels" is **A, B, C, S.** In CPR, you memorized ABC for Airway, Breathing, and Circulation. Now just add an S and it becomes: **A**scending Aorta, **B**rachiocephalic, **C**arotid (LEFT), and **S**ubclavian. **There could be an argument that the Lt and Rt. main coronary arteries are the 1st branches off aorta.

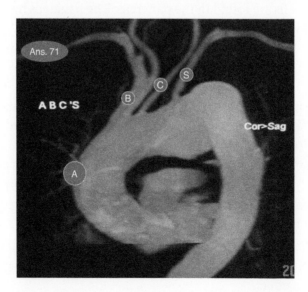

72. **True.**

73. **D.** Glomular filtration.

74. **D.** The choroid plexus makes CSF. All ventricles have choroid plexus.

75. **B.** The cruciate ligaments "cross" and are best seen in the sagittal plane.

76. **A.** The right ventricle is the most anterior chamber in the mediastinum.

77. **B.** The left ventricle is the most posterior.

78. **D.** STIR is the sequences of choice to differentiate gray/white matter **in the pediatric brain** as myelination of white matter is not complete until about 36–40 months of age.

79. **D.** The coronal plane in a spine with scoliosis can be helpful in counting and identifying the vertebral bodies. Some site routinely run a T1 coronal when scoliosis is seen.

80. **D.** The cerebellar tonsils drop down off the cerebellum and can herniate down through the foramen magnum possibly causing/leading to hydrocephalus.

81. **D.**

82. **C.** The body reacts to infection by processing more WBC's to fight the infection.

83. **C.** Typical lumbar plexus coverage is from T12 to L5.

84. **C.**

85. **A.**

86. **A.** Inability to speak is called aphagia. **A** means "not" or "without," **phagia** to speak.

87. **C.** The vertebral arteries are branches off the subclavian arteries.

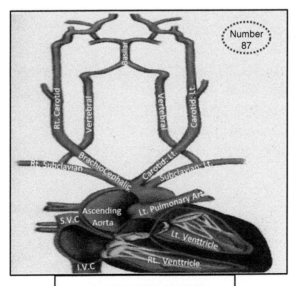

**GREAT VESSEL ANATOMY**

88. **B.** A tangled mass or collection of blood vessels is called a "Hemangioma."

89. **A.** Bell's palsy affects the 5th or trigeminal nerve. ** **know your Cranial Nerves****.

90. **A.** Of all the cranial nerves, the 1st and 2nd (olfactory and optic) are the biggest.

91. **A.** Anosmia is the loss of sense of smell. Smell comes from the 1st C.N. or olfactory.

92. **C.** Bowel and bladder function comes from the nerves originating from the thoraco-lumbar region of the spine. "Cauda Equina Syndrome" includes back/leg pain, either uni or bilateral combined with bowel and bladder symptoms.

93. **B.** Think P.A.D. for **P**ia, **A**rachnoid, and **D**ura. From brain to skull: B.S.P.A.D.

94. **D.** P**i**a is the inner (PIA has an I in it, so think **I** for inner) and Dura.

95. **B.**

96. **D.** The vagus or vagal nerve controls the diaphragm.

97. **D.** All of these may be the patient's response to a stressful situation or trigger.

98. **C.** Fainting.

99. **D.**

100. **C.** Pulmonary arteries are the only arteries in the body to carry **DE-Oxygenated blood.**

101. **B.**

102. **B.**

103. **C.** Patent means OPEN.

104. **True.** Oxygen is considered a drug/medication requiring an MD order for administration.

105. **C.** This position is called the Sims/Recovery position, and is used for comfort, and airway management.

106. **C.** Besides a HIPPA violation, it is also an invasion of someone's privacy.

107. **C.**

108. **A.**

109. **D.** Four zones comprise the area around an MRI scanner.

110. **True.** Zone one is open to the general public.

111. **A.** A PA or Waters view with lateral view is the standard or care to R/O FB in the orbits for prescreen for an MRI.

112. **D.** There are three categories to describe implants. Safe, Conditional, and Unsafe.

113. **D.** MR safe means safe at all fields, under either low SAR conditions with no conditions as to coil, or patient position.

114. **B.** MR conditional means that there are some restrictions usually with regard to which coils should be used and or SAR limitations.

115. **C.** Cannot be scanned or brought into the room regardless of field strength.

116. **C.** The FDA limits clinical imaging to 4 T.

117. **B.** Doubling the flip angle will 4× the RF deposition in the patient.

118. **D.** Hypo means low, Glycemia is the presence of glucose in the blood.

119. **C.** The pulmonary veins carry oxygenated blood.

120. **True.** Department policies vary on this value. Always follow your department's policy on administering IV contrast in regards to the eGFR.

121. **B.** The eGFR calculation that is performed uses various factors of age, gender, race, and a current serum creatinine. The "e" means it is an estimate which also means there can be a significant margin for error. The eGFR can be inaccurate in people with an extreme body habitus like limb amputations, malnutrition, or the morbidly obese. The eGFR calculation has changed over time to now include options for body surface adjustment of height and weight. eGFR is calculated by the abbreviated MDRD equation: **186 × (Creatinine/88.4)−1.154 × (Age)-0.203 × (0.742 if female) × (1.210 Afro-American)**. Have the eGFR value calculated by a local laboratory.

122. **C.** A nosocomial infection is actually acquired from within the hospital or medical facility. A common pathogen is Clostridium Difficile (C Diff.) that is the most common cause of nosocomial GI infections.

123. **D.** While all four of these tasks are important and should be performed, doing the correct exam on the correct patient is always number 1.

124. **D.** Most institutes have a two-identifier system for patient identification such as Name and D.O.B.

125. **A.** Root word is benefit.

126. **D.** Both A and B. Basically doing something good while doing no more harm.

127. **C.** Hypo = low, Glycemia is to have sugar in the blood.

128. **B.** The classic signs of an anaphylactic reaction are paleness, hives, difficulty in swallowing/breathing, and nausea.

129. **C.** A hack of enough oxygen to support bodily functions is the textbook definition of hypoxia. Hypoxia or Hypoxic is often and usually used in referring to affecting the brain.

130. **C.** Foley catheters should be kept below the level of the bladder to lessen or reduce the chance of urine re-entering the bladder and possibly causing an infection.

131. **D.** A patent airway is vital for patient survival.

132. **B.** Bradycardia means a slow heart rate and is opposite to tachycardia.

133. **D.** Get the patient out of the scan room. During a "Code," a lot of people show up trying to help out and each one is a potential accident looking for a place to happen. Close the scan room door and guard it. No unscreened personnel going into the room.

134. **B.** Febrile means "Feverish," Afebrile is the opposite meaning without a fever.

135. **B.** False. Chances of PNS increase with increased field strength.

136. **A.** True. Away from isocenter is where there is the highest amount of magnetic field change from the time-varying magnetic fields (TVMF).

137. **B.** False. Gradient intense sequences like DWI, EPI, and perfusion are the most likely to cause PNS.

138. **B.** False. PNS is not usually painful and does not cause long-term medical affects. IF PNS is painful, the sequence should be stopped and factors changed to lessen the PNS.

139. **A.** True. PNS stops when the TVM fields stop. Remember, PNS is an effect caused by Faraday's law of induction which states that a varying magnetic field passing through a conductor will cause current to flow in that conductor. The peripheral nerves in the hands and feet are the "conductors." So, let us tear apart Faraday's law as it applies to the human body. The equation is: $\Delta V = \Delta B / \Delta T$. It is not that bad. First of all, the "$\Delta$" means change or in Greek: Delta, whose symbol is $\Delta$. Now in English: the change in voltage $\Delta V$, (amount of flow) equals the change magnetic field ($\Delta B$)/ (over) change in time $\Delta T$. So, stronger gradients applied faster = more PNS.

140. **D.** M.R. Cholagio-pancreatography. Is used for anatomical detail of the hepatic, bile ducts, gall bladder, and pancreatic ducts. Stones do not give any signal while the bile gives a lot of signal. The Rad is looking for filling defects in the biliary tree.

141. **B.** Aseptic technique applies to I.V. starts as well as access a patient's infusion port.

142. **D.** Obliques coronal.

143. **B.** All are pathogens.

144. **B.** Losing a lot of blood means you lost a large volume of blood. Hypovolemic.

145. **A.** See Figure 1.1+2 for illustrations.

146. **B.**

**147. D.**

**148. B.**

**149. C.**

**150. C.**

**151. C.** The largest of the cranial nerves are the olfactory and the optic. They are the largest in "Caliber" meaning diameter.

**152. B.** Respondeat Superior. This is Latin for "Let the Master Speak." The radiologist calls the shots.

**153. False.** I HATE THOSE DOUBLE NEGATIVE QUESTIONS!!! **Stop!!!** Think, for a second, right now your BBB is intact so Gad WILL NOT cross it. *Gad will cross a non-intact BBB.* Consider the BBB a filter that only lets certain things through. Tumors, infections, and trauma put a hole in the BBB and the Gad molecule gets through causing pathology to enhance.

**154. A.** The infundibulum is an extension of the pituitary gland, and is important for internal secretion of oxytocin and antidiuretic hormones. Infundibulum actually means funnel shaped. It is not B: The optic nerves are actually an extension of the brain, so do not normally enhance with unless there is pathology.

**155. D.** A bolus, as in IV contrast, is a rapidly administered dose that can be thought of a "Rounded" mass that flows in the blood stream for MRA exams.

**156. C.** During a Code, lots of people show up. The scan room should be secured to keep unscreened staff and unsafe equipment out of the scan room.

**157. A.**

**158. A.**

**159. B.**

**160. A.**

**161. C.** As in an intervertebral disc. When there is a lack of signal (from loss of water) especially on T2 and STIR images, they are thought to be "desiccated."

**162. C.** When a blood vessel does not follow a normal course or path, it is described as being an "aberrant" vessel.

**163. C.**

**164. B.**

**165. D.**

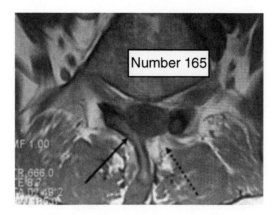

Number 165

166. **D.** When a patient has had spinal surgery to remove herniated intervertebral disc material, a surgeon will remove the lamina of vertebral body, thus performing a "Laminectomy." Solid arrow normal lamina, dotted laminectomy.

167. **B.**

168. **B.**

169. **A.**

170. **E.**

171. **B.**

172. **A.**

173. **D**

174. **C.** Careful, when you here "CO" you instantly think "two" like "Co-conspirator," but not here. You will hear this term referring often to the aorta as in "Coarctation of the Aorta" meaning a **short narrowing of the vessel.**

175. **C.** You could transpose Stricture and Coarctation and you would be mostly correct as both terms refer to a narrowing, but stricture or constriction is mostly used to refer to a narrowing caused by a muscle(s) that constricts an opening or passageway like in the urethra or esophagus.

176. **D.** "BI" means two as in **Bifurcate**, "DI" also means two as in **Di**oxide or **Di**plopia (to see double), and finally "TRI" as in triangle or **Trifurcate**: to split into three. The popliteal artery **Trifurcates** into the anterior tibial, posterior tibial, and the fibular arteries.

# Enlarged Pictures

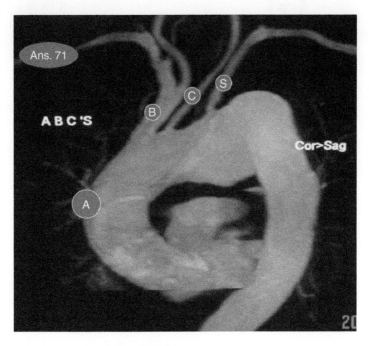

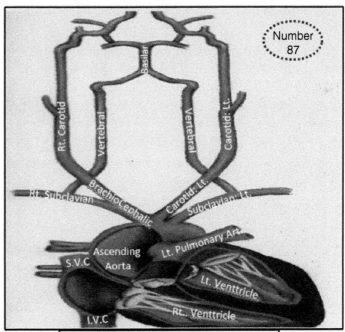

**GREAT VESSEL ANATOMY**

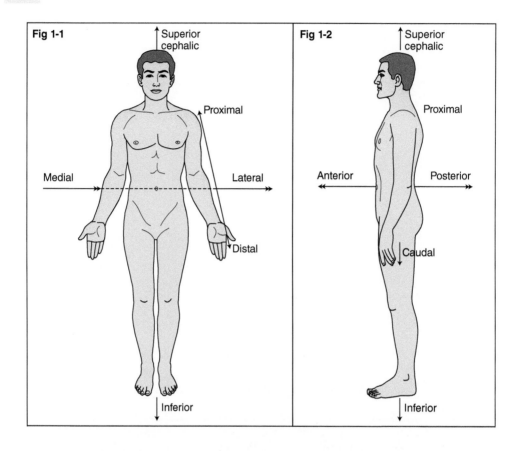

Answer number 165: The solid arrow points to an intact lamina. The dotted arrow points to a surgically absent lamina from a laminectomy.

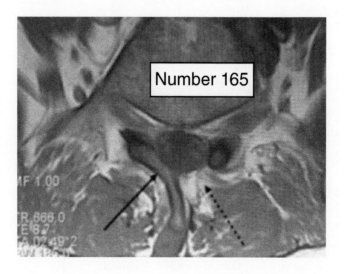

# 2 Parameters, Image Formation, Data Acquisition

These questions will simulate questions that might be seen in the ARRT Advanced MR Registry. These questions are designed to test your knowledge in the basic aspects of MR: Magnets, Nuclear Precession, RF, and Relaxation and Signal generation. Remember, select the *best* answer to the question. That answer may not be the exact answer in your head, but the best answer to the question being asked.

The general breakdown of questions on this subject is:

- Principles of image formation ≈ 35–40
- Sequence parameters ≈ 36
- Data acquisition ≈ 30

1. What is the difference in precessional frequency between fat and water?

| | |
|---|---|
| **A.** 3.5 ppm | ☐ |
| **B.** 35.5 ppm | ☐ |
| **C.** 220 MHz | ☐ |
| **D.** A or C | ☐ |

2. A revolving/alternating magnetic field causing current to flow in a coil is called.

| | |
|---|---|
| **A.** Ferric induction | ☐ |
| **B.** Faraday's law of induction | ☐ |
| **C.** Chemical shift | ☐ |
| **D.** Faraday's law of reduction | ☐ |

*MRI Registry Review: Tech to Tech Questions and Answers*, First Edition. Stephen J. Powers.
© 2021 John Wiley & Sons Ltd. Published 2021 by John Wiley & Sons Ltd.

3. What system is used to produce spatial signal localization?

| | |
|---|---|
| **A.** Fourier transform | ☐ |
| **B.** RF power amplifiers | ☐ |
| **C.** The main magnetic field | ☐ |
| **D.** Magnetic field gradients | ☐ |

4. An RF pulse applied long and or strong enough to flip the longitudinal NMV into the X/Y is called a _____?

| | |
|---|---|
| **A.** TE | ☐ |
| **B.** 180° | ☐ |
| **C.** 45° | ☐ |
| **D.** 90° | ☐ |

5. A transmitted range of frequencies is called a _____.

| | |
|---|---|
| **A.** Frequency readout | ☐ |
| **B.** Phase encode | ☐ |
| **C.** Bandwidth | ☐ |
| **D.** None of these | ☐ |

6. At equilibrium, the amount of transverse magnetization is _____.

| | |
|---|---|
| **A.** 100% | ☐ |
| **B.** 50% | ☐ |
| **C.** 90° | ☐ |
| **D.** Zero | ☐ |

7. What is the Larmor frequency of hydrogen at a $B_0$ of 0.75?

| | |
|---|---|
| **A.** 15.75 MHz | ☐ |
| **B.** 42.57 MHz | ☐ |
| **C.** 220 MHz | ☐ |
| **D.** 31.92 MHz | ☐ |

**8.** The signal generated immediately after an excitation pulse is called _____.

|  |  |
|---|---|
| **A.** Gyromagnetic ratio | ☐ |
| **B.** Decay summations | ☐ |
| **C.** Free induction decay | ☐ |
| **D.** Precessional frequency | ☐ |

**9.** One T1 time is the time it takes for _____ of the longitudinal NMV to _____.

|  |  |
|---|---|
| **A.** 63, decay | ☐ |
| **B.** 37, regrow | ☐ |
| **C.** 37, decay | ☐ |
| **D.** 63, regrow | ☐ |

**10.** One T2 time is the time it takes for the transverse NMV to _____ to _____.

|  |  |
|---|---|
| **A.** Decay, 37% | ☐ |
| **B.** Decay, 63% | ☐ |
| **C.** Regrow, 37% | ☐ |
| **D.** Regrow, 63% | ☐ |

**11.** Equilibrium is a term used to describe:

|  |  |
|---|---|
| **A.** Lose of all energy | ☐ |
| **B.** In phase | ☐ |
| **C.** Out of phase | ☐ |
| **D.** Precession | ☐ |

**12.** Spins that attain alignment anti-parallel to $B_0$ are at a _____.

|  |  |
|---|---|
| **A.** High energy state | ☐ |
| **B.** Low energy state | ☐ |
| **C.** Equilibrium | ☐ |
| **D.** Entropy | ☐ |

**13.** Nuclei rotate their axis. The amount of "wobble" or angle off perpendicular is called the _____.

|   |   |
|---|---|
| **A.** Flip angle | ☐ |
| **B.** Torque | ☐ |
| **C.** Magnetic field strength | ☐ |
| **D.** Magnetic dipole moment | ☐ |

**14.** A vector has what two attributes?

|   |   |
|---|---|
| **A.** Direction and magnetism | ☐ |
| **B.** Magnitude and deviation | ☐ |
| **C.** Direction and magnitude | ☐ |
| **D.** Magnitude and duration | ☐ |

**15.** What does F.I D. stand for?

|   |   |
|---|---|
| **A.** Free induction decay | ☐ |
| **B.** Free inflection decay | ☐ |
| **C.** Fourier induction decay | ☐ |
| **D.** Free inclusion direction | ☐ |

**16.** Difference in signal intensity between two or more tissues describes what?

|   |   |
|---|---|
| **A.** Relaxation | ☐ |
| **B.** Signal to noise | ☐ |
| **C.** Contrast | ☐ |
| **D.** F.I.D. | ☐ |

**17.** Another name for the main magnetic field is _____?

|   |   |
|---|---|
| **A.** $B_1$ | ☐ |
| **B.** NMV | ☐ |
| **C.** $B_2$ | ☐ |
| **D.** $B_0$ | ☐ |

**18.** $B_1$ is used to describe what application?

|   |   |
|---|---|
| **A.** The magnet after it is quenched | ☐ |
| **B.** The field during ramp up | ☐ |
| **C.** An RF field parallel to $B_0$ | ☐ |
| **D.** An RF field perpendicular to $B_0$ | ☐ |

**19.** Which is the Larmor equation?

| | |
|---|---|
| **A.** $W_0 = 57.42 \times \text{Tesla}$ | ☐ |
| **B.** $W_0 = 42.57 \times \text{Tesla}$ | ☐ |
| **C.** $W_0 = 42.57 \times \text{FOV}$ | ☐ |
| **D.** None of these | ☐ |

**20.** Faraday's law of induction states a moving a coil of wire through a magnetic field induces _____?

| | |
|---|---|
| **A.** Magnetism | ☐ |
| **B.** Contrast | ☐ |
| **C.** Signal to noise | ☐ |
| **D.** Current | ☐ |

**21.** An NMV pointing at the coil at TE will produce signal.

| | |
|---|---|
| **A.** False | ☐ |
| **B.** True | ☐ |

**22.** Another name for T2 relaxation is _____.

| | |
|---|---|
| **A.** Spin lattice | ☐ |
| **B.** Spin density | ☐ |
| **C.** Hydrogen density | ☐ |
| **D.** Spin-spin | ☐ |

**23.** Relaxation or dephasing caused by magnetic susceptibilities is called _____.

| | |
|---|---|
| **A.** RID | ☐ |
| **B.** NMV | ☐ |
| **C.** Spin-Lattice | ☐ |
| **D.** T2* | ☐ |

**24.** Rephasing is caused by _____.

| | |
|---|---|
| **A.** A 180 RF pulse | ☐ |
| **B.** The excitation pulses | ☐ |
| **C.** Slice select gradient | ☐ |
| **D.** Gradient timing pulses | ☐ |

**25.** Echoes caused by a refocusing RF pulse are called a spin echo while an echo from a gradient reversal is a gradient echo.

|   |   |   |
|---|---|---|
| **A.** True | | ☐ |
| **B.** False | | ☐ |

**26.** Relaxation is described as.

|   |   |
|---|---|
| **A.** Protons returning to the X/Y plane | ☐ |
| **B.** Protons returning to the Z plane | ☐ |
| **C.** Protons going to a lower energy state | ☐ |
| **D.** B and C | ☐ |

**27.** If allowed to relax for a sufficient amount of time, protons will eventually reach what state?

|   |   |
|---|---|
| **A.** Magnetism | ☐ |
| **B.** $B_0$ | ☐ |
| **C.** Equilibrium | ☐ |
| **D.** Spin lattice | ☐ |

**28.** After the RF excitation pulse, the NMV flips into the X/Y and acquires phase.

|   |   |
|---|---|
| **A.** False | ☐ |
| **B.** True | ☐ |

**29.** Another name for T1 relaxation is _____.

|   |   |
|---|---|
| **A.** Spin lattice | ☐ |
| **B.** Spin density | ☐ |
| **C.** Hydrogen density | ☐ |
| **D.** Spin–spin | ☐ |

**30.** T1 and T2 are relaxation processes and proton density is a tissue _____.

|   |   |
|---|---|
| **A.** Attitude | ☐ |
| **B.** Characteristic | ☐ |
| **C.** Thermo-dynamic characteristic | ☐ |
| **D.** Aptitude | ☐ |

**31.** T1 relaxation is considered a _____ process.

| | |
|---|---|
| **A.** Decay | ☐ |
| **B.** Degree | ☐ |
| **C.** Regrowth | ☐ |
| **D.** Rephasing | ☐ |

**32.** Tissues must T2 relax completely before T1 relaxation can start.

| | |
|---|---|
| **A.** True | ☐ |
| **B.** False | ☐ |

**33.** Spatial resolution is the ability to define small structures. Factors contributing to spatial resolution include:

| | |
|---|---|
| **A.** Field of view | ☐ |
| **B.** Scan matrix | ☐ |
| **C.** Slice thickness | ☐ |
| **D.** A, B and C | ☐ |

**34.** The $B_1$ field is at what orientation to $B_0$?

| | |
|---|---|
| **A.** Parallel | ☐ |
| **B.** Perpendicular | ☐ |
| **C.** Quadrilateral | ☐ |
| **D.** Oblique | ☐ |

**35.** There are two kinds of or states of protons. Free and Bound.

| | |
|---|---|
| **A.** False | ☐ |
| **B.** True | ☐ |

**36.** An example of bound protons would be?

| | |
|---|---|
| **A.** Cortical bone | ☐ |
| **B.** Normal tendon | ☐ |
| **C.** Normal ligaments | ☐ |
| **D.** All the above | ☐ |

**37.** Describing a magnet as a "Dipole" means it has _____.

| | |
|---|---|
| **A.** Two poles | ☐ |
| **B.** East and West poles | ☐ |
| **C.** North and South poles | ☐ |
| **D.** A and C | ☐ |

**38.** The gyromagnetic ratio of hydrogen is 42.57 MHz at 1 T. 42.57 MHz is a _____.

| | |
|---|---|
| **A.** Decay | ☐ |
| **B.** Degree | ☐ |
| **C.** Constant | ☐ |
| **D.** None of these | ☐ |

**39.** The gyromagnetic ratio of hydrogen at 3 T is?

| | |
|---|---|
| **A.** 63.86 MHz | ☐ |
| **B.** 21.28 MHz | ☐ |
| **C.** 127.71 MHz | ☐ |
| **D.** 42.57 MHz | ☐ |

**40.** When scanning at 3 T, the gyromagnetic ratio of hydrogen is?

| | |
|---|---|
| **A.** 57.42 MHz | ☐ |
| **B.** 63.85 MHz | ☐ |
| **C.** 42.57 MHz | ☐ |
| **D.** 127.71 MHz | ☐ |

**41.** 1 T is equal to _____ gauss.

| | |
|---|---|
| **A.** 100 | ☐ |
| **B.** 1000 | ☐ |
| **C.** 10 000 | ☐ |
| **D.** 100 000 | ☐ |

**42.** 5000 gauss equals to 0.5 T

| | |
|---|---|
| **A.** False | ☐ |
| **B.** True | ☐ |

**43.** How many Gauss are in a 7T magnet?

A. 700 ☐
B. 70 000 ☐
C. 700 ☐
D. 70 ☐

**44.** 0.5 mT (5 G) is equal to _____ T?

A. 0.5 T ☐
B. 0.05 T ☐
C. 0.005 T ☐
D. 0.0005 T ☐

**45.** The gyromagnetic ratio of hydrogen is 42.57 MHz at 1 T. 42.57 MHz is a _____.

A. Decay ☐
B. Degree ☐
C. Does not change ☐
D. None of these ☐

**46.** The gyromagnetic ratio of hydrogen at 0.5 T is?

A. 63.86 MHz ☐
B. 21.28 MHz ☐
C. 127.71 MHz ☐
D. 42.57 MHz ☐

**47.** The amount of signal in an image divided by the amount of background noise is called the _____?

A. SNR ☐
B. CNR ☐
C. Contrast ☐
D. Spatial resolution ☐

**48.** Contrast is defined as signal intensity differences between tissues enabling the tissues to be seen as different or distinct from each other.

A. True ☐
B. False ☐

**49.** Using different TR's and TE's to bring out varying inherent signal intensities between tissues is:

A. SNR ☐
B. CNR ☐
C. Contrast ☐
D. Spatial resolution ☐

**50.** A transmitted range of radiofrequencies is called a _____.

A. Phase encoding ☐
B. Gradient slope ☐
C. Bandwidth ☐
D. 180° pulse ☐

**51.** A material that weakly repels a magnetic field with no measurable magnetic properties of its own is called _____?

A. Paramagnetic ☐
B. Ferromagnetic ☐
C. Dipole ☐
D. Diamagnetic ☐

**52.** In a conventional bore scanner, with the patient headfirst, supine, the long axis of the patient and the long axis of the scanner are parallel.

A. True ☐
B. False ☐

**53.** In a gradient echo sequence, what factor can be varied in order to change image contrast?

A. TR ☐
B. TI ☐
C. Flip angle ☐
D. Transmitter B/W ☐

**54.** Hydrogen density is a tissue characteristic.

A. True ☐
B. False ☐

**55.** The magnetic moment possessed by a hydrogen proton comes from the proton having _____.

| | |
|---|---|
| **A.** Spin | ☐ |
| **B.** Resonance | ☐ |
| **C.** Phase | ☐ |
| **D.** Spin echo | ☐ |

**56.** How many RF pulses are needed to produce an FID echo?

| | |
|---|---|
| **A.** 0 | ☐ |
| **B.** 1 | ☐ |
| **C.** 2 | ☐ |
| **D.** 3 | ☐ |

**57.** Why is hydrogen used in MR medical imaging?

| | |
|---|---|
| **A.** It is the abundant in the body | ☐ |
| **B.** It is easily flipped into the X/Y plane | ☐ |
| **C.** It has wobble | ☐ |
| **D.** All the above | ☐ |

**58.** The gyromagnetic ratio of hydrogen is measured in _____?

| | |
|---|---|
| **A.** MHz | ☐ |
| **B.** KHz | ☐ |
| **C.** PHz | ☐ |
| **D.** PPM | ☐ |

**59.** How many RF pulses are needed to produce a single spin echo?

| | |
|---|---|
| **A.** 0 | ☐ |
| **B.** 1 | ☐ |
| **C.** 2 | ☐ |
| **D.** 3 | ☐ |

**60.** One T1 time is the time it takes for 63% of the transverse NMV to return to $B_0$. True or False.

**61.** One T2 time is the amount of time it takes for 37% of the transverse NMV to decay to its original value. True or False.

**62.** True or False: Noise is present in all electronic equipment.

**63.** Temporal resolution is the ability to scan _____ over _____.

| | |
|---|---|
| **A.** slowly, a large area | ☐ |
| **B.** quickly, a large FOV | ☐ |
| **C.** quickly, time | ☐ |
| **D.** quickly, small pixels | ☐ |

**64.** Examples of free protons are:

| | |
|---|---|
| **A.** Fat | ☐ |
| **B.** Muscle | ☐ |
| **C.** Marrow | ☐ |
| **D.** All of these | ☐ |

**65.** Magnetic susceptibility is what?

| | |
|---|---|
| **A.** A tissue's ability to be excited by RF | ☐ |
| **B.** A tissue's inability to be flipped | ☐ |
| **C.** A tissue's ability to relax | ☐ |
| **D.** A tissue's ability to be magnetized | ☐ |

**66.** The $B_1$ Field is produced by the _____.

| | |
|---|---|
| **A.** Head coil | ☐ |
| **B.** RF transmission | ☐ |
| **C.** Slice select gradient | ☐ |
| **D.** Receiver coil | ☐ |

**67.** There are three magnetic states of material. Ferrous, Diamagnetic, and _____.

| | |
|---|---|
| **A.** Dipole | ☐ |
| **B.** Solid | ☐ |
| **C.** Liquid | ☐ |
| **D.** Paramagnetic | ☐ |

**68.** Components of the Larmor equations are: Precessional frequency, Gyromagnetic ratio, and _____.

| | |
|---|---|
| **A.** Field length | ☐ |
| **B.** Field strength | ☐ |
| **C.** Phase ratio | ☐ |
| **D.** Spin ratio | ☐ |

**69.** How many 90 RF pulses are needed to produce an FSE Seq?

**A.** Less than 5  ☐
**B.** 2 or more  ☐
**C.** 1  ☐
**D.** More than 20  ☐

**70.** Why is hydrogen used in MR medical imaging?

**A.** It is abundance in the body  ☐
**B.** It is easily flipped into the X/Y plane  ☐
**C.** It has wobble  ☐
**D.** All the above  ☐

**71.** Another name for T2 relaxation is _____?

**A.** Spin lattice  ☐
**B.** Spin density  ☐
**C.** Hydrogen density  ☐
**D.** Transverse  ☐

**72.** Why does air not give signal on MR images?

**A.** Lack of RF  ☐
**B.** Too much RF  ☐
**C.** Lack of hydrogen  ☐
**D.** Lack of electrons  ☐

**73.** Another name for T2 relaxation is _____?

**A.** Spin lattice  ☐
**B.** Spin density  ☐
**C.** Hydrogen density  ☐
**D.** Spin–spin  ☐

**74.** Another name for T1 relaxation is _____?

**A.** Longitudinal Relaxation  ☐
**B.** Spin density  ☐
**C.** Hydrogen density  ☐
**D.** Spin–spin  ☐

**75.** Another name for proton density is _____?

- **A.** Spin lattice ☐
- **B.** Spin density ☐
- **C.** Hydrogen density ☐
- **D.** B and C ☐

**76.** Noise can be described as?

- **A.** Random ☐
- **B.** Varying ☐
- **C.** Always present ☐
- **D.** A, B, and C ☐

**77.** The inherent body coil is a _____ coil.

- **A.** Transmit ☐
- **B.** Receive ☐
- **C.** Transmit/Receive ☐
- **D.** None of these ☐

**78.** Coils that are arranged in a long row is called or described as _____?

- **A.** Body array ☐
- **B.** Linear ☐
- **C.** Quadrature ☐
- **D.** Phase array ☐

**79.** Coils are orientated at what angle to the NMV?

- **A.** Parallel ☐
- **B.** Orthogonal ☐
- **C.** Perpendicular ☐
- **D.** B or C ☐

**80.** In general, a quadrature coil improves SNR over a linear coil by approximately _____ %.

- **A.** 20 ☐
- **B.** 30 ☐
- **C.** 40 ☐
- **D.** 60 ☐

**81.** In general, you do not need anti-aliasing options on a _____ coil.

| | |
|---|---|
| **A.** Volume | ☐ |
| **B.** Linear | ☐ |
| **C.** Receive only | ☐ |
| **D.** Transmit/Receive | ☐ |

**82.** After an excitation pulse, the initial signal or echo that is produced is called the _____?

| | |
|---|---|
| **A.** Induced | ☐ |
| **B.** Simulated | ☐ |
| **C.** F.I.D. | ☐ |
| **D.** Stimulated | ☐ |

**83.** The liquid helium used to cool the magnetics' coil has a temperature of _____.

| | |
|---|---|
| **A.** −452 °F | ☐ |
| **B.** −32 °K | ☐ |
| **C.** −32°F | ☐ |
| **D.** 0°C | ☐ |

**84.** _____ material will slightly repel a magnetic field while a _____ will strongly attract.

| | |
|---|---|
| **A.** Diamagnetic/Paramagnetic | ☐ |
| **B.** Ferromagnetic/Paramagnetic | ☐ |
| **C.** Diamagnetic/Ferromagnetic | ☐ |
| **D.** Ferromagnetic/Diamagnetic | ☐ |

**85.** Which one of the following will Fourier transform be applied to?

| | |
|---|---|
| **A.** The FID | ☐ |
| **B.** Transmitted B/W | ☐ |
| **C.** Contrast | ☐ |
| **D.** k-Space | ☐ |

**86.** Signal in a coil is _____ through _____.

| | |
|---|---|
| **A.** situated, Faraday's law | ☐ |
| **B.** generated, induction | ☐ |
| **C.** generated, convection | ☐ |
| **D.** stimulated, conduction | ☐ |

**87.** Resolution is the ability to decern or define _____ structures.

A. Small ☐
B. Bright ☐
C. Large ☐
D. Dark ☐

**88.** The process of tissues giving off energy to the _____ is called _____?

A. lattice, T2 ☐
B. lattice, T1 ☐
C. tissue, proton density ☐
D. tissue, hydrogen density ☐

**89.** The distribution or concentration of hydrogen spins describes what?

A. T1 ☐
B. T2 ☐
C. TR ☐
D. PD ☐

**90.** Which RF pulse imparts the largest amount of energy into a tissue?

A. 60° ☐
B. 40° ☐
C. 90° ☐
D. 180° ☐

**91.** The time when the majority of protons have realigned with $B_0$ is called _____.

A. Saturation ☐
B. T2 ☐
C. Anti-parallel ☐
D. Equilibrium ☐

**92.** The result of the excitation pulse is _____.

A. Protons precess in phase ☐
B. Protons precess randomly ☐
C. Protons precess aligned anti-parallel ☐
D. Protons precess in the Z direction ☐

**93.** Which RF pulse imparts the largest amount of transverse net magnetization?

> **A.** 60° ☐
> **B.** 45° ☐
> **C.** 80° ☐
> **D.** 180° ☐

**94.** A vector has what two properties?

> **A.** Direction and Magnetism ☐
> **B.** Amplitude and Direction ☐
> **C.** Direction and Magnitude ☐
> **D.** B and C ☐

**95.** Current flowing in the same direction in two parallel wires produces magnetism which will _____.

> **A.** Cancel the other ☐
> **B.** Add together ☐
> **C.** No magnetism is generated ☐
> **D.** Equals 4× the NMV ☐

**96.** What is it called when a time-varying magnetic field produces voltage in a coil?

> **A.** Faraday's law ☐
> **B.** Ohm's law ☐
> **C.** Larmor's law ☐
> **D.** DaVinci's law ☐

**97.** When a conductor loses electrical resistance at low temperatures, it means it is a _____?

> **A.** Resistor ☐
> **B.** Conductor ☐
> **C.** Superconductor ☐
> **D.** Director ☐

**98.** How many pairs of gradients are there?

| | |
|---|---|
| **A.** 3 | ☐ |
| **B.** 2 | ☐ |
| **C.** 1 | ☐ |
| **D.** 4 | ☐ |

**99.** An increased size in a coil will _____ noise therefore _____ the SNR?

| | |
|---|---|
| **A.** increase, increase | ☐ |
| **B.** increase, decrease | ☐ |
| **C.** decrease, decrease | ☐ |
| **D.** decrease, increase | ☐ |

**100.** Which best describes a surface coil?

| | |
|---|---|
| **A.** Seldon used in imaging | ☐ |
| **B.** Works best when 2× the diameter away from the body part | ☐ |
| **C.** Works to increase the S/N of a specific ROI | ☐ |
| **D.** Generally smaller than volume coils | ☐ |

**101.** What_____ percent of longitudinal relaxation has occurred after one T1 time?

| | |
|---|---|
| **A.** 37% | ☐ |
| **B.** 63% | ☐ |
| **C.** 100% | ☐ |
| **D.** 36% | ☐ |

**102.** Photo-phosphenes are the result of _____.

| | |
|---|---|
| **A.** $B_0$ | ☐ |
| **B.** Alternating magnetic fields | ☐ |
| **C.** $B_1$ | ☐ |
| **D.** 3T | ☐ |

**103.** Hydrogen density is determined by _____.

| | |
|---|---|
| **A.** T2×T1 | ☐ |
| **B.** Amounts of hydrogen protons in a tissue | ☐ |
| **C.** Fat content in a tissue | ☐ |
| **D.** Lack of fat in a tissue | ☐ |

**104.** Protons in a magnetic field that are aligned anti-parallel are?

> **A.** In a higher energy state ☐
> **B.** Will counteract the parallel protons ☐
> **C.** A and B ☐
> **D.** None of these ☐

**105.** The condition when there are more parallel aligned protons than anti-parallel is called a/an _____.

> **A.** NMV ☐
> **B.** X/Y plane ☐
> **C.** Inversion plane ☐
> **D.** $B_1$ ☐

**106.** What is the condition reached very quickly by protons after being placed in the magnetic field?

> **A.** Phase coherence ☐
> **B.** FID ☐
> **C.** Equilibrium ☐
> **D.** Resonant ☐

**107.** When in the equilibrium state, protons precess _____.

> **A.** At the Larmor frequency ☐
> **B.** Below the Larmor frequency ☐
> **C.** In-phase ☐
> **D.** Above the Larmor frequency ☐

**108.** Maximum SNR is achieved when the NMV is at _____ to a receiver coil.

> **A.** 60° ☐
> **B.** 45° ☐
> **C.** 90° ☐
> **D.** 180° ☐

**109.** A grouping of four or more coils is called or referred to as.

> **A.** Linear ☐
> **B.** Circular ☐
> **C.** Transmit/Receive ☐
> **D.** Quadrature ☐

**110.** What sequence relies on a series of phase shifts for image contrast?

> **A.** GRE ☐
> **B.** FSE ☐
> **C.** DWI ☐
> **D.** Phase contrast ☐

**111.** In a TSE/FSE sequence, which factor is most responsible for image contrast?

> **A.** ETE ☐
> **B.** TR ☐
> **C.** ETL ☐
> **D.** Echo spacing ☐

**112.** What sequence relies on a Venc to produce tissue contrast?

> **A.** GRE ☐
> **B.** FSE ☐
> **C.** DWI ☐
> **D.** Phase contrast ☐

**113.** What sequence is a perfusion sequence based upon?

> **A.** GRE ☐
> **B.** FSE ☐
> **C.** DWI ☐
> **D.** Phase contrast ☐

**114.** A Fat-Sat sequence has a _____ applied prior to excitation?

> **A.** Sat pulse ☐
> **B.** Inversion pulse ☐
> **C.** Preparatory pulse ☐
> **D.** Gradient reversal pulse ☐

**115.** What parameter would you adjust if the image showed blurring, but the patient was not moving.

> **A.** TR ☐
> **B.** ETE ☐
> **C.** Slice thickness ☐
> **D.** Echo train length ☐

**116.** What is a minor concern when scanning on a permanent magnet?

| | |
|---|---|
| **A.** Patient weight | ☐ |
| **B.** Screening | ☐ |
| **C.** Fringe magnetic field | ☐ |
| **D.** FOV | ☐ |

**117.** Identify this curve in Figure 2.1

| | |
|---|---|
| **A.** T2 | ☐ |
| **B.** T2* | ☐ |
| **C.** T1 | ☐ |
| **D.** PD | ☐ |

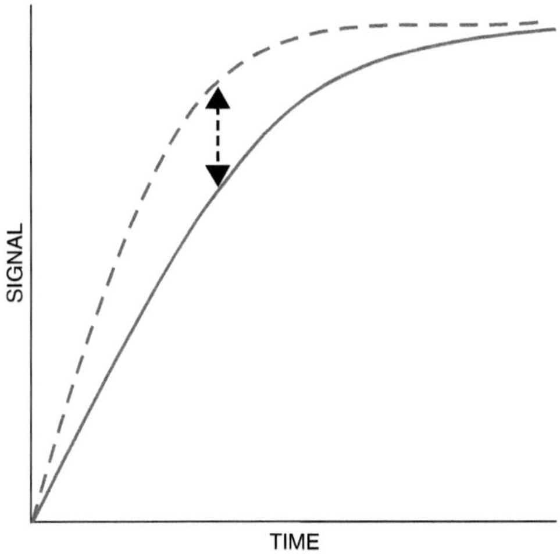

TIME

Fig 2-1

**118.** In Figure 2.1, the tissue represented by the dashed line would be _____ intense to the solid line

| | |
|---|---|
| **A.** Hypo | ☐ |
| **B.** Iso | ☐ |
| **C.** Hyper | ☐ |
| **D.** None of these | ☐ |

**119.** The difference in signal intensity between tissues is called _____.

| | |
|---|---|
| **A.** Signal | ☐ |
| **B.** Noise | ☐ |
| **C.** Contrast | ☐ |
| **D.** Decay | ☐ |

**120.** In Figure 2.1, which tissue has a shortest relaxation time?

| | |
|---|---|
| **A.** Dashed line tissue | ☐ |
| **B.** Solid line tissue | ☐ |

**121.** In Figure 2.1, represents tissues doing what?

| | |
|---|---|
| **A.** Dephasing | ☐ |
| **B.** Regrowing | ☐ |
| **C.** Aligning with $B_1$ | ☐ |
| **D.** None | ☐ |

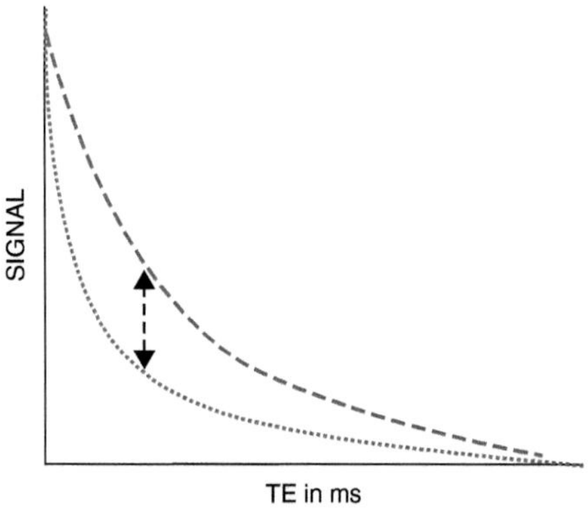

TE in ms

Fig 2-2

**122.** Identify the curve in Figure 2.2

| | |
|---|---|
| **A.** T2 | ☐ |
| **B.** T2* | ☐ |
| **C.** T1 | ☐ |
| **D.** PD | ☐ |

**123.** In Figure 2.2, which tissue has the shortest relaxation time?

| | |
|---|---|
| **A.** Dashed line tissue | ☐ |
| **B.** Dotted line tissue | ☐ |

**124.** In Figure 2.2, at the far right where the curves are very close, the signal intensity of both tissues would be _____.

| | |
|---|---|
| **A.** High | ☐ |
| **B.** Low | ☐ |
| **C.** Isointense | ☐ |
| **D.** B and C | ☐ |

**125.** In Figure 2.2 at the far right where the curves are very close the contrast between these two tissues would be _____.

A. High ☐
B. Low ☐
C. Isointense ☐
D. B and C ☐

**126.** In Figure 2.2, represents tissues doing what?

A. Decaying ☐
B. Regrowing ☐
C. Aligning with $B_0$ ☐
D. Returning to the X/Y plane ☐

**127.** Both relaxations represented in Figures 2.1 and 2.2 occur simultaneously.

A. True ☐
B. False ☐

**128.** What is the chemical shift between fat and water?

A. 223 Hz ☐
B. 42.57 MHz ☐
C. 3.5 ppm ☐
D. Depends on the slice thickness ☐

**129.** What is the chemical shift between fat and water at 3 T?

A. 223 MHz ☐
B. 42.57 MHz ☐
C. 3 ppm ☐
D. 446 Hz ☐

**130.** As the TE is increased, what can be said about the image contrast?

A. It is more PD ☐
B. It is more T1 ☐
C. It is less T1 ☐
D. It is more T2 ☐

**131.** In a hydrogen density weighted image, the short TE will decrease the
_____ and a long TR will decrease the _____.

**A.** T1, T2 ☐
**B.** T2, T1 ☐
**C.** T2, PD ☐
**D.** PD, T2 ☐

**132.** A change in which factor will not increase the SNR of the image?

**A.** ↑FOV ☐
**B.** ↑Slice thickness ☐
**C.** ↑TE ☐
**D.** ↓Rec. B/W ☐

**133.** Which matrix will give the smallest pixel size?

**A.** $256 \times 128$ ☐
**B.** $192 \times 256$ ☐
**C.** $256^2$ ☐
**D.** $128 \times 192$ ☐

**134.** Which matrix will give an isotropic pixel size?

**A.** $256 \times 128$ ☐
**B.** $192 \times 256$ ☐
**C.** $256^2$ ☐
**D.** $128 \times 192$ ☐

**135.** A slice's location in the slice select direction is determined by the _____?

**A.** Slope of the FEG ☐
**B.** Transmitted B/W ☐
**C.** Receiver B/W ☐
**D.** Duration of the SSG ☐

**136.** What is the voxel size with a FOV of 220 mm, a scan matrix of 224×320, and a slice thickness of 5 mm?

> **A.** 5×0.89×0.86 mm  ☐
> **B.** 5×0.86×0.98 mm  ☐
> **C.** 5×0.98×0.68 mm  ☐
> **D.** 5×1.06×0.98 mm  ☐

**137.** Of the above pixel dimensions in Number 136, which one if the most isotropic?

> **A.** 5 × 0.89 × 0.86 mm  ☐
> **B.** 5 × 0.86 × 0.98 mm  ☐
> **C.** 5 × 0.98 × 0.68 mm  ☐
> **D.** 5 × 1.06 × 0.98 mm  ☐

**138.** What is the voxel volume of a voxel measuring:
5 mm × 0.86 mm × 1.06 mm?

> **A.** 4.55 mm³  ☐
> **B.** 5.55 mm³  ☐
> **C.** 5.44 mm³  ☐
> **D.** 5.72 mm³  ☐

**139.** SNR is related to the number of signal averages with the equation of?

> **A.** $NSA^2$  ☐
> **B.** $\sqrt{NSA}$  ☐
> **C.** NSA×1.4  ☐
> **D.** $\sqrt{NSA}/2$  ☐

**140.** Decreasing the FOV results in _____.

> **A.** ↓SNR, ↑ Resolution, Smaller pixels  ☐
> **B.** ↑SNR, ↓ Resolution, Smaller pixels  ☐
> **C.** ↓SNR, ↑ Resolution, Same size pixels  ☐
> **D.** ↓SNR, ↓ Resolution, Smaller pixels  ☐

**141.** A change in which factor will change pixel size?

| | |
|---|---|
| **A.** FOV | ☐ |
| **B.** Slice thicknessTE | ☐ |
| **C.** Rec. B/W | ☐ |

**142.** What is the in-plane resolution with a FOV of 220 a scan matrix of 224×320, slice thickness of 5 mm?

| | |
|---|---|
| **A.** 5.0 mm | ☐ |
| **B.** 5.5 mm | ☐ |
| **C.** 5.44 mm | ☐ |
| **D.** 5.72 mm | ☐ |

**143.** What is the opposite of time of flight (flow-related enhancement)?

| | |
|---|---|
| **A.** Motion | ☐ |
| **B.** Inherent phase shift | ☐ |
| **C.** Flow void | ☐ |
| **D.** Flow comp | ☐ |

**144.** 2D TOF angiography is a better choice for slow flow over 3D TOF because of the chance of?

| | |
|---|---|
| **A.** Motion | ☐ |
| **B.** Coherent phase shifts | ☐ |
| **C.** Flow void | ☐ |
| **D.** In-plane saturation | ☐ |

**145.** 3D TOF because of the _____ typically has higher resolution than a 2D TOF?

| | |
|---|---|
| **A.** Voxel volume | ☐ |
| **B.** FOV | ☐ |
| **C.** Flip angle | ☐ |
| **D.** Slab coverage | ☐ |

**146.** Another name or term for flow void is _____.

A. Flow compensation ☐
B. Gradient motion nulling ☐
C. High-velocity signal loss ☐
D. In-plane saturation ☐

**147.** Flip angle is determined by _____.

A. How long the SSG is applied ☐
B. How long the FEG is applied ☐
C. How long the $B_0$ field is applied ☐
D. How long the $B_1$ field is applied ☐

**148.** Slice thickness is determined by _____.

A. Amplitude of SSG ☐
B. Transmitted B/W ☐
C. Amplitude of FEG ☐
D. A and B ☐

**149.** What sequence captures slices simultaneously?

A. Interleaved ☐
B. 2D TOF ☐
C. 3D TOF ☐
D. Phase contrast ☐

**150.** What is the condition reached very quickly by protons after being removed from the magnetic field?

A. Phase coherence ☐
B. FID ☐
C. Equilibrium ☐
D. Resonance ☐

**151.** In a magnetic field and at the equilibrium state, protons precess _____.

> **A.** Faster than the Larmor frequency ☐
> **B.** At the Larmor frequency ☐
> **C.** In-phase ☐
> **D.** Out of phase ☐

**152.** Minimum SNR is achieved when the NMV is at _____ to a receiver coil.

> **A.** 60° ☐
> **B.** 45° ☐
> **C.** 90° ☐
> **D.** 180° ☐

**153.** T1 relaxation is also known as _____.

> **A.** Spin–spin ☐
> **B.** F.I.D. ☐
> **C.** Spin-lattice ☐
> **D.** Dephasing ☐

**154.** T2 relaxation is also known as _____.

> **A.** Spin–spin ☐
> **B.** F.I.D. ☐
> **C.** Spin-lattice ☐
> **D.** Rephasing ☐

**155.** Eddy currents are _____.

> **A.** Localized electric currents induced by a varying magnetic field ☐
> **B.** Opposing magnetic fields from alternating current ☐
> **C.** Swirling RF fields ☐
> **D.** Both A and B ☐

**156.** What is a dipole–dipole interaction?

> **A.** An interaction between protons ☐
> **B.** An interaction between a proton and an electron ☐
> **C.** An interaction between two magnets ☐
> **D.** All of these ☐

**157.** What coil would best be used for large FOV images of the spine?

| | |
|---|---|
| **A.** Helmholtz | ☐ |
| **B.** Linear array | ☐ |
| **C.** Body coil | ☐ |
| **D.** Receive only | ☐ |

**158.** What tissue has a Long T1 and Long T2?

| | |
|---|---|
| **A.** Fat | ☐ |
| **B.** Gad | ☐ |
| **C.** CSF | ☐ |
| **D.** White matter | ☐ |

**159.** Precession is defined as?

| | |
|---|---|
| **A.** Random spinning of nuclei in a magnetic field | ☐ |
| **B.** Ordered spinning of nuclei in a magnetic field | ☐ |
| **C.** Protons tumbling in a magnetic field | ☐ |
| **D.** Protons spinning at the Larmor frequency | ☐ |

**160.** In one T1 Time, how much of the NMV is still in the X/Y plane?

| | |
|---|---|
| **A.** 63% | ☐ |
| **B.** 37% | ☐ |
| **C.** 50% | ☐ |
| **D.** 22% | ☐ |

**161.** An IR (STIR or FLAIR) sequence starts off with a _____.

| | |
|---|---|
| **A.** 60° | ☐ |
| **B.** 45° | ☐ |
| **C.** 90° | ☐ |
| **D.** 180° | ☐ |

**162.** An FSE sequence ends with a _____.

| | |
|---|---|
| **A.** 60° | ☐ |
| **B.** Echo | ☐ |
| **C.** 90° | ☐ |
| **D.** 180° | ☐ |

**163.** In a spin-echo sequence with 20 Slice, 2 nex, 500 ms TR, 15 ms TE, 5 mm thick slice, and a 192×256 scan matrix, how many TRs will be needed to fill the k-Space.

|  |  |
|---|---|
| **A.** 192 | ☐ |
| **B.** 256 | ☐ |
| **C.** 512 | ☐ |
| **D.** 384 | ☐ |

**164.** When the TR is shorter than T2/T2* of a tissue in a GRE sequence, a _____ will develop.

|  |  |
|---|---|
| **A.** Spin–spin | ☐ |
| **B.** Steady state | ☐ |
| **C.** Spin-lattice | ☐ |
| **D.** Rephasing | ☐ |

**165.** To produce a gradient echo, the sequence lacks a _____.

|  |  |
|---|---|
| **A.** 180° inversion | ☐ |
| **B.** 180° | ☐ |
| **C.** Gradient reversal | ☐ |
| **D.** Saturation pulse | ☐ |

Match the RF pulse pattern on the left with the pulse sequence on the right.

| Matches for Questions 166 to 169: |
|---|
| 1: FSE 2: GRE 3: IR 4: SE |

**166.** (A) 90°-180° Echo: _____

**167.** (B) 180°-90°-180° Echo: _____

**168.** (C) 90°-180° Echo-180° Echo-180° Echo: _____

**169.** (D) 90°-Echo: _____

**170.** A conventional spin-echo sequence is able to produce two different contrasts, PD and T2 per slice.

| | |
|---|---|
| **A.** False | ☐ |
| **B.** True | ☐ |

**171.** Gadolinium ions are considered to be _____?

| | |
|---|---|
| **A.** Iron oxide | ☐ |
| **B.** Paramagnetic | ☐ |
| **C.** Diamagnetic | ☐ |
| **D.** Supramagnetic | ☐ |

**172.** Gadolinium will shorten the _____ and the _____ of a tissue.

| | |
|---|---|
| **A.** T1, Spin-lattice | ☐ |
| **B.** T1, Spin–spin | ☐ |
| **C.** PD, T1 | ☐ |
| **D.** PD, T2 | ☐ |

**173.** For an TOF MRA of the carotids, the saturation pulse is placed _____ to the slices/slab.

| | |
|---|---|
| **A.** Inferior | ☐ |
| **B.** Parallel | ☐ |
| **C.** Superior | ☐ |
| **D.** Lateral | ☐ |

**174.** In a peripheral TOF MRA of say the hand or foot, the sequence of choice would be.

| | |
|---|---|
| **A.** 3D TOF | ☐ |
| **B.** 2D TOF | ☐ |
| **C.** 3D MOTSA | ☐ |
| **D.** Post contrast T1 spin-echo | ☐ |

**175.** High-resolution imaging includes all of the following except _____.

A. High matrix ☐
B. Thin slices ☐
C. Small FOV ☐
D. Short TE ☐

**176.** Which sequence could best diagnose bone bruise, avascular necrosis, or infection _____?

A. STIR ☐
B. GRE ☐
C. FSE ☐
D. Spin-echo ☐

**177.** An MRCP sequence typically has what scan factors?

A. Long TR, Short TE, and Fat-Sat ☐
B. Short TR, Short TE ☐
C. Long TR, Very Long TE, and Fat-Sat ☐
D. Very Short TR and TE with large Flip angle ☐

**178.** Halving the FOV would result in a drop in SNR to _____.

A. 1/2 ☐
B. 1/3 ☐
C. 1/4 ☐
D. 1/5 ☐

**179.** The correct way to identify (number) vertebral bodies is to count starting at _____.

A. C1 ☐
B. C2 ☐
C. T1 ☐
D. L5/S1 ☐

**180.** When is phase encoding performed?

**A.** During the 90° ☐
**B.** In between the 90° and 180° ☐
**C.** After excitation but before the echo ☐
**D.** After frequency encoding ☐

**181.** The excitation pulse is applied simultaneously with the _____.

**A.** Slice select gradient ☐
**B.** Phase encoding gradient ☐
**C.** Frequency encoding gradient ☐
**D.** None of these ☐

**182.** The echo forms at _____.

**A.** 1TAU ☐
**B.** 2TAU ☐
**C.** TE/2 ☐
**D.** Half the TR ☐

**183.** In a TOF MRA of foot, the saturation pulse should be placed where in relation to the slices?

**A.** Above ☐
**B.** Below ☐
**C.** Parallel ☐
**D.** Lateral ☐

**184.** Another name for a "SPOILED" GRE sequence is _____?

**A.** Coherent ☐
**B.** Incoherent ☐
**C.** Re-Phased ☐
**D.** De-Phased ☐

**185.** How are the slices or "LOCS" produced in a 3D sequence?

| | |
|---|---|
| **A.** A series of 90° RFs in the slice select gradient | ☐ |
| **B.** Ramp sampling of RF | ☐ |
| **C.** A second slice encoding gradient is applied | ☐ |
| **D.** Fourier transform is applied twice | ☐ |

**186.** Longitudinal is _____ to the transverse plane?

| | |
|---|---|
| **A.** Parallel | ☐ |
| **B.** 45° | ☐ |
| **C.** Perpendicular | ☐ |
| **D.** Oblique | ☐ |

**187.** An excitation pulse will flip the longitudinal NMV into the _____ if the RF pulse has the same _____ as the slice.

| | |
|---|---|
| **A.** X/Y, Precessional frequency | ☐ |
| **B.** Transverse, Amplitude | ☐ |
| **C.** $B_0$, Amplitude | ☐ |
| **D.** $B_1$, Larmor frequency | ☐ |

**188.** At 1 T, which three correctly describes the precessional frequency of hydrogen? _____.

| | |
|---|---|
| **A.** 42.6 and Gyromagnetic ratio, Constant | ☐ |
| **B.** Gyromagnetic ratio, 127.89, Constant | ☐ |
| **C.** 42.6, Gyromagnetic ratio, 3 T | ☐ |
| **D.** 63%, Constant, 1.5 T | ☐ |

**189.** What is being described? An accumulation of vectors aligned with an external static external magnetic field.

| | |
|---|---|
| **A.** $B_0$ | ☐ |
| **B.** The X/Y plane | ☐ |
| **C.** A NMV | ☐ |
| **D.** Ohm's law | ☐ |

**190.** In a T1 weighted image, which choice is correct for brightest to darkest tissue _____.

|   |   |
|---|---|
| **A.** Fat, Gad, Protein | ☐ |
| **B.** Fat, Gad, Muscle | ☐ |
| **C.** Fat, Muscle, Water | ☐ |
| **D.** Fat, Gray matter, Gad | ☐ |

**191.** The precessional frequency of hydrogen is _____ at a field strength of

_____.

|   |   |
|---|---|
| **A.** 42.6, 3T | ☐ |
| **B.** 42.6, 1.5T | ☐ |
| **C.** 42.6, 1T | ☐ |
| **D.** 127.89, 1.5T | ☐ |

**192.** The ability to locate in space the position from which a signal originated is called.

|   |   |
|---|---|
| **A.** Spatial resolution | ☐ |
| **B.** Temporal resolution | ☐ |
| **C.** Spatial localization | ☐ |
| **D.** Temporal localization | ☐ |

**193.** Protons spin on an axis in the presence of an applied external magnetic field.

|   |   |
|---|---|
| **A.** True | ☐ |
| **B.** False | ☐ |

**194.** Protons spin on an axis in the presence of an applied external magnetic field but are not fully perpendicular to that applied field. The deviation off perpendicular is called.

|   |   |
|---|---|
| **A.** Lattice angle | ☐ |
| **B.** Angular momentum | ☐ |
| **C.** Flip angle | ☐ |
| **D.** Ernst angle | ☐ |

**195.** The RF pulses used in MR imaging are considered to be.

A. Ionizing and low energy ☐
B. Non-ionizing and low energy ☐
C. High energy and ionizing ☐
D. Low energy and ionizing ☐

**196.** Which of the following factors will NOT affect the patient's SAR?

A. Increased TR ☐
B. Decreased echo train length ☐
C. Parallel imaging ☐
D. Echo spacing ☐

**197.** When compared to a wide rec. B/W, a narrow receiver B/W has a _____ SNR and a _____ min. TE.

A. lower, longer ☐
B. lower, shorter ☐
C. higher, longer ☐
D. shorter, lower ☐

**198.** The flip angle of a spin-echo is _____.

A. 180° ☐
B. 75° ☐
C. 90° ☐
D. It does not have one ☐

**199.** Saturation pulses are frequently used to:

A. Decrease motion ☐
B. Reduce pulsatile flow artifacts ☐
C. Increase scan time ☐
D. A and B ☐

**200.** A Sat. pulse is applied when?

A. Between the 90° and 180° ☐
B. After the 180° ☐
C. Before the echo ☐
D. Before the 90° ☐

**201.** Gradient echo sequences use partial flip angles that are _____.

> **A.** 45° ☐
> **B.** 90° ☐
> **C.** 12° ☐
> **D.** usually less than 90° but can be up to 90° ☐

**202.** A tissue can be saturated when _____.

> **A.** The TR is very short ☐
> **B.** There is insufficient time to T1 relax ☐
> **C.** Saturation pulses are applied ☐
> **D.** All of these ☐

**203.** An increase in TE will affect all of the following except:

> **A.** SNR ☐
> **B.** Echo spacing ☐
> **C.** Image contrast ☐
> **D.** SAR ☐

**204.** Increasing the flip angle while keeping the TR constant will cause?

> **A.** An increase in SAR ☐
> **B.** Saturation ☐
> **C.** Increased T2 ☐
> **D.** Both A and B ☐

**205.** The TE in ms can be affected by all the following except.

> **A.** FOV ☐
> **B.** Frequency matrix ☐
> **C.** Receiver bandwidth ☐
> **D.** Slice thickness ☐

**206.** In an inversion recovery sequence, the time from the inversion pulse to the 90° is the.

> **A.** Time of inversion ☐
> **B.** Interruption time ☐
> **C.** Inversion time ☐
> **D.** A and C ☐

**207.** Another name for Time is _____.

| | |
|---|---|
| **A.** Temporal | ☐ |
| **B.** Tempus | ☐ |
| **C.** TAU | ☐ |
| **D.** All of these | ☐ |

**208.** An increase in the FOV will _____ the resolution and _____ the SNR

| | |
|---|---|
| **A.** Decrease, Increase | ☐ |
| **B.** Decrease, Decrease | ☐ |
| **C.** Increase, Increase | ☐ |
| **D.** Increase, Increase | ☐ |

**209.** Narrowing the receiver bandwidth results in a _____,_____, and _____.

| | |
|---|---|
| **A.** Higher SNR and Resolution, Increased blur | ☐ |
| **B.** Lower SNR, Less chemical shift, Wrap | ☐ |
| **C.** Higher SNR, More chem. shift, Increased TE | ☐ |
| **D.** More chem. shift, Higher SNR, More T1 | ☐ |

**210.** In a coherent GRE, residual transverse NMV is _____ while in a spoiled GRE it is _____.

| | |
|---|---|
| **A.** Dephased, Dephased | ☐ |
| **B.** Rephased, Rephased | ☐ |
| **C.** Rephased, Dephased | ☐ |
| **D.** Dephased, Rephased | ☐ |

**211.** The initial RF pulse in an IR sequence moves the longitudinal NMV from 0° to _____.

| | |
|---|---|
| **A.** 90° | ☐ |
| **B.** 180° | ☐ |
| **C.** 270° | ☐ |
| **D.** 180/2 | ☐ |

**212.** Another name for the frequency encoding gradient is the _____.

A. ADC ☐
B. Readout gradient ☐
C. Phase encoding gradient ☐
D. Slice select gradient ☐

**213.** Gadolinium is well seen on a short tau inversion recovery sequence.

A. True, IR sequences enhanced the effects of Gado multiple times ☐
B. False, you only see the effects of Gado on spoiled GRE's ☐
C. Correct, Gado enhances all types of sequences ☐
D. False, STIR suppresses multiple short T1 relaxing tissues. Gado is one of them. ☐

**214.** Contrast in an IR sequence is controlled by the _____ and _____.

A. TR, TE ☐
B. TR, TI ☐
C. TE, TI ☐
D. TR, Flip angle ☐

**215.** The length of time the readout gradient is applied is related to the _____, _____, and _____.

A. FOV, Rec. B/W, and Phase matrix ☐
B. Frequency matrix, Rec. B/W, and TE ☐
C. FOV, Frequency matrix, and Rec. B/W ☐
D. ETL, ETS, and the TE ☐

**216.** Tripling the nex/AQC will increase in the SNR by a factor of _____.

A. 3 ☐
B. 6 ☐
C. 1.7 ☐
D. 1.4 ☐

**217.** An IR sequence with a TR of 3500 ms, TE 42 ms, and a TI of 150 ms will show fat as dark, CSF bright, and not show the gadolinium you just gave. This sequence is _____ weighted.

A. T2 ☐
B. PD ☐
C. T1 ☐
D. SPGR ☐

**218.** Increasing the number of phase steps will increase the patient's SAR dose.

A. True ☐
B. False ☐

**219.** SNR in a 3D sequence increases with the number of _____ and is equal to the _____.

A. Slices, √ of the number of slices/Locs ☐
B. Phase steps, √ of the number of slices ☐
C. Flip angle, Voxel volume ☐
D. Slab thickness, FOV ☐

**220.** Increasing the number of phase steps results in an image with better _____ but _____.

A. Resolution, more chemical shift ☐
B. Motion, lower SNR ☐
C. Resolution, lower SNR ☐
D. Smaller pixels, higher SNR ☐

**221.** A factor to consider when swapping phase and frequency directions is:

A. Which direction is the shortest axis ☐
B. Where is the motion coming from ☐
C. Will I get wrap ☐
D. All of these ☐

**222.** The effective TE in an FSE sequence is placed where in the k-Space

A. Edges ☐
B. Left side ☐
C. Right side ☐
D. Center ☐

**223.** What are eddy currents?

| | |
|---|---|
| **A.** a.k.a. Foucault currents | ☐ |
| **B.** They result from rapidly changing magnetic fields | ☐ |
| **C.** Opposing polarity magnetic fields causing distortion | ☐ |
| **D.** All of these | ☐ |

**224.** In order to double the SNR by using nex or Acq., you would have to _____ the nex:

| | |
|---|---|
| **A.** Double | ☐ |
| **B.** Triple | ☐ |
| **C.** Half | ☐ |
| **D.** Quadruple | ☐ |

**225.** Why is the TR in a proton density weighted image usually/often 3000+ ms?

| | |
|---|---|
| **A.** To increase SNR | ☐ |
| **B.** To increase T1 | ☐ |
| **C.** To increase T2 | ☐ |
| **D.** To decrease T1 | ☐ |

**226.** Motion on your images can be lessened by:

| | |
|---|---|
| **A.** All of these | ☐ |
| **B.** Immobilization | ☐ |
| **C.** Motion suppression sequences | ☐ |
| **D.** Scan faster | ☐ |

**227.** If scanning faster when your patient won't hold still usually results in _____.

| | |
|---|---|
| **A.** Lower resolution | ☐ |
| **B.** Higher SNR | ☐ |
| **C.** Better T1 | ☐ |
| **D.** A and C | ☐ |

**228.** A short TI suppresses a long T1 tissue while a long TI suppresses a short T1 tissue.

| | |
|---|---|
| **A.** False | ☐ |
| **B.** True | ☐ |

**229.** As slice thickness increases, what IQ factor also increases?

|   |   |
|---|---|
| **A.** Resolution | ☐ |
| **B.** Noise | ☐ |
| **C.** T1 contrast | ☐ |
| **D.** Partial volume | ☐ |

**230.** All factors remaining the same, as TR increases, _____ also increases.

|   |   |
|---|---|
| **A.** Resolution | ☐ |
| **B.** Signal | ☐ |
| **C.** T2 contrast | ☐ |
| **D.** Noise | ☐ |

**231.** All factors remaining the same, as TE increases, _____ decreases.

|   |   |
|---|---|
| **A.** Resolution | ☐ |
| **B.** Signal | ☐ |
| **C.** T2 contrast | ☐ |
| **D.** Noise | ☐ |

**232.** All factors remaining the same, as flip angle increases, _____ also increases.

|   |   |
|---|---|
| **A.** Resolution | ☐ |
| **B.** Signal | ☐ |
| **C.** T2 contrast | ☐ |
| **D.** Noise | ☐ |

**233.** Each line of k-Space contains information for the entire image.

|   |   |
|---|---|
| **A.** True | ☐ |
| **B.** False | ☐ |

**234.** All factors remaining the same, the higher the parallel imaging factor SNR is _____.

|   |   |
|---|---|
| **A.** Higher | ☐ |
| **B.** Lower | ☐ |
| **C.** Not affected | ☐ |

**235.** Due to the way data are acquired/processed with parallel imaging, wrap/ aliasing is always seen _____ in the image.

A. Left/Right ☐
B. Top/Bottom ☐
C. Ant./Post. ☐
D. Middle ☐

**236.** What is the opposite of T.O.F. (F.R.E.) angiography?

A. FSE ☐
B. CE-MRA ☐
C. Flow void ☐
D. DWI ☐

**237.** All other factors remaining the same, with higher and higher the parallel imaging factors, resolution is _____.

A. Higher ☐
B. Lower ☐
C. Not affected ☐

**238.** Auto pre-scan operations include Adjusting the receiver, Precessional frequency, and _____?

A. TR ☐
B. Transmitter gain ☐
C. TE ☐
D. Iso-center ☐

**239.** What is the effect on IQ when the ETL is very long?

A. Higher SNR ☐
B. Increased resolution ☐
C. Scan time is longer ☐
D. Increased blurring ☐

**240.** What is the effect on IQ when the echo spacing is increased?

| | |
|---|---|
| **A.** Lower SNR | ☐ |
| **B.** Higher resolution | ☐ |
| **C.** Scan time is shorter | ☐ |
| **D.** Increased T2 contrast | ☐ |

**241.** What two scan parameters can affect echo spacing?

| | |
|---|---|
| **A.** Phase and Frequency matrix | ☐ |
| **B.** Phase matrix and Transmitter B/W | ☐ |
| **C.** Frequency matrix and Receiver B/W | ☐ |
| **D.** Parallel imaging factor and Receiver B/W. | ☐ |

**242.** As echo spacing increases, the echoes will be more:

| | |
|---|---|
| **A.** Spin lattice | ☐ |
| **B.** Spin–spin | ☐ |
| **C.** Spin density | ☐ |
| **D.** DWI | ☐ |

**243.** An example of areas where there are high differences in magnetic susceptibility?

| | |
|---|---|
| **A.** Sinuses and Brain | ☐ |
| **B.** Peri-orbital fat and the Orbit | ☐ |
| **C.** Gray and White matter | ☐ |
| **D.** Dural sinuses and Brain | ☐ |

**244.** Areas of magnetic field inhomogeneity appear as _____ on a GRE sequence.

| | |
|---|---|
| **A.** High signal | ☐ |
| **B.** Signal loss with warping | ☐ |
| **C.** Signal warping but no Signal loss | ☐ |
| **D.** There is no effect on I.Q. | ☐ |

**245.** Areas of decreased diffusion on a DWI sequence appear as _____.

> **A.** High signal ☐
> **B.** Low signal ☐
> **C.** Iso intense signal ☐
> **D.** Not well seen ☐

**246.** On a DWI sequence, Image contrast comes from?

> **A.** T1 differences ☐
> **B.** PD differences ☐
> **C.** T2 differences ☐
> **D.** Differences in diffusion ☐

**247.** Which of the following will not affect a sequence's minimum TE?

> **A.** Number of slices ☐
> **B.** Frequency matrix ☐
> **C.** FOV ☐
> **D.** Rec. B/W ☐

**248.** To find the TI to null a tissue, the equation used is _____.

> **A.** TR/2 ☐
> **B.** TR/TE ☐
> **C.** T1×0.69 ☐
> **D.** TR×0.69 ☐

**249.** What is the effect on IQ on shortening the TR to approximately 200 ms on a T1 at 3T?

> **A.** Low T1 contrast ☐
> **B.** Low T2 contrast ☐
> **C.** Low SNR ☐
> **D.** SAR limits may be exceeded ☐

**250.** What is the effect on T1 contrast when the ETL is lengthened?

A. Less T1 contrast ☐
B. More T2 contrast ☐
C. Low SNR ☐
D. None of these ☐

**251.** Which parameter will not change voxel size?

A. FOV ☐
B. Rec. bandwidth ☐
C. Slice thickness ☐
D. Frequency matrix ☐

**252.** Of the following sequences, which is the least sensitive to magnetic susceptibility?

A. Turbo spin-echo ☐
B. D.W.I. ☐
C. Spin-echo ☐
D. Gradient echo ☐

**253.** There are two kinds of shimming. They are?

A. Wooden and Plastic ☐
B. Active and Plastic ☐
C. Active and Passive ☐
D. Auto and Standard ☐

**254.** A STIR sequence is used to suppress _____ tissue while a T2 FLAIR suppresses _____ tissue.

A. Short T1, short T2 ☐
B. Long T2, short T1 ☐
C. Short T1, long T1 ☐
D. Long T2 and long T1 ☐

**255.** From the following parameters, which will give the best T1 contrast image?

| | |
|---|---|
| **A.** 3500 TR, 35 TE | ☐ |
| **B.** 450 TR, 100 TE | ☐ |
| **C.** 5555 TR, 100 TE | ☐ |
| **D.** 567 TR, 10 TE | ☐ |

**256.** Good I.Q. in soft tissue fat sat imaging of the neck, larynx, and brachial plexus can be made difficult by?

| | |
|---|---|
| **A.** Scan coverage | ☐ |
| **B.** Air/Tissue interfaces | ☐ |
| **C.** Field inhomogeneities | ☐ |
| **D.** B and C | ☐ |

**257.** What is being described: With a constant TR and an increasing flip angle, the point at which signal begins to decrease is the?

| | |
|---|---|
| **A.** Gradient echo dephasing | ☐ |
| **B.** Miramar effect | ☐ |
| **C.** Ernst angle | ☐ |
| **D.** Pleisiodynamic effect | ☐ |

**258.** What does the 180° pulse not correct for?

| | |
|---|---|
| **A.** Main mag. field inhomogeneities | ☐ |
| **B.** Local mag. field inhomogeneities | ☐ |
| **C.** Motion | ☐ |
| **D.** Magnetic susceptibilities | ☐ |

**259.** Of the MRA sequences listed below, which one has the best background suppression?

| | |
|---|---|
| **A.** 2D TOF | ☐ |
| **B.** Phase contrast | ☐ |
| **C.** 3D TOF | ☐ |
| **D.** CE-MRA | ☐ |

**260.** Which sequence will produce the brightest fat?

> **A.** T1 ☐
> **B.** T2 ☐
> **C.** Partial flip angle GRE ☐
> **D.** STIR ☐

**261.** How is pixel size determined?

> **A.** FOV ÷ Frequency × Phase ☐
> **B.** FOV ÷ Scan Matrix ☐
> **C.** Scan Matrix ÷ Slice Thickness ☐
> **D.** FOV × Scan Matrix ☐

**262.** What artifact would you expect to see due to the differences in frequency between fat and water?

> **A.** Wrap ☐
> **B.** Poor fat sat ☐
> **C.** Chemical shift ☐
> **D.** Aliasing ☐

**263.** What is being described: An RF pulse is applied off resonance to water in order to lessen signal from another.

> **A.** Water excitation ☐
> **B.** Magnetization transfer ☐
> **C.** Dixon technique ☐
> **D.** Fat saturation ☐

**264.** What imaging method can be thought of as imaging multiple slices simultaneously?

> **A.** 2D ☐
> **B.** Interleaved ☐
> **C.** Dixon technique ☐
> **D.** 3D ☐

**265.** Hydrogen is the only element that can be used in MR Imaging. True or False?

The chart below is for you to practice what will happen to the images if you made a change to the protocol. Many of the questions you may see are designed to test if you know the consequences of your actions.

| Parameter | Change | SNR | Resolution |
|---|---|---|---|
| FOV | ↑ | | |
| Slice Thickness | ↑ | | |
| GAP | ↓ | | |
| Phase Matrix | ↓ | | |
| NSA/NEX/ACQ | ↑ | | |
| Receiver Bandwidth | Narrow | | |
| Frequency Matrix | ↑ | | |
| Surface Coil | Go Smaller | | |

| | | Weighting | | |
|---|---|---|---|---|
| | Change | T1 | T2 | Scan time |
| TR | ↓ | | | |
| TE | ↑ | | | |
| ETL | ↑ | | | |

\* Use arrows to indicate the direction of change.

I encourage you to copy this chart and practice. For the answers you get wrong, go to the corresponding section in MRI Physics: Tech to Tech Explanations and re-review to improve your understanding. *Work on your weaknesses not your strengths.* The answer sheet for this chart is at the end of the section answers.

# Section 2: Parameters, Image Formation, Data Acquisition: Answers

1. **A.** The ppm means that for every 1 million rotations that water does, fat does 3.5 less. Water is at 1 000 000, so fat rotates 999 996.5 rotations.
2. **A.** The moving magnetic field causes electrons to flow-inducing current in the coil.

3. **D.** Gradients are key in "Spatial Localization."

4. **D.** The 90°, X/Y, and transverse plane are all pretty interchangeable.

5. **C.** An RF pulse is not just a "single" frequency but a range frequencies or bandwidth. The RF that excites a slice is a transmitted B/W. Do not let the B/W term confuse you. 2 B/W's: a transmitted B/W to excite the slice, and a receiver B/W that samples at TE.

6. **D.** Equilibrium is the system returning to the lowest energy level possible.

7. **D.** $W_0 = B_0 y$. In this question, I substituted for $B_0$ for Tesla. Hopefully you picked up on this. It is not uncommon to substitute/swap terms. You need to know the terminology.

8. **C.** F.I.D. Free Induction Decay. This means DECAY of signal because the protons are FREE of the INDUCTION from the RF.

9. **D.** Know that T1 is a REGROWTH process. The protons will return (REGROW) back toward $B_0$.

10. **A.** T2 is a DECAY process which means that transverse (X/Y) NMV is spreading out or decaying.

11. **A.** Another equilibrium question.

12. **A.**

13. **D.** Magnetic moment or Angular momentum.

14. **C.**

15. **A**

16. **C.** Contrast is an unbelievably important concept that you must grasp.

17. **D**

18. **D**

19. **B.** The Larmor equation is as stated number 7. The Gyromagnetic Ratio × Field strength = Precessional Frequency.

20. **D.** This question is nothing more the Faraday's law stated in reverse. Here the coil is moving through a magnetic field instead of the typical moving magnetic passing a coil. It is also the answer to Question 2. Remember one question can answer another.

21. **B**

22. **D**

23. **D.** T2*.

24. **A**

25. **A**

26. **D.** Both B + C. Know the different terms and how they may be substituted. So, why is "A" not correct? The Protons do not go back to the X/Y without an RF pulse being applied.

27. **C.** Another equilibrium question, number 6, 11, and 27. I point this out because so far there have been three equilibrium questions, all the same answer. Number 6 and 11 are rather similar.

28. **B**

29. **A**

30. **B.** I put the term "Thermo-Dynamic Characteristic" in to make you think. Do not let the question "lead" you. PD is a tissue characteristic. Answers A and D, are out-right wrong leaving B and C making it a 50/50 Gauss. Even though C is tempting because of the word Characteristic, have you ever really seen that term in an MR text book? No. When tissues T1 and T2 relax, they are releasing energy which could in a Quantum Physics context be called a Thermo-Dynamic Characteristic. This question is a PD question not a T1 or T2 question. Try not to read into it.

31. **C.** Before the excitation pulse, 100% of the NMV is aligned with $B_0$, after excitation, it is all in the transverse. Over time the NMV returns over time to $B_0$, so it is considered a REGROWTH process.

32. **B**

33. **D**

34. **B.** The $B_1$ field is orientated at 90° or orthogonal to $B_0$.

35. **B**

36. **D**

37. **D.** Di means 2. Dipole means two poles. A magnet has a North and South pole so is a "Dipole."

38. **C.** 42.57 is a CONSTANT and never changes regardless of the magnetic field strength.

39. **D.** Make sure you practice the Larmor equation math multiple times.

40. **C.** Another "Constant" question.

| Gauss | to mT | G ÷ by 10 = mT | mT ÷ by 1000 = Tesla |
| --- | --- | --- | --- |
| 1 G | 1.G ÷ 10 = | 0.1 mT | 0.0001 T |
| 5 G | 5.G ÷ 10 = | 0.5 mT | 0.0005 T |
| 10 000 G | 10 000.G ÷ 10 = | 1000 mT | 1 T |

G to mT, ÷ by 10 or move decimal point 1 place left; mT to T, ÷ by 1000 or move decimal point 3 places to left

| mTesla | to Gauss | mT × 10 = G |
| --- | --- | --- |
| 0.1 mT | 0.1 × 10 = | 1 G |
| 0.5 mT | 0.5 × 10 = | 5 G |

mT to G, multiply by 10 or move decimal point 1 place

## Section 2 Question 41–54

41. **C**
42. **B**
43. **B**
44. **D**
45. **C**
46. **B**
47. **A**
48. **A.** True.
49. **C.** This is a rather worthy version of Question 16.
50. **C**
51. **D.** Water is diamagnetic, Gado is paramagnetic, Ferrous is strongly attracted, Dipole is a magnet.
52. **A**
53. **C**
54. **A.** Interchangeable terms: Hydrogen density, Proton density, and Spin density.
55. **A.** Protons behave like magnetic because they have "Spin" or rotate on their axis.
56. **B.** Immediately after the RF (Excitation pulse) is turned off, protons start to return to $B_0$ (going from transverse to longitudinal). What is happening is a magnetic field is passing by or through the coils thus inducing current (Faraday's Law). This causes a small amount of signal which happens very quickly. That small quick signal is called the F.I.D.
57. **D**
58. **A**
59. **C**
60. True.
61. True.
62. True.
63. **C. Temporal** Res.= scanning over **TIME**, **Spatial** Resolution = scanning over a Distance or **SPACE**. "T" for Time, and "S" for Space.
64. **D.** All of these tissues have protons that can be aligned and "flipped" by RF so can give signal vs. Tendon/Cortical bone that contain protons, that cannot be flipped so give very little to no signal.

65. **D**

66. **B**

67. **D**

68. **B**

69. **C.** You only need one 90° RF but more then two 180°s to make a FSE.

70. **D**

71. **D.** Transverse also known as "Spin-Spin Relaxation."

72. **C**

73. **D**

74. **A**

75. **D**

76. **D**

77. **C**

78. **D**

79. **D**

80. **C**

81. **D**

82. **C**

83. **A.** Liquid helium is at −452 °F. (very close to absolute zero). Absolute zero is −459 °F or 0 °K. This extremely cold temperature lowers the resistance in the wires that carry the electric current that makes $B_0$.

84. **C.** Diamagnetic, water, weakly repels $H_2O$, a ferrous material is strongly attracted.

85. **D.** k-Space holds the raw data acquired during the scan, then FT will process the data.

86. **B.** We generate signal during a scan. Noise is a random entity that is also received by the coil. A bigger coil lowers the SNR. More noise is received which lowers the overall SNR.

87. **A.** Seeing a tissue as brighter or darker compared to another is contrast.

88. **B.** T1 is Spin-lattice while T2 is Spin–spin.

89. **D.** MRI has a lot of interchangeable terms. You need to be familiar with them.

90. **D**

91. **D**

92. **A**

93. **C**

94. D

95. B

96. A

97. C. Any substance that at low temperatures, lose both electrical resistance and magnetic flux fields is a superconductor. The alloy niobium-titanium is an example.

98. A

99. B

100. C

101. B

102. B

103. B

104. C

105. A. A) Phase coherence B) FID C) Equilibrium D) Resonant

106. C. It is not "A," as protons do not attain phase coherence until the excitation pulse ($B_1$) is applied. Not B, FID only happens after RF pulses, no RF is mentioned, and not D as resonance happens after RF. The best answer is equilibrium even though equilibrium is thought to occur with energy loss not being put into a magnetic field.

107. A

108. C. When a tissue's NMV is at 90° to the coil, then Max. Signal (brightness) will be generated in the coil by that tissue. A tissue that simultaneously is at say 45° to the coil will generate less signal and not be as bright (gray). One tissue being bright, another not so bright equals *CONTRAST*. I cannot stress enough the importance of the concept of contrast in MRI and all the other modalities.

109. D. QUAD = 4.

110. D

111. A. It is not C even though the ETL will and does affect image contrast. To long of an ETL on a T1 weighted sequence and you leave T1 land. Also, if the echo spacing is too long, the later echoes of the ETL will have progressively T2 in them and this will also affect the image contrast.

112. D

113. A

114. C

115. D

**116. C**

*Questions 117–126 cover relaxation curves. Additional information on interpreting relaxation curves can be found in Chapter 3 of MRI Physics: Tech to Tech Explanations.*

**117. C.** T1 regrows, so lines go up and to the right. As two or more lines converge upon each other, T1 image contrast decreases. The lines represent signal intensity over time. The area in between the lines is or can be considered image contrast.

**118. C.** The bright tissue is always the top line. Note that the signal amplitude is noted on the left. Isointense means the curves are very close together.

**119. C.** Again, difference in signal intensity is CONTRAST.

**120. A**

**121. B**

**122. A**

**123. B**

**124. D**

**125. D**

**126. A**

**127. A**

**128. C.** 3.5 is the stock answer to what is the PF difference between fat and water.

**129. D.** Hopefully you have memorized the frequency differences by Field strength: at 1.5 T it is 223 and 444 at 3 T.

**130. D**

**131. B.** See the Weighting Triangles in Chapter 3 of *MRI Physics: Tech to Tech Explanations.*

**132. C**

**133. C**

**134. C**

**135. B**

**136. C**

**137. A**

**138. A**

**139. B.** While scan time doubles, the SNR ↑'s by a factor of the square root of the number of nex. The number of nex/NSA in how many times each line is filled by successive TR's. By that I mean that in say a 2 nex sequence, TR number 1 fills line 1, and TR number 2 fills line 1 again, TR number 3 fills line 2, TR number 4 fills line 2 again, and so on until each line is filled twice. Filling a line twice requires the PEG is applied at the same amplitude on successive TR's.

140. **A.** It is not B as a FOV will ↓ Pixel size which = fewer Hydrogen protons per pixel which = lower SNR. Remember, Signal is the number of protons in a pixel, and a quality image has lots of pixels. We must balance between SNR, resolution, and scan time.

141. **A.** It is not "B" as thickness is related to voxel size or volume.

142. **A.** "In-Plane resolution" is another/fancy way to say Slice Thickness.

143. **D.** Flow void (or HVSL) displays as black vessels whereas TOF (flow-related enhancement) is seen as bright vessels.

144. **D.** During an MRA, the longer blood is in a slice or slab, the more RF's it receives and is more likely to saturate causing losing signal.

145. **A.** If you hear "Voxel Volume," think thickness. A pixel is a DOT, a voxel is a dot with VOLUME.

146. **C**

147. **D.** It is not C as $B_1$ is always on, a slice (SSG) does have a flip angle which comes from $B_1$, and the FEG has no RF at all.

148. **D.** Both A and B: The amplitude of the SSG with a constant transmitter B/W will alter the slice thickness and alternately, a constant SSG and by varying the trans. B/W will alter the slice thickness.

149. **C**

150. **C.** All systems want to be at the lowest possible energy state.

151. **B.** The Larmor frequency of tissues is governed by $B_1$.

152. **A**

153. **C**

154. **A**

155. **A**

156. **C.** A magnet has two (Di) poles. North and South.

157. **B**

158. **C**

159. **D**

160. **B**

161. **D.** A PSD of 180°- 90° - 180° is an inversion recovery.

162. **B**

163. **D.** The number of phase encodes needed for a sequence is the Phase matrix times the number of nex (or NSA or Acquisitions), so $192 \times 2 = 384$. You could ask the same question as to how many TR's are needed for the same sequence. It would be the same answer. As on a SE, there is one PEG per TR.

164. **B**

165. **B**

166. 4. 90°/180° echo: Basic SE RF pattern.

167. 3. 180°/90°/180° echo: Inversion recovery RF pattern.

168. 1. 90°/180° echo, °180 echo, °180 echo is a fast spin-echo RF pattern.

169. 2. 90°/Echo is a gradient echo pattern. **Of note here is that a GRE does not usually start with a 90° RF excitation pulse but they can.**

170. **D.** True. A dual echo spin-echo still an option today, though seldom used. Years ago, it was used in the brain and spine to evaluate for multiple sclerosis.

171. **B**

172. **B.** T1 is spin-lattice and T2 is spin–spin. We almost always combine T1 with T2. Seldom do you change it up to say T1 with spin–spin, or spin-lattice with T2. What they sometimes do is use the interchangeable terms in an uncommon order: like T2, then T1. When referring to those two weightings, you always say T1 and then T2. It is just what we do. We do not say it the other way around.

173. **C**

174. **B.** 2D is better for slow flow as it decreases the likelihood of in-plane saturation. Blood only has to get through a 2, 3, or 4 mm slice vs. in a 3D where blood has to travel 30–50 mm. While both 2D and 3D have very short TR's, it is the distance that needs to be traveled to get out of the slice before the multiple RF's cause saturation.

175. **D.** TE is not a scan parameter that has anything to do with the geometry of the pixels. It is the geometry (size) of the pixels that make it a "High Resolution vs. Standard Resolution" scan.

176. **A.** STIR. While T2 fat sat and STIR sequences have very similar contrasts (dark fat and bright fluid), STIR is usually the "go to" sequence for marrow edema in MSK studies while T2 F/S is a bit more common for soft tissue structures, especially in the brain. **Authors note**: This last statement is not a rule, just an observation. As far as F/S vs. STIR, if you cannot get a good T2 F/S, STIR becomes your plan B. STIR's are far less sensitive to field inhomogeneities than is F/S.

177. **C**

178. **C.** FOV is a huge contributor to or killer of SNR. Half the FOV and you are left with 1/4th the original SNR. Easy math here: $\frac{1}{2} \times \frac{1}{2} = \frac{1}{4}$. Remember you are halving in two directions.

179. **B**

180. **B.** Know your basic PSD's. Remember S.P.F. Slice, Phase, Frequency.

181. **A**

182. **B.** 1 TAU is the time from excitation to refocus and 1 TAU from refocus to TE this = 2TAU.

183. **B**

184. **B**

185. **C**

186. **C**

187. **A**

188. **A**

189. **C**

190. **C**

191. **C**

192. **C**

193. **A**

194. **B**

195. **B**

196. **D**

197. **C**

198. **C**

199. **D**

200. **D**

201. **D**

202. **B**

203. **D**

204. **D**

205. **D**

206. **A**

207. **D**

208. **A**

209. **C**

210. **C**

**211. B**

**212. B**

**213. D.** STIR, because of its short TI, will suppress all tissues with similarly T1 relaxation times. If you know the T1 of any tissue, multiply it by 0.69 and use that TI to suppress it.

**214. C**

**215. C.** This is a 2 for 1 kind of question. 1st. do you know what the "Read-out Gradient" is and 2nd. what does the Frequency Encoding Gradient affect. Remember the longer a gradient is applied, the more time in ms of the TR it eats up, and how much it increases the TE in ms.

**216. C.** All things being equal, SNR is a factor of the square root ($\sqrt{}$) of the # of nex/acq.

**217. C**

**218. A.** More phase steps equal more 180's in an FSE. (SAR is seldom a concern with GRE's)

**219. A**

**220. C.** Better resolution is good, but without signal to see it with there is really no net gain.

**221. D**

**222. D.** Remember **C-C. C**enter lines of k-Space give image **C**ontrast

**223. D.** Foucault Currents is another name for Eddy Currents

**224. D.** Adding nex/acq is an inefficient way to add signal from a time perspective.

**225. D.** Long TR is to minimize T1 contrast in an image. It's not "A" even though a longer TR will ↑ SNR. It's not "C", T2's you do have a long TR to lessen T1, but T2 comes from a long TE

**226. A**

**227. A**

**228. False.** Long TI will suppress Long T1 tissue and Short TI suppresses Short T1 Tissue.

**229. D.** Of the 4 answers, "B" is the best choice. As slice thickness ↑'s resolution goes down but SNR goes up. Slice thickness does not affect weighting. However, as slice thickness goes up, "Partial Volume affect" increases. Partial Volume is an oblique way of saying Resolution. If the IACs are 2mm's thick and you scan them with a 10 mm thick slice you are not going to see them very well.
You only "partially" see them. They blend or average themselves into the slice. Section 2: #232: T2 axials of IAC's at 5mm and 3 mm. You see the IAC's better on the 3's as there is less Partial volume effect.

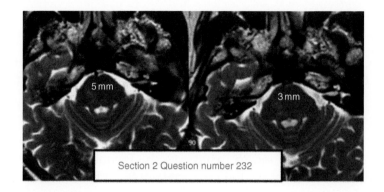

5 mm    3 mm

Section 2 Question number 232

230. **B.** When more protons re-align with $B_0$, there will be more signal. It's opposite to using to short of a TR which causes tissue saturation (low signal).

231. **B**

232. **B.** Check out ERNST Angle on pg. 77 of Tech-to-Tech Explanations.

233. **B.**

234. **B.** As the PI factor ↑'s, less phase lines as actually filled. Less Phase steps = less RF's = ↓ SAR. Increasing the PI factor may not be the 1st choice in lowering SAR but if that's all you have then you have to do what you have to do.

235. **D**

236. **C**

237. **B**

238. **B.** Transmitter Gain is a factor that tells how much RF power is needed to push/flip the NMV into the X/Y plane.

239. **D**

240. **D**

241. **C**

242. **B.** Remember another name for T2 can be Spin-Spin.

243. **A**

244. **B**

245. **A**

246. **D**

247. **A**

248. **C**

249. **C.** If tissues are not given enough time to T1 relax (which comes from the TR) and they get another excitation pulse to soon they will not

give max. signal at TE. Images become grainy. **Grainy images always mean low SNR**. The contrast may be there but with very low signal you just can't see it. You need balance between Contrast, SNR and Resolution, the IQ Triangle. See MRI Physics Tech to Tech Explanations, in Chapter 3, Image Optimization for more on the IQ Triangle. Also, you may have thought answer D. No. While SAR limits may get exceeded with a very short TR, SAR is not an IQ concern.

250. **B.** While keeping the ETL short (2 or 3 echoes) on a T1 weighted image is a golden rule, the reason to keep it short is to keep T2 out of your k-Space. A short ETL doesn't make it more T1, it makes it less T2. Remember TR is T1, TE is for T2.

251. **B.** of the 4 listed scan parameters, Rec. B/W is the only one that will not change the geometry of the pixel or voxel.

252. **A.** The least sensitive to Susceptibility is the FSE or Turbo Spin Echo. This question of often asked backwards to this one. Like: Which sequence is the most sensitive to Magnetic susceptibility. (Substitute METAL for the word Magnetic Susceptibility).

253. **C.** Aside for the Manual Shim that most systems allow the user to do, there are 2 other ways/options for magnetic field shimming: Active and Passive

254. **C.**

255. **D.** Short TR and Short TE. "A" will have lousy T1 contrast due to the long TE, "B" will be who knows what contrast wise as You'll maximize both T1 and T2 with that combo, and "C" is a T2.

256. **D.** Soft tissue imaging of the Neck, Larynx and Brachial Plexus can be difficult to get good Fat Sat images due to the Field Inhomogeneities caused by the Air/tissue interfaces with in the FOV.

257. **C**

258. **C**

259. **B.**

260. **A.** Of the listed contrasts, T1 will have the brightest fat. T2, yes, fat is bright but pound for pound, T1 has brighter fat. STIR, (Short Time Inversion Recovery) by its nature suppresses short T1 relaxing tissues due the short TI. As far as the "Partial Flip Angle GRE" goes, insufficient data. The first question when hear "GRE" is, what's the flip angle? The F/A tells you a lot about the weighting as will the TE. In GRE land, High F/A and **Short TE = T1**, a Low F/A and **long TE= T2**.

261. **B.** The FOV is ÷ by the scan matrix (Phase and Freq matrix.) You may need to do that math twice. For example, if the FOV is 240 and the matrix is 192 × 256. 240 ÷ 192 = 1.25 and 240 ÷ 256= .93. if the matrix is square, i.e. $256^2$ then it's .93×.93 or $.93^2$.

262. **C.** The differences in PF between Fat and Water at any given field strength is actually called Chemical Shift. If you think about it, even though both contain Hydrogen, they are both different "chemicals" and are shown with their peaks at different places along the MR Spectrum. When you manually tune for a Fat sat, you are seeing a spectrum of the 2 chemicals with the space between the peaks is the "Chemical Shift". See Below: Note the denotation of the PF on the bottom in boxes.

263. **B.** Mag. Transfer is used most often in Brain MRA to suppress signal from white matter to increase contrast between the WM and the vessels. It is also used in T1 weighted post gad Brain imaging to again suppress white matter and bring out enhancing M.S. lesions.

264. **D.** 2D and 3D will, due to the vert short TR and TE suppress the background some, CE-MRA does a pretty good job if you subtract the pre for the post (but Subtraction was not a listed option and don't assume it.) Just because your site does sub's, that's not the case everywhere. So, Phase contrast does the best job of background suppression right out of the box. The 3D Pulse Sequence excites the entire volume with RF and then partition it into "slices or Locs" multiple slice encodings.

*Please be advised that different manufactures display the fat and water peaks reversed. This means that the fat may be shown on the left with water on the right.*

Note the Hz (frequency) at bottom of the image.

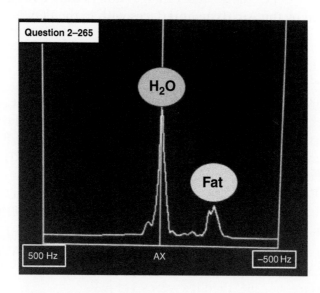

265. **False.** Hydrogen is used because of its shear abundance and ease of being flipped into the Transverse Plane. There are many other elements/Isotopes such as: $^3$He, $^{13}$Carbon, $^{19}$Flourine, and $^{31}$ Phosphorus. Note that these elements have an odd number of Protons in their nucleus, are unbalanced, will have a Magnetic Moment and able to give signal during an MR Sequence.

# Section 2: Enlarged Illustrations

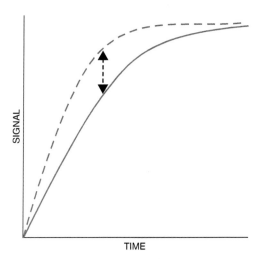

**Figure 2.1** T1 relaxation curves. Shown are curves for two different tissues. The tissue represented by the dashed line has a shorter or faster T1 relaxation time when compared to the solid line tissue with a longer or slower T1 relaxation time. The space between them is signal intensity from each at any given time. Note that the spacing between the two is small early on in time and late at the top right. *Remember* that the difference in signal intensity between two tissues is **CONTRAST**. The dashed line will be brighter at any given time than the solid line tissue. Early and late in the curves, contrast is small. The arrow shows the maximum amount of T1 contrast between the two tissues.

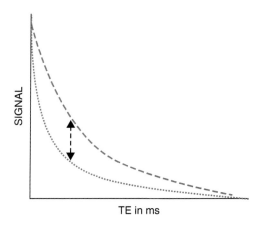

**Figure 2.2** T2 Relaxation curves. Shown are curves for two different tissues. The tissue represented by the dotted line has a shorter or faster T2 relaxation time when compared to the dashed line tissue with a longer or slower T2 relaxation time. The space between them is signal intensity from each at any given time. Note that the spacing between the two is small early on in time and late at the top right. *Remember* that the difference in signal intensity between two tissues is **CONTRAST**. The dashed line will be brighter at any given time than the solid line tissue. Early and late in the curves, contrast is small. The arrow shows the maximum amount of T2 contrast between the two tissues.

| Gauss | to mT | G ÷ by 10 = mT | mT ÷ by 1000 = Tesla |
|---|---|---|---|
| 1 G | 1.G ÷ 10 = | 0.1 mT | 0.0001 T |
| 5 G | 5.G ÷ 10 = | 0.5 mT | 0.0005 T |
| 10000 G | 10000.G ÷ 10 = | 1000 mT | 1 T |

G to mT; ÷ by 10 or move decimal point 1 place left. mT to T; ÷ by 1000 or move decimal point 3 places to Left

| mTesla | to Gauss | mT × 10 = G |
|---|---|---|
| 0.1 mT | 0.1 × 10 = | 1 G |
| 0.5 mT | 0.5 × 10 = | 5 G |

mT to G; multiply by 10 or move decimal point 1 place

# Section 2 Questions 41–54

**Section 2: Question 41–45:** Gauss conversion: A commonly asked question is about the 5 Gauss line. These are highlighted in yellow. Note that Gauss to mTesla is a division of 10. Move decimal over one place to left. You will very likely be asked in mT's, the equivalent of Gauss of vice versa.

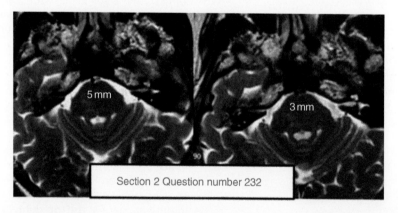

**Section 2: Question 232.** The images are axial through the posterior fossa at the levels of the IAC's. The left image is 5 mm's thick, right are 3 mm's thick. The thinner slices show the IAC's better. This is due to a lessening of the "Partial Volume Effect"

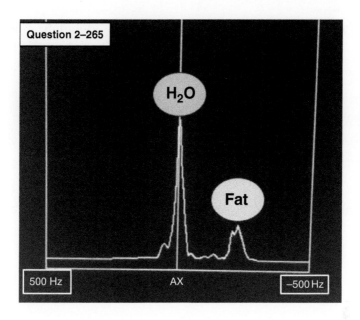

**Section 2: Question 265.** These two peaks are positioned, from left to right due to their respective precessional frequencies. The space between the two peaks is called the "Chemical Shift." The artifact that is seem when these two peaks are further apart is of course called Chemical Shift. Chemical Shift artifact is made worse by the scan factor: Receiver Bandwidth.

An easy way to remember this is that when you NARROW the B/W, you WIDEN the Chemical shift.

# Chapter 2: Parameters, Image Formation, Data Acquisition

The idea of this advanced examination, besides testing your general knowledge or MRI, is to see if you know the **consequences of your actions.** If you do X or Y, then how will G and H be affected. Below is a common fill in the blank chart that hits the most commonly changed scan parameters. **These affects are something you need to know both for the Advanced Registry and in real-life scanning**. I urge you to photocopy this chart and practice. Try talk it out with a coworker or another student technologist. By explaining it to someone else, you will be surprised how much you learn by teaching. See Chapter 11 in *MRI Physics: Tech to Tech Explanations* for extra information.

The chart below has an added column from the previous chart. It states the direction of change of the pixel size/volume as the top eight parameters will change the geometry of the pixel/voxels.

| Paratmeter | CHANGE | SNR | Resolution | Pixel volume |
|---|---|---|---|---|
| FOV | ↑ | ↑ | ↓ | ↑ |
| Slice Thickness | ↑ | ↑ | ↓ | ↑ |
| GAP | ↓ | θ | θ | θ |
| Phase Matrix | ↓ | ↑ | ↓ | ↑ |
| NSA/NEX/ACQ | ↑ | ↑ | θ | θ |
| Receiver Bandwidth | Narrow | ↑ | θ | θ |
| Frequency Matrix | ↑ | ↓ | ↑ | ↓ |
| Surface Coil | Go Smaller | ↑ | θ | θ |

| | | Contrast | | |
|---|---|---|---|---|
| | Change | T1 | T2 | Scan Time |
| TR | ↓ | ↑ | θ | ↑ |
| TE | ↑ | ↓ | ↑ | θ |
| ETL | ↑ | ↓ | ↑ | ↓ |

The θ means no effect on I.Q.

| 2 | Parameter | PRO | CON | T1 contrast | T2 contrast | PD |
|---|---|---|---|---|---|---|
| 3 | Increased TR | Higher number of slices, Lower SAR, Increased SNR | Increased Scan Time, Less T1 | Less T1 | Less T1 | Less T1 |
| 4 | Increased TE | More T2 | Decreased SNR | More T2 | More T2 | More T2 |
| 5 | Increased NEX | Increased SNR, Mild motion suppression | Increased Scan time | | | |
| 6 | Increased Slice thickness | More Coverage, Increased SNR | Less Resolution | | | |
| 7 | Increased FOV | Higher SNR, shorter Min. TE, Less Wrap, Increased Coverage | Less Resolution, | | | |
| 8 | Increased Freq. Matrix | Higher Resolution | Less SNR, Longer Min. TE and bigger ETS | | | |
| 9 | Increased Phase Matrix | Higher Res. | Lower SNR, Longer Scan time | | | |
| 10 | Increased Flip Angle (GRE) | More T1, Increased SNR | Higher SAR | | | |
| 11 | Increase Echo Train** | Shorter Scan time, More T2 | More Blurring, Higher SAR, Higher mix of Contrasts | | | |
| 12 | | | | T1 Contrast | T2 Contrast | PD |
| 13 | Decreased TR | Decreased SNR, Less Slices, More T1 | Higher SAR | More t1 | More Sat | More t1 |
| 14 | Decreased TE | Increased SNR, Less T2 | Less T2 | θ | → | θ |

| 2 | Parameter | PRO | CON | T1 contrast | T2 contrast | PD |
|---|---|---|---|---|---|---|
| 15 | Decreased NEX | Decreased SNR | Decreased SNR | | | |
| 16 | Decreased Slice thickness | Increased Resolution | Lower SNR | | | |
| 17 | Decreased FOV | Higher Resolution | Lower SNR, Longer Min. TE, More wrap | | | |
| 18 | Decreased Freq Matrix | Higher SNR, Lower Min. TE and smaller ETS | Less Res. | | | |
| 19 | Decrease Echo Train** | Less T2, Longer scan time, more T1, Less SAR, Less mix of contrasts | Less Blur | | | |
| 20 | Decreased Phase Matrix | Higher SNR | Lower Res | | | |
| 21 | Decreased Flip Angle (GRE) | More T2* | Lower SAR, lower SNR | | | |
| 22 | Wide Receiver B/W | Shorter Min. TE and ETS, Less Chem. Shift Artifact | Lower SNR | | | |
| 23 | Narrow Receiver B/W | Higher SNR | Longer Min. TE and ETS, more Chem. Shift Artifact | | | |
| 24 | Large Coil | More Anatomical Coverage and penetration | Overall lower SNR | | | |
| 25 | Small Coil | Overall Higher SNR | Less Coverage and depth of penetration | | | |

**Long ETLs means more echoes with increasing amounts of T2, (more contrasts) but a shorter ETL means fewer contrasts going into k-space.
**Long ETL has TE's of say: 10, 20, 30, 40, 50, 60, 70, 80, 90, 100, 110, 120, 130 = a bigger mix. A short ETL has TE's of say: 10, 20, 30. Is less of a mix.
Note: If you can get the Pros/Cons of increasing each factor, than logically the opposite is true for decreasing each factor.

# 3 Pulse Sequences and MRI Math

In this section, I will ask you to identify the various pulse sequences as well as some of the components of a PSD. I consider this an extension of Section 2. There will also be math involved in calculating scan times, pixel size, and voxel volume. Even though, the ARRT groups Sequences in with Image Production, I decided to make Section 3 heavy on Pulse Sequence identification and MRI Math. There you will find Chapters 4–10 useful. The questions in this section will follow in order, Chapters 4 through 10. I will start with CSE, move to FSE, Tissue Suppression, GRE, move onto k-Space, and finally EPI sequences.

There will be other questions related to sequences, math, and general I.Q.

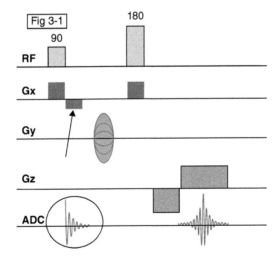

*MRI Registry Review: Tech to Tech Questions and Answers*, First Edition. Stephen J. Powers.
© 2021 John Wiley & Sons Ltd. Published 2021 by John Wiley & Sons Ltd.

**1.** Identify the sequence in Figure 3.1:

|   |   |
|---|---|
| **A.** Gradient echo | ☐ |
| **B.** Fast spin-echo | ☐ |
| **C.** Inversion recovery | ☐ |
| **D.** Conventional spin-echo | ☐ |

**2.** What gradient is applied during both the 90° and 180° RF pulses?

|   |   |
|---|---|
| **A.** Phase encoding | ☐ |
| **B.** Slice select | ☐ |
| **C.** Frequency encoding | ☐ |

**3.** In Figure 3.1, what gradient is applied during echo formation?

|   |   |
|---|---|
| **A.** Phase | ☐ |
| **B.** Frequency | ☐ |
| **C.** Slice select | ☐ |
| **D.** ADC | ☐ |

**4.** The partial echo (circled) in Figure 3.1 that forms from the 90° is called the _____?

|   |   |
|---|---|
| **A.** TE | ☐ |
| **B.** Fourier echo | ☐ |
| **C.** Hahn echo | ☐ |
| **D.** F.I.D. | ☐ |

**5.** What gradient is applied between the 90 and 180° RF pulses?

|   |   |
|---|---|
| **A.** Phase | ☐ |
| **B.** Frequency | ☐ |
| **C.** Slice select | ☐ |
| **D.** ADC | ☐ |

**6.** What is the purpose of the 180°?

|   |   |
|---|---|
| **A.** Re-phase vectors in the X/Y plane | ☐ |
| **B.** Increase the SAR | ☐ |
| **C.** De-phase vectors in the X/Y plane | ☐ |
| **D.** Cause the FID to form | ☐ |

7. What is the purpose of the small negative polarity SSG (Arrow) after the 90°?

   **A.** Acts to re-phase vectors de-phased by the initial SSG ☐
   **B.** Increase the SAR ☐
   **C.** De-phase vectors in the X/Y plane ☐
   **D.** Assist the phase encoding gradient ☐

8. What time is the 180° applied?

   **A.** ½ the TE ☐
   **B.** TE/2 ☐
   **C.** 1 TAU ☐
   **D.** A, B, and C ☐

9. What is the prime difference between a GRE and a spin-echo sequence?

   **A.** Better T1 contrast ☐
   **B.** Lower resolution ☐
   **C.** Spin-echo has a 180° ☐
   **D.** No FID is produced ☐

10. Usually, the TE in a spin-echo is longer than in a typical GRE, WHY?

    **A.** The presence of a 90° ☐
    **B.** No FID ☐
    **C.** The presence of a 180° ☐
    **D.** Short TR ☐

11. The frequency encoding gradient is sometimes called the _____?

    **A.** Read-Out ☐
    **B.** Oscillating ☐
    **C.** Iteration ☐
    **D.** Periotic ☐

12. Why is the phase gradient applied at different amplitudes from TR to TR?

    **A.** To re-phase the X/Y plane ☐
    **B.** To de-phase the X/Y plane ☐
    **C.** To alter the echo's phase ☐
    **D.** Re-phase the echo at TE ☐

**13.** The RF applied by the 180° is actually _____ times the RF as the 90°?

A. 2 ☐
B. 3 ☐
C. 4 ☐
D. 8 ☐

**14.** The 90° and the 180° pulses both have the same _____

A. Phase ☐
B. Frequency ☐
C. Amplitude ☐
D. Fourier constant ☐

**15.** The sequence in Figure 3.1 is a _____?

A. 1D ☐
B. 2D ☐
C. 3D ☐
D. None of these ☐

**16.** In a spin-echo seq., changing the TE from 15 to 10 ms causes the 180° to be applied at ____?

A. 7.5 ms ☐
B. 5 ms ☐
C. Does not change ☐
D. You cannot change the TE ☐

**17.** How many times is the phase encoding gradient applied?

A. $256 \times 2$ ☐
B. 224/2 ☐
C. The phase steps in the matrix $\times$ the nex ☐
D. Half the TR ☐

**18.** All geometric factors being the same, the SAR delivered to a patient during a SE when compared to a gradient echo would be _____.

A. The same ☐
B. Less ☐
C. More ☐
D. None of these ☐

**19.** What is the scan time: TR 3500, TE 90, $192 \times 256$ matrix, nex = 1, 22 slices, 5 mm thick with a FOV = 230?

A. 7:25 minutes ☐
B. 4:45 minutes ☐
C. 11:12 minutes ☐
D. 8:54 minutes ☐

**20.** Identify the Sequence in Figure 3.2.

A. Inversion recovery ☐
B. Gradient echo ☐
C. Dual echo spin-echo ☐
D. Echo planar ☐

**21.** The second echo in the sequences has a lower signal amplitude due to its _____?

A. TI ☐
B. TR ☐
C. TE ☐
D. Matrix ☐

**22.** The images in Figure 3.2 would be an:

A. Axial ☐
B. Coronal ☐
C. Sagittal ☐
D. Oblique ☐

**23.** Why is the phase gradient changed for each echo?

A. To change the TE ☐
B. To change the TR ☐
C. To place it in a different line of k-Space ☐
D. To reduce the patient's SAR ☐

**24.** The Sequence in Figure 3.2 is used to give what two weightings?

A. T1, T2 ☐
B. T2 and PD ☐
C. T1 and PD ☐
D. Both are T1 ☐

**25.** The first echo would be _____ and the second which would be more _____?

A. T1, PD ☐
B. T2, T1 ☐
C. PD, T2 ☐
D. Both have equal weighting ☐

**26.** The sequence in Figure 3.2 is an older sequence option previously used to aid in the diagnosis of what condition?

A. Alzheimer's ☐
B. Dementia ☐
C. Multiple Sclerosis ☐
D. CVA ☐

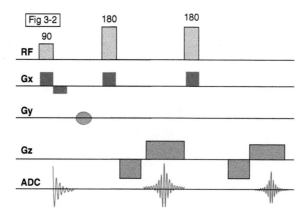

**27.** Identify the Sequence in Figure 3.3.

A. Inversion recovery ☐
B. Gradient echo ☐
C. Turbo spin-echo ☐
D. Double or Dual echo spin-echo ☐

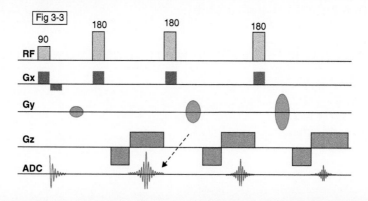

**28.** As the Echo train increases, SAR will _____.

| | |
|---|---|
| **A.** Decrease | ☐ |
| **B.** Increase | ☐ |
| **C.** Not change | ☐ |
| **D.** Unknown | ☐ |

**29.** By virtue of the amplitude of the first Phase encoding gradient, with a short TR, the first echo would go into the _____ of k-Space and make the image more _____.

| | |
|---|---|
| **A.** Center lines, PD | ☐ |
| **B.** Outer lines, T1 | ☐ |
| **C.** Center lines, T1 | ☐ |
| **D.** Center lines, T2 | ☐ |

**30.** All scan parameters remaining the same, the sequence shown in Figure 3.3 would have a shorter scan time than the sequence in Figure 3.1 by a factor of _____.

| | |
|---|---|
| **A.** 1/2 | ☐ |
| **B.** 1/3 | ☐ |
| **C.** 1/4 | ☐ |
| **D.** No time change | ☐ |

**31.** All scan parameters remaining the same, the sequence shown in Figure 3.3 would have a _____ SAR than the sequence in Figure 3.1 by a factor of _____.

| | |
|---|---|
| **A.** Higher, 2× | ☐ |
| **B.** Lower, 3× | ☐ |
| **C.** Higher, 3× | ☐ |

**32.** The echo in Figure 3.3 pointed out by a dashed arrow will be placed where in the k-Space? (note amplitude of the phase encoding gradient.)

| | |
|---|---|
| **A.** Center lines | ☐ |
| **B.** Outer lines | ☐ |
| **C.** The third line | ☐ |
| **D.** Does not matter | ☐ |

**33.** The echo pointed to (dashed arrow) will contribute mostly _____ to the image.

| | |
|---|---|
| **A.** TE | ☐ |
| **B.** Contrast | ☐ |
| **C.** Edge detail | ☐ |
| **D.** T1 | ☐ |

**34.** As the Echo train increases, _____ can/will _____.

| | |
|---|---|
| **A.** Blur, decrease | ☐ |
| **B.** Resolution, increase | ☐ |
| **C.** T2, decrease | ☐ |
| **D.** Blur, increase | ☐ |

**35.** The _____ will need to be _____ as Echo train increases.

| | |
|---|---|
| **A.** TE, decreased | ☐ |
| **B.** TE, increased | ☐ |
| **C.** TR, decreased | ☐ |
| **D.** TR, increased | ☐ |

**36.** As ETL increases, image contrast becomes more _____ and less _____.

| | |
|---|---|
| **A.** T1, T2 | ☐ |
| **B.** PD, T2 | ☐ |
| **C.** T2, PD | ☐ |
| **D.** T2, T1 | ☐ |

**37.** The _____ makes the sequence in Figure 3.3 a _____.

| | |
|---|---|
| **A.** TE, GRE | ☐ |
| **B.** TR, GRE | ☐ |
| **C.** ETL, FSE | ☐ |
| **D.** ETL, IR | ☐ |

**38.** The time in ms in between echoes in Figure 3.3 is called the _____.

> **A.** Echo train ☐
> **B.** min. TE ☐
> **C.** Echo spacing ☐
> **D.** Both B and C ☐

**39.** What is the ETL in Figure 3.3?

> **A.** 1 ☐
> **B.** 2 ☐
> **C.** 3 ☐
> **D.** There is no Echo train ☐

**40.** All factors being the same, a SE is less sensitive to metal when compared to a gradient echo.

> **A.** True ☐
> **B.** False ☐

**41.** In Question 40, if you double your nex, SNR will increase by: _____

> **A.** Double ☐
> **B.** Triple ☐
> **C.** .41 ☐
> **D.** 1.73 ☐

**42.** The central lines of k-Space are filled by the _____ in a _____ sequence.

> **A.** Echo spacing, Spin-echo ☐
> **B.** Echo train, FSE ☐
> **C.** Effective TE, Fast spin-echo ☐
> **D.** Receiver B/W, FSE ☐

**43.** True or False: In a Fast Spin-Echo, the later echoes in the Echo train have a higher SNR than the early echoes.

> **A.** True ☐
> **B.** False ☐

**44.** What is the pixel size with a 230 mm FOV, 192×256 matrix, and 5 mm thick slices?

A. 1.6×1.2 mm ☐
B. 1.19×0.98 mm ☐
C. 1.19×0.89 mm ☐
D. 5×5 mm ☐

**45.** What would the voxel volume be from Question 44?

A. 5 mm$^3$ ☐
B. 5.29 mm$^3$ ☐
C. 3.65 mm$^3$ ☐
D. 4.21 mm$^3$ ☐

**46.** What is the scan time for the sequence in Figure 3.3: 2345 TR, TE-97, 25 slices, 256×224 matrix, 2 nex, 4 mm thick slices, FOV-320 mm, ETL = 3. 5.8

A. 5:48 minutes ☐
B. 5.8 minutes ☐
C. 349 seconds ☐
D. All of these ☐

**47.** The image contrast in Question 47 is:

A. T1 ☐
B. T2 ☐
C. PD ☐
D. STIR ☐

**48.** Which of the three echoes in Figure 3.3 is the effective TE ___.

A. 1st. ☐
B. 2nd. ☐
C. 3rd. ☐
D. None of them ☐

**49.** All scan parameters remaining the same, the sequence shown in Figure 3.2 would have a shorter scan time than the sequence in Figure 3.1 by a factor of_____

| | |
|---|---|
| **A.** 1/2 | ☐ |
| **B.** 1/3 | ☐ |
| **C.** 1/4 | ☐ |
| **D.** No time change | ☐ |

**50.** All scan parameters remaining the same, the sequence shown in Figure 3.2 would have a _____ SAR than the sequence in Figure 3.1 by a factor of_____

| | |
|---|---|
| **A.** 2 | ☐ |
| **B.** 3 | ☐ |
| **C.** 4 | ☐ |
| **D.** No SAR change | ☐ |

**51.** What is the scan time: TR 550, TE 11, Acq = 2 Matrix $320 \times 224$, FOV 280, ETL = 2 with 32 coronal slices that are 5 mm thick with a 10% gap?

| | |
|---|---|
| **A.** 2:48 minutes | ☐ |
| **B.** 123 seconds | ☐ |
| **C.** 2.35 minutes | ☐ |
| **D.** None of these | ☐ |

**52.** What is the in-plane resolution in Question 49?

| | |
|---|---|
| **A.** $0.87 \times 1.25$ | ☐ |
| **B.** $0.87 \times 1.25 \times 5$ mm | ☐ |
| **C.** 280 mm | ☐ |
| **D.** 5 mm | ☐ |

**53.** Identify the sequence in Figure 3.4.

| | |
|---|---|
| **A.** STIR | ☐ |
| **B.** FLAIR | ☐ |
| **C.** Inversion recovery | ☐ |
| **D.** GRE | ☐ |

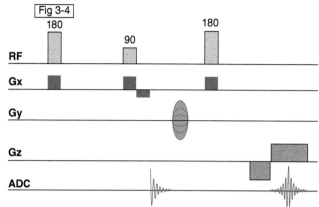

**54.** In the sequence of Figure 3.4, fluid will be bright and fat will be dark.

> **A.** False ☐
> **B.** True ☐
> **C.** Cannot be determined ☐

**55.** The time interval between the 90° and the 180° is called _____?

> **A.** TE ☐
> **B.** TR ☐
> **C.** TI ☐
> **D.** 1 TAU ☐

**56.** The time interval between the 180° and the 90° is called _____?

> **A.** 1 TAU ☐
> **B.** TI ☐
> **C.** TR ☐
> **D.** 2 TAU ☐

**57.** What is the scan time in a sequence with these scan factors: TR = 3245 ms, TE = 45 ms, FOV 255, Matrix 224×224, TI = 150 ms, 2 nex, ETL = 7?

> **A.** 3:46 minutes ☐
> **B.** 3:57 minutes ☐
> **C.** 207 seconds ☐
> **D.** 4:36 minutes ☐

**58.** With the scan factors in number 55, fluid will be bright and fat will be dark.

| | |
|---|---|
| **A.** False | ☐ |
| **B.** True | ☐ |
| **C.** Cannot determine | ☐ |
| **D.** Fluid dark and Fat bright | ☐ |

**59.** The basic scan time formula is:

| | |
|---|---|
| **A.** TR × Phase × nex ÷ 60 000 = scan time in ms | ☐ |
| **B.** TR × Phase × nex + TE ÷ 60 000 = scan time in ms | ☐ |
| **C.** TR × Phase × Frequency × nex ÷ 60 000 = scan time in ms | ☐ |
| **D.** None of these | ☐ |

**60.** Increasing the ETL in the factors in number 55 would _____ the scan time.

| | |
|---|---|
| **A.** Increase | ☐ |
| **B.** Decrease | ☐ |
| **C.** Not change | ☐ |

**61.** TR = 3245 ms, TE = 45 ms, FOV 255, Matrix 224 × 224, TI = 150 ms, 2 nex, ETL = 7. Changing the FOV to 300 mm would _____ the SNR, _____ the resolution, and _____ the scan time.

| | |
|---|---|
| **A.** decrease, increase, not change | ☐ |
| **B.** increase, increase, increase | ☐ |
| **C.** increase, decrease, increase | ☐ |
| **D.** increase, decrease, not change | ☐ |

**62.** Isotropic voxels are required. Which set of factors listed below would yield them?

| | |
|---|---|
| **A.** 360 FOV, 288 × 288 matrix, 1.4 mm slice | ☐ |
| **B.** 360 FOV, 256 × 224 matrix, 1.4 mm slice | ☐ |
| **C.** 360 FOV, 256 × 384 matrix, 1.2 mm slice | ☐ |
| **D.** 360 FOV, 256 × 256 matrix, 1.4 mm slice | ☐ |

**63.** Isotropic voxels give optimum image quality when reformatting 3D data sets.

A. True    ☐
B. False    ☐

**64.** With the scan factors in number 57, fluid will be bright.

A. False    ☐
B. True    ☐
C. Cannot determine    ☐
D. Fluid dark and Fat bright    ☐

**65.** Decreasing the TR to 1200 in number 57, fluid will be bright and fat will be dark.

A. False    ☐
B. True    ☐
C. Cannot determine    ☐
D. Fluid dark and Fat bright    ☐

**66.** Decreasing the TI allows less time for _____ relaxation.

A. T2    ☐
B. T1    ☐
C. PD    ☐
D. None of these    ☐

**67.** A short TI suppresses short T1 relaxing tissue while long TI's suppress long T1 tissue.

A. True    ☐
B. False    ☐

**68.** Identify the sequence in Figure 3.5.

A. Spin-echo with STIR    ☐
B. GRE    ☐
C. Fat-Sat spin-echo    ☐
D. FLAIR    ☐

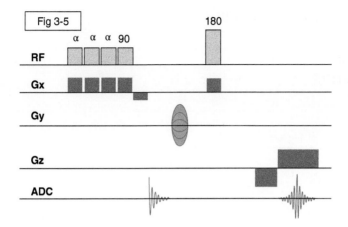

**69.** What is the scan time formula for FSE?

> **A.** TR × Phase × nex ÷ ETL ÷ 60 000 = scan time in ms □
> **B.** TR × Phase × nex ÷ 60 000 = scan time in ms □
> **C.** TR × Phase × Frequency × nex ÷ 60 000 = scan time in ms □
> **D.** None of these □

**70.** If the images are blurry but the patient is NOT moving, what scan factor can be adjusted?

> **A.** nex □
> **B.** ETS □
> **C.** ETL □
> **D.** Transmitter B/W □

**71.** What is the scan time formula for a Fat-Sat FSE?

> **A.** TR × Phase × nex ÷ ETL ÷ 60 000 = scan time in ms □
> **B.** TR × Phase × nex ÷ 60 000 = scan time in ms □
> **C.** TR × Phase × Frequency × nex ÷ 60 000 = scan time in ms □
> **D.** None of these □

**72.** What scan parameter is the cause of chemical shift artifact?

> **A.** A wide Transmitter B/W □
> **B.** An odd number TE □
> **C.** High phase matrix □
> **D.** A narrow rec. bandwidth □

**73.** Identify the sequence in Figure 3.6.

- **A.** DWI ☐
- **B.** FSE ☐
- **C.** 2D GRE ☐
- **D.** EPI ☐

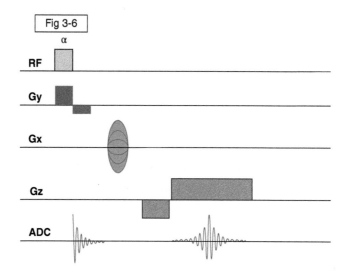

**74.** Figure 3.6 will yield a _____ slice.

- **A.** Axial ☐
- **B.** Coronal ☐
- **C.** Sagittal ☐
- **D.** Oblique coronal ☐

**75.** Phase runs in which direction in Figure 3.6?

- **A.** Right–Left ☐
- **B.** A/P ☐
- **C.** S/I ☐

**76.** What is the purpose if the dual opposing gradients coming from Gz?

- **A.** Make it a coronal ☐
- **B.** Lengthen the TE ☐
- **C.** De-phase then re-phase the X/Y plane ☐
- **D.** Shorten the TR ☐

**77.** ADC stands for what?

> **A.** Anterior Di-Com. Coil ☐
> **B.** Axial to Digital Converter ☐
> **C.** Anti-Di-com Converter ☐
> **D.** Analog to Digital Converter ☐

**78.** Figure 3.6 is a _____ because it has no _____.

> **A.** Spin-echo, Bandwidth ☐
> **B.** STIR, TI ☐
> **C.** GRE, 180 ☐
> **D.** SE, ETL ☐

**79.** The scan time formula for 2D GRE sequence:

> **A.** TR × Phase × nex ÷ 60000 = scan time in ms ☐
> **B.** TR × Phase × nex + TE ÷ 60 000 = scan time in ms ☐
> **C.** TR × Phase × Frequency × nex ÷ 60 000 = scan time in ms ☐
> **D.** None of these ☐

**80.** What is the flip angle in Figure 3.6?

> **A.** 90° ☐
> **B.** 180° ☐
> **C.** 45° ☐
> **D.** Unknown, not stated ☐

**81.** The flip angle in a GRE is usually something less than 90° but can be as high as 90°.

> **A.** True ☐
> **B.** False ☐

**82.** As the frequency matrix is increased, the TE will also lengthen.

> **A.** True ☐
> **B.** False ☐

**83.** The frequency direction in Figure 3.6 is?

A. A/P ☐
B. R/L ☐
C. S/I ☐

**84.** A narrow receiver bandwidth will _____ the SNR, increase _____ and may cause the _____ to lengthen.

A. Decrease, Aliasing, FOV ☐
B. Increase, Cross Talk, ETL ☐
C. Increase, Chemical shift, TE ☐
D. Decrease, Motion, TE ☐

**85.** As the flip angle is increased in a GRE, there is more chance of _____?

A. Motion ☐
B. Aliasing ☐
C. Tissue saturation ☐
D. Chemical shift ☐

**86.** As the TE is increased in a GRE, the image weighting is more _____?

A. T2* ☐
B. T1 ☐
C. PD ☐
D. MRA ☐

**87.** As the TR is increased in a GRE, there in less chance of _____?

A. Motion ☐
B. Aliasing ☐
C. Tissue saturation ☐
D. Chemical shift ☐

**88.** Identify the sequence in Figure 3.7.

A. DWI ☐
B. FSE ☐
C. 3D GRE ☐
D. EPI ☐

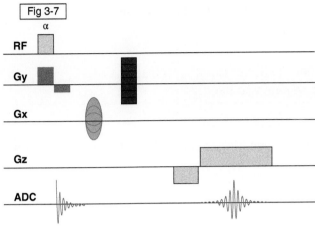

Fig 3-7

**89.** Figure 3.7 will yield a _____ slice.

| | |
|---|---|
| **A.** Axial | ☐ |
| **B.** Coronal | ☐ |
| **C.** Sagittal | ☐ |
| **D.** Oblique coronal | ☐ |

**90.** What makes Figure 3.7 a 3D sequence?

| | |
|---|---|
| **A.** It is an MRA | ☐ |
| **B.** The extra gradient pulses in the slice direction | ☐ |
| **C.** The flip angle | ☐ |
| **D.** The TR is short | ☐ |

**91.** As the flip angle is decreased, the images will be more _____?

| | |
|---|---|
| **A.** T1 | ☐ |
| **B.** T2 | ☐ |
| **C.** PD | ☐ |
| **D.** DWI | ☐ |

**92.** In 3D sequences, SNR increases with the number of "LOCS" or partitions by a factor of.

| | |
|---|---|
| **A.** SNR = LOCS/2 | ☐ |
| **B.** SNR = √ number of LOCs | ☐ |
| **C.** SNR = √ of Phase Matrix | ☐ |
| **D.** SNR = Number of LOCS × Thickness | ☐ |

**93.** The number of "LOCs" comes from the _____.

> **A.** Phase matrix ☐
> **B.** TR ☐
> **C.** Number of slice gradient applications ☐
> **D.** The coverage you need ☐

**94.** 3D sequences have higher resolution compared to a 2D with similar scan factors.

> **A.** True ☐
> **B.** False ☐

**95.** What is the scan time? TR = 45, TE = 4, Matrix 320×224, slice thickness 2 mm, 1 nex, partitions = 50, FOV = 230

> **A.** 8:24 minutes ☐
> **B.** 7:11 minutes ☐
> **C.** 4:55 minutes ☐
> **D.** 6:13 minutes ☐

**96.** What kind of pixels will the above sequence yield?

> **A.** Square ☐
> **B.** Isotropic ☐
> **C.** Anisotropic ☐
> **D.** Oblique ☐

**97.** What is the pixel size in Question 93?

> **A.** 0.71 × 0.88 mm ☐
> **B.** 0.88 × 1.0 mm ☐
> **C.** 0.71 × 1.02 mm ☐
> **D.** 1.0 × 1.0 mm ☐

**98.** What is the voxel volume in Question 93?

> **A.** 1.45 mm³ ☐
> **B.** 2.11 mm³ ☐
> **C.** 3.71 mm³ ☐
> **D.** 1.37 mm³ ☐

**99.** As the number of partitions increase in a 3D sequence, SNR will _____, resolution will _____, and scan time will _____.

| | |
|---|---|
| **A.** Decrease, Decrease, Decrease | ☐ |
| **B.** Increase, Increase, Decrease | ☐ |
| **C.** Increase, Increase, Increase | ☐ |
| **D.** Decrease, Increase, Decrease | ☐ |

**100.** As the slab thickness increase in a 3D MRA, there is more chance of _____?

| | |
|---|---|
| **A.** Motion | ☐ |
| **B.** Aliasing | ☐ |
| **C.** In-Plane saturation | ☐ |
| **D.** Chemical shift | ☐ |

**101.** In any TOF MRA sequence, ideally the blood flow _____ to the slices/slab?

| | |
|---|---|
| **A.** Should be parallel | ☐ |
| **B.** Should be perpendicular | ☐ |
| **C.** at 90° | ☐ |
| **D.** B or C | ☐ |

**102.** 2D TOF MRA's can be run post gadolinium as long as you have superior and inferior saturation pulses.

| | |
|---|---|
| **A.** True | ☐ |
| **B.** False | ☐ |
| **C.** Saturation pulses would not help post gado | ☐ |
| **D.** B and C | ☐ |

**103.** TR = 45, TE = 4, Matrix 320×224, slice thickness 2 mm, 1 nex, partitions = 50, FOV = 230. How many nex are needed to double the SNR in the sequence?

| | |
|---|---|
| **A.** 2 | ☐ |
| **B.** 4 | ☐ |
| **C.** 6 | ☐ |
| **D.** 8 | ☐ |

**104.** Increasing the TE on a sequence will _____.

|   |   |
|---|---|
| **A.** Decrease T1 | ☐ |
| **B.** Decrease SNR | ☐ |
| **C.** Decrease chemical shift artifact | ☐ |
| **D.** Decrease T2 | ☐ |

**105.** On non-MRA sequences, the blood vessels are dark, this phenomenon is called?

|   |   |
|---|---|
| **A.** Saturation | ☐ |
| **B.** Flow void | ☐ |
| **C.** Flow compensation | ☐ |
| **D.** In-Plane saturation | ☐ |

**106.** Flow compensation/Gradient motion nulling should be applied in long TR sequences to help decrease _____.

|   |   |
|---|---|
| **A.** Respiratory motion | ☐ |
| **B.** Eye motion | ☐ |
| **C.** Muscle spasm | ☐ |
| **D.** Pulsatile ghosting from blood vessels | ☐ |

**107.** Increasing the flip angle increases the patient's SAR. True or False?

**108.** An increase in the flip angle yields an image with _____.

|   |   |
|---|---|
| **A.** More T2 contrast | ☐ |
| **B.** More PD contrast | ☐ |
| **C.** Less T2 contrast | ☐ |
| **D.** More T1 contrast | ☐ |

**109.** Increasing flip angle and shortening the TR in a sequence can cause _____?

|   |   |
|---|---|
| **A.** Motion | ☐ |
| **B.** Tissue saturation | ☐ |
| **C.** In-plane saturation | ☐ |
| **D.** Chemical shift | ☐ |

**110.** The central lines of k-Space are filled by the _____ in a _____ sequence.

| | |
|---|---|
| **A.** Echo spacing, Spin-echo | ☐ |
| **B.** Echo train, FSE | ☐ |
| **C.** Effective TE, Fast spin-echo | ☐ |
| **D.** Receiver B/W, FSE | ☐ |

**111.** True or False: In a fast spin-echo, the later echoes in the Echo train have a higher SNR than the early echoes.

| | |
|---|---|
| **A.** True | ☐ |
| **B.** False | ☐ |

**112.** How is the TR affected in a 3D GRE sequence by increasing the number of partitions?

| | |
|---|---|
| **A.** May need to be longer | ☐ |
| **B.** Can be shortened | ☐ |
| **C.** It is not affected | ☐ |
| **D.** Increases with the $\sqrt{}$ of the number of partitions | ☐ |

**113.** Identify the sequence in Figure 3.8.

| | |
|---|---|
| **A.** 3D Dual echo GRE | ☐ |
| **B.** 3D Dual echo spin-echo | ☐ |
| **C.** Dual echo fast spin-echo | ☐ |
| **D.** Spoiled GRE | ☐ |

**114.** What scan plane would Figure 3.8 show?

| | |
|---|---|
| **A.** Axial | ☐ |
| **B.** Coronal | ☐ |
| **C.** Sagittal | ☐ |
| **D.** Oblique | ☐ |

**115.** Frequency is in what direction in Figure 3.8?

| | |
|---|---|
| **A.** A/P | ☐ |
| **B.** S/I | ☐ |
| **C.** R/L | ☐ |
| **D.** Oblique sag. | ☐ |

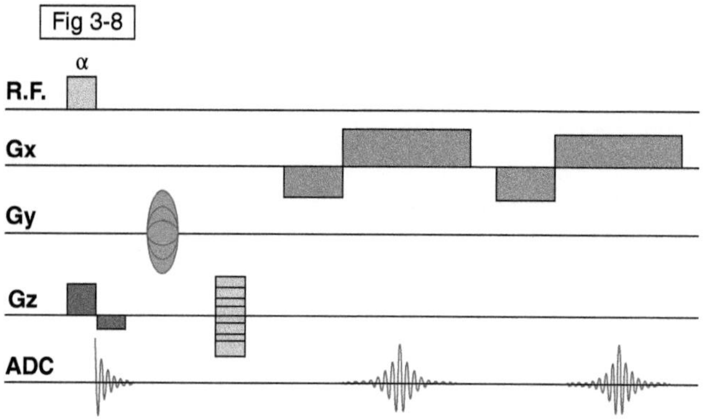

Fig 3-8

**116.** Flow compensation is applied sequence in Figure 3.8?

A. True ☐
B. False? ☐

**117.** The sequence in Figure 3.8 is also known as _____.

A. Dixon ☐
B. Opposed phase ☐
C. In and Out of phase ☐
D. All the above ☐

**118.** An out of phase echo can only be acquired with a _____ sequence.

A. Spin-echo ☐
B. Turbo spin-echo ☐
C. STIR ☐
D. GRE ☐

**119.** The out of phase TE changes with field strength.

A. False ☐
B. True ☐

**120.** Identify the sequence in Figure 3.8A.

A. 3D Dual echo GRE ☐
B. 3D Dual echo spin-echo ☐
C. 2D Dual echo fast spin-echo ☐
D. Spoiled GRE ☐

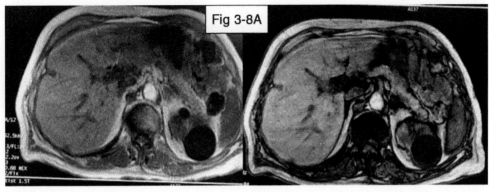

Fig 3-8A

**121.** The out of phase TE is on the right:

| | |
|---|---|
| **A.** False | ☐ |
| **B.** True. | ☐ |

**122.** What artifact is demonstrated in the image to the right?

| | |
|---|---|
| **A.** Out of phase | ☐ |
| **B.** Intra voxel phase cancellation | ☐ |
| **C.** Chemical shift of the 2nd kind | ☐ |
| **D.** All the above | ☐ |

**123.** What sequence can be used to get fat saturation at low fields?

| | |
|---|---|
| **A.** FLAIR | ☐ |
| **B.** GRE with Water saturation | ☐ |
| **C.** DIXON | ☐ |
| **D.** All the above | ☐ |

**124.** The artifact seen in image Figure 3.8a is only seen is which sequence?

| | |
|---|---|
| **A.** Fast spin-echo | ☐ |
| **B.** STIR | ☐ |
| **C.** DWI | ☐ |
| **D.** GRE | ☐ |

**125.** This type of sequence is often used to evaluate what body part?

| | |
|---|---|
| **A.** Basil ganglia | ☐ |
| **B.** Cervical cord | ☐ |
| **C.** The Uterus | ☐ |
| **D.** Adrenals | ☐ |

**126.** At 1.5 T, the first out of phase TE is _____ and the first in-phase TE is _____.

| | |
|---|---|
| **A.** 2.2, 4.4 | ☐ |
| **B.** 4.4, 2.2 | ☐ |
| **C.** 4.4, 8.8 | ☐ |
| **D.** 4.4, 6.6 | ☐ |

**127.** k-Space is thought to be made up of three sections, the _____ lines are for image contrast while the two outer lines contribute to the images _____.

| | |
|---|---|
| **A.** Center, Edge detail | ☐ |
| **B.** Outer, Contrast | ☐ |
| **C.** T1, T2 | ☐ |
| **D.** T2, T1 | ☐ |

**128.** When doing a CSE sequence, k-Space filling is _____ while a fast spin-echo uses _____ k-Space filling method.

| | |
|---|---|
| **A.** Reversed linear, Re-ordered | ☐ |
| **B.** Re-ordered, Linear | ☐ |
| **C.** Elliptical, Centric | ☐ |
| **D.** Linear, Re-ordered | ☐ |

**129.** The Effective TE (ETE) in a turbo spin-echo goes into the _____ lines due to the _____ amplitude of the _____ encoding gradient.

| | |
|---|---|
| **A.** Edges, high, Frequency | ☐ |
| **B.** Center, low, Slice | ☐ |
| **C.** Center, low, Phase | ☐ |
| **D.** Edges, high, Phase | ☐ |

**130.** In a CE-MRA, for optimum image quality, it is desired to be filling the
_____ lines of k-Space when the gadolinium reaches the _____.

| | |
|---|---|
| **A.** Edges, Heart | ☐ |
| **B.** Center, Heart | ☐ |
| **C.** Center, Target vessel | ☐ |
| **D.** 1st to 55th, Target vessels | ☐ |

**131.** There are multiple methods to correctly time the arrival of IV contrast.
These include all the following except:

| | |
|---|---|
| **A.** Care-bolus | ☐ |
| **B.** Timing bolus | ☐ |
| **C.** 20 Mississippi | ☐ |
| **D.** Smart prep | ☐ |

**132.** Temporal resolution is scanning quickly over time. True or False?

**133.** Spatial resolution is the ability to discern _____ structures over

_____.

| | |
|---|---|
| **A.** small, time | ☐ |
| **B.** large, time | ☐ |
| **C.** small, distance | ☐ |
| **D.** bright, dark | ☐ |

**134.** Temporal resolution is affected by a number of scan factors that include:
Select all that do not apply.

| | |
|---|---|
| **A.** FOV | ☐ |
| **B.** TR | ☐ |
| **C.** TE | ☐ |
| **D.** Phase matrix | ☐ |
| **E.** Frequency matrix | ☐ |
| **F.** Rec. B/W | ☐ |
| **G.** Nex | ☐ |
| **H.** Number of slices | ☐ |
| **I.** Fractional echo | ☐ |
| **J.** Fat-Sat | ☐ |
| **K.** Imaging plane | ☐ |
| **L.** Sat pulses | ☐ |
| **M.** Inject. rate | ☐ |

**135.** In a non-contrast 2D or 3D MRA, vessels are bright due to the _____ effect, while the background tissue appears dark due to _____.

A. Saturation, IV contrast ☐
B. Phase contrast, Saturation ☐
C. Time of flight, Saturation pulses ☐
D. Time of flight, Tissue saturation ☐

**136.** A 2D TOF MRA is better at imaging _____ when compared to a 3D.

A. Stagnant flow ☐
B. Fast flow ☐
C. Slow flow ☐
D. Post contrast ☐

**137.** Another name for "Parabolic" flow is _____?

A. Vortex ☐
B. Turbulent flow ☐
C. Laminar flow ☐
D. Stagnant flow ☐

**138.** Two major advantages of 3D TOF MRA over 2D are _____ and ability to image _____.

A. Higher resolution, without IV Contrast ☐
B. Better MIP's and image faster flow ☐
C. Higher resolution, faster flow ☐
D. Higher resolution, slow flow ☐

**139.** Cutting or carving out the background tissue leaving the bright vessels in an MRA/V is called _____?

A. Multi Planar Reconstruction ☐
B. Min. Intensity Projection ☐
C. Maximum Intensity Projection ☐
D. Segmentation ☐

**140.** Creating images in other planes different than the one that the data set was acquired at is called a _____.

| | |
|---|---|
| **A.** Multi Planar Reconstruction | ☐ |
| **B.** Min. Intensity Projection | ☐ |
| **C.** Maximum Intensity Projection | ☐ |
| **D.** Segmentation | ☐ |

**141.** A "collapsed"/projection image generated by the scanner of a TOF seq. is a _____

| | |
|---|---|
| **A.** Multi Planar Reconstruction | ☐ |
| **B.** Min. Intensity Projection | ☐ |
| **C.** Maximum Intensity Projection | ☐ |
| **D.** Segmentation | ☐ |

**142.** In an MRA sequence, the TR and TE need to be short to avoid _____.

| | |
|---|---|
| **A.** Motion | ☐ |
| **B.** Flow-related enhancement | ☐ |
| **C.** Flow void | ☐ |
| **D.** None of these | ☐ |

**143.** What is being described? When a data set is transformed from signal intensities over time into signal intensities of frequency.

| | |
|---|---|
| **A.** Fourier transform | ☐ |
| **B.** Reverse Fourier transform | ☐ |
| **C.** Faraday transform | ☐ |
| **D.** Ohm's interpretations | ☐ |

**144.** k-Space can be filled in a circular/spiral fashion from the inner to outer lines called?

| | |
|---|---|
| **A.** Centric | ☐ |
| **B.** Elliptical centric | ☐ |
| **C.** Reversed elliptical centric | ☐ |
| **D.** Rectilinear filling | ☐ |

**145.** When you acquire ½ (60%) of the data and interpolate the unfilled half is called?

A. Fractional Fourier ☐
B. Partial Fourier ☐
C. Half Fourier ☐
D. All of these ☐

**146.** Using a Half Fourier technique affects IQ with a _____.

A. Higher SNR ☐
B. Lower SNR ☐
C. No change in IQ ☐
D. More motion ☐

**147.** k-Space is thought to have two directions, they are:

A. Slice and Phase ☐
B. Slice and Frequency ☐
C. Frequency and Phase ☐

**148.** In conventional SE imaging, one line of k-Space is filled per _____.

A. TE ☐
B. TR ☐
C. Phase ☐
D. TI ☐

**149.** In conventional SE imaging, each line of k-Space has the same _____.

A. TE ☐
B. TR ☐
C. Phase ☐
D. TI ☐

**150.** T = 4356, 12 5 mm thick slices, ETE = 120, ETS is 12 ms, Matrix is 256², FOV = 235, ETL = 19 with 2 Acq. What is the scan time?

A. 185 seconds ☐
B. 3:05 minutes ☐
C. 3.09 minutes ☐
D. Any of these ☐

**151.** In Question 151, how many lines of k-Space are filled per slice per slice?

| | |
|---|---|
| **A.** 11 | ☐ |
| **B.** 19 | ☐ |
| **C.** 256 | ☐ |
| **D.** 1 | ☐ |

**152.** From Question 151, how many lines of k-Space are filled per TR?

| | |
|---|---|
| **A.** 11 | ☐ |
| **B.** 12 | ☐ |
| **C.** 256 | ☐ |
| **D.** 228 | ☐ |

**153.** In Question 151, the Echo train length in ms runs from _____ to _____.

| | |
|---|---|
| **A.** 10–190 ms | ☐ |
| **B.** 19–144 ms | ☐ |
| **C.** 12–228 ms | ☐ |
| **D.** Cannot be determined | ☐ |

**154.** Identify the sequence in Figure 3.9.

| | |
|---|---|
| **A.** 2D GRE with flow comp | ☐ |
| **B.** 3D Steady-state GRE | ☐ |
| **C.** 3D PC | ☐ |
| **D.** Spoiled GRE | ☐ |

**155.** The two extra pulses at the end of the PSD in Figure 3.9 are to?

| | |
|---|---|
| **A.** Spoil any residual transverse NMV | ☐ |
| **B.** Refocus any residual transverse NMV | ☐ |
| **C.** Apply Sat pulses | ☐ |
| **D.** Shorten the TE | ☐ |

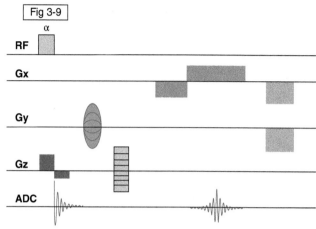

Fig 3-9

**156.** The extra gradient pulses applied after the TE are sometimes called:

| | |
|---|---|
| **A.** Spoiler pulses | ☐ |
| **B.** Rewinder pulses | ☐ |
| **C.** Sat. bands | ☐ |
| **D.** Con-joined pulses | ☐ |

**157.** Sequences like that seen in Figure 3.9 are used to get images that are more _____ like.

| | |
|---|---|
| **A.** T1 | ☐ |
| **B.** T2 | ☐ |
| **C.** PD | ☐ |
| **D.** MRA | ☐ |

**158.** Figure 3.9 would give you a _____ plane image.

| | |
|---|---|
| **A.** Coronal | ☐ |
| **B.** Sagittal | ☐ |
| **C.** Axial | ☐ |
| **D.** Para-Sagittal | ☐ |

**159.** Images from a steady-state GRE sequence are used when _____ is desired.

| | |
|---|---|
| **A.** Bright fat | ☐ |
| **B.** Bright fluids | ☐ |
| **C.** Dark fluids | ☐ |
| **D.** Bright IV contrast | ☐ |

**160.** Identify the sequence in Figure 3.10.

| | |
|---|---|
| **A.** 2D GRE with flow comp | ☐ |
| **B.** 3D steady-state GRE | ☐ |
| **C.** 2D PC | ☐ |
| **D.** Spoiled GRE | ☐ |

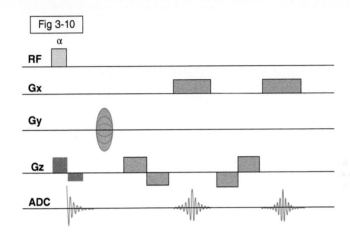

**161.** What sequence provides tissue contrast based on acquired phase differences?

| | |
|---|---|
| **A.** GRE | ☐ |
| **B.** 3D TOF | ☐ |
| **C.** Phase contrast | ☐ |
| **D.** T2* | ☐ |

**162.** Phase contrast produces images can show the _____.

| | |
|---|---|
| **A.** Slowing of flow | ☐ |
| **B.** Direction of flow | ☐ |
| **C.** Amount of turbulence | ☐ |
| **D.** Phase changes over distance | ☐ |

**163.** Phase contrast can also produce images can show the _____.

| | |
|---|---|
| **A.** Slowing of flow | ☐ |
| **B.** Velocity of flow | ☐ |
| **C.** Displacement of a vessel | ☐ |
| **D.** Bright background | ☐ |

**164.** Phase contrast MRA produces a _____ background which aids in post-processing.

| | |
|---|---|
| **A.** Bright | ☐ |
| **B.** Dark | ☐ |
| **C.** Gray | ☐ |
| **D.** Uniform | ☐ |

**165.** Phase contrast can run post gadolinium because _____.

| | |
|---|---|
| **A.** PC is sensitive to the T1 relaxation of blood | ☐ |
| **B.** PC is not sensitive to the T1 relaxation of blood | ☐ |
| **C.** PC is based in the T2* of blood | ☐ |
| **D.** B and C | ☐ |

**166.** Identify the sequence in Figure 3.11.

| | |
|---|---|
| **A.** GRE | ☐ |
| **B.** 2D GRE | ☐ |
| **C.** 3D Spoiled GRE | ☐ |
| **D.** 3D MRA | ☐ |

Fig 3-11

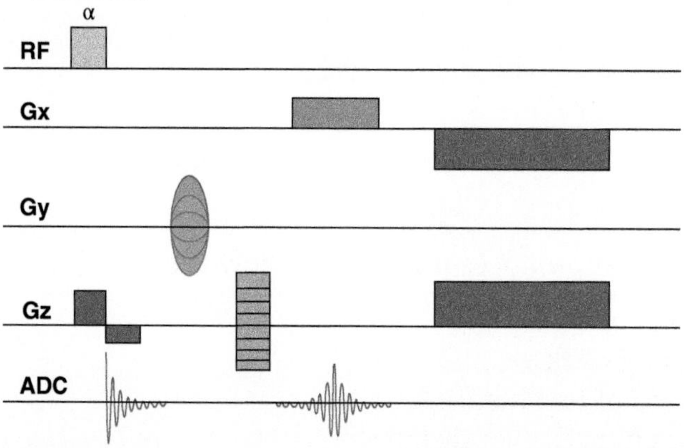

**167.** What is the purpose of the two extra gradient pulses applied at the end of the echo?

| | |
|---|---|
| **A.** To re-phase residual NMV in the X/Y plane | ☐ |
| **B.** To de-phase residual NMV in the X/Y plane | ☐ |
| **C.** Act as flow comp gradients | ☐ |
| **D.** Sagittal and axial saturation pulses | ☐ |

**168.** Image contrast displayed from Figure 3.11 would be?

> **A.** T2    ☐
> **B.** T2*    ☐
> **C.** T1    ☐
> **D.** PD    ☐

**169.** IV Contrast would display as _____ Figure 3.11?

> **A.** Dark    ☐
> **B.** Bright    ☐
> **C.** A flow void    ☐

**170.** Identify the sequence in Figure 3.12.

> **A.** Spin echo    ☐
> **B.** Fast spin echo    ☐
> **C.** Spin echo-based EPI    ☐
> **D.** B and C    ☐

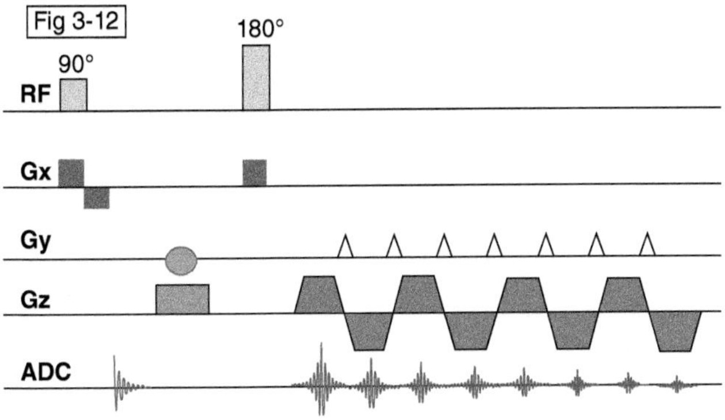

Fig 3-12

**171.** Image contrast in a sequence like that in Figure 3.12 can be?

> **A.** T1    ☐
> **B.** T2    ☐
> **C.** PD    ☐
> **D.** All of these    ☐

**172.** Another name for Figure 3.12 is a?

- **A.** Fast GRE ☐
- **B.** Single shot EPI ☐
- **C.** Single shot fast spin echo ☐
- **D.** DWI ☐

**173.** A typical use for the sequence in Figure 3.12 is:

- **A.** Cardiac ☐
- **B.** Breath hold abdomens ☐
- **C.** Fetal imaging ☐
- **D.** All of these ☐

**174.** The term Single Shot means:

- **A.** Only 1 TR is needed ☐
- **B.** The TR is thought to be infinite ☐
- **C.** Scan time are very short ☐
- **D.** All of these ☐

**175.** All factors remaining the same, the SAR levels in an EPI versus an FSE is _____:

- **A.** The same ☐
- **B.** Less ☐
- **C.** Higher ☐

**176.** A drawback to the EPI sequence is its sensitivity to magnetic susceptibility.

- **A.** True ☐
- **B.** False ☐

**177.** Peripheral nerve stimulation is not a concern in EPI imaging.

- **A.** True ☐
- **B.** False ☐

**178.** Identify the sequence in Figure 3.13.

| | |
|---|---|
| **A.** Spin echo | ☐ |
| **B.** Fast spin echo | ☐ |
| **C.** Spin echo-based EPI | ☐ |
| **D.** DWI | ☐ |

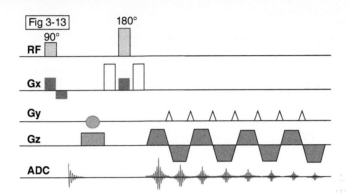

**179.** The above sequence is commonly used in the brain for detection of?

| | |
|---|---|
| **A.** Stroke | ☐ |
| **B.** Infection | ☐ |
| **C.** M.S. | ☐ |
| **D.** Tumor | ☐ |

**180.** Areas of restricted cellular diffusion appear _____ on a DWI?

| | |
|---|---|
| **A.** Dark | ☐ |
| **B.** Bright | ☐ |
| **C.** Gray | ☐ |
| **D.** Iso-intense to brain | ☐ |

**181.** Areas of un-restricted cellular diffusion appear darker due to:

| | |
|---|---|
| **A.** Lack of a blood supply | ☐ |
| **B.** De-phasing due to the applications of gradients | ☐ |
| **C.** Re-phasing due to the applications of gradients | ☐ |
| **D.** The cells are filling with water | ☐ |

**182.** The term Single Shot also means:

| | |
|---|---|
| **A.** Relatively motion insensitive | ☐ |
| **B.** A gradient intense sequence | ☐ |
| **C.** All lines of phase are collected in 1 TR | ☐ |
| **D.** All of these | ☐ |

**183.** The sequence in Figure 3.13 starts off as a _____ but ends as a _____.

| | |
|---|---|
| **A.** STIR, FSE | ☐ |
| **B.** Spin echo, FSE | ☐ |
| **C.** Fast spin echo, GRE | ☐ |
| **D.** CSE, GRE | ☐ |

**184.** In Figure 3.13, due to the gradient reversals from the frequency gradient, k-Space is filled how?

| | |
|---|---|
| **A.** At an angle | ☐ |
| **B.** Rectilinearly | ☐ |
| **C.** Centric | ☐ |
| **D.** Linearly | ☐ |

**185.** What is the chemical shift of fat and water at 3.0 T?

| | |
|---|---|
| **A.** 3.55 ppm | ☐ |
| **B.** 2.2 ms | ☐ |
| **C.** 4.4 ppm | ☐ |
| **D.** There is no chemical shift above 1.5 T | ☐ |

**186.** Because the EPI sequence is very much GRE based even though it starts off a spin-echo RF pulse profile, it is important to _____ before running the sequence.

| | |
|---|---|
| **A.** Reboot the system | ☐ |
| **B.** Reset the center frequency of the system | ☐ |
| **C.** Shim | ☐ |
| **D.** Lower the ETL | ☐ |

**187.** In a conventional GRE sequence when a dark area is seen in the parenchyma of the brain is seen it is likely to be either _____ or _____?

A. Blood, I.V. Contrast ☐
B. A blood vessel, Calcification ☐
C. Blood, Calcification ☐
D. CSF, Hydrocephalus ☐

**188.** If you could acquire an echo at a 0ms, the protons would be _____?

A. In phase ☐
B. Out of phase ☐
C. Half out of phase ☐
D. Half in phase ☐

**189.** In actuality, scanning Fat Sat images are a form of _____?

A. In phase ☐
B. Chemical shift ☐
C. Out of phase ☐
D. Off center FOV ☐

**190.** There are two kinds of parameters in MRI: _____ and _____.

A. Intrinsic, External ☐
B. Intrinsic, Extraneous ☐
C. Extrinsic, Intrinsic ☐
D. Interior, Exterior ☐

**191.** Intrinsic parameters are those that affect image contrast such as:

A. TR, TE ☐
B. ETL, ETS ☐
C. TI and Flip angle ☐
D. All of these ☐

**192.** Extrinsic parameters are those that affect sequence geometry such as:

> **A.** Slice thickness/Gap ☐
> **B.** Number of Partitions, FOV ☐
> **C.** Matrix, Acquisitions ☐
> **D.** All of these ☐

**193.** A Saturation pulse or Band is really a wide transmitted B/W RF pulse placed either within or outside the FOV in order to reduce artifacts such as Wrap, Pulsatile, or Breathing motion.

> **A.** True ☐
> **B.** False ☐

**194.** Figure 3.14 demonstrates what?

> **A.** Fat + Water peaks ☐
> **B.** Chemical shift ☐
> **C.** Tuning of a surface coil ☐
> **D.** A and B ☐

**195.** As field strength increases, the peaks shown in Figure 3.14 will _____.

> **A.** Get closer ☐
> **B.** Get further apart ☐
> **C.** Get smaller ☐
> **D.** Invert ☐

**196.** In Figure 3.14, knowing that fat has a slower precessional frequency than water, the peak on the right is _____?

> **A.** Fat ☐
> **B.** Gad ☐
> **C.** Water ☐
> **D.** Protein ☐

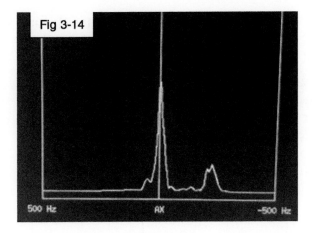

Fig 3-14

500 Hz      AX      -500 Hz

**197.** A patient presents for a breast exam but is not sure what kind of implants were implanted. From the graph shown in Figure 3.15, what kind of implants are likely present?

| | |
|---|---|
| **A.** Saline | ☐ |
| **B.** Silicone | ☐ |
| **C.** Dual lumen | ☐ |
| **D.** All of these | ☐ |

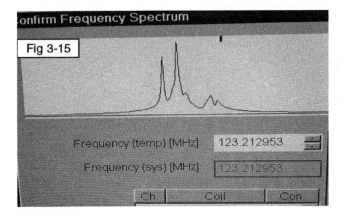

Confirm Frequency Spectrum

Fig 3-15

Frequency (temp) [MHz] 123.212953

Frequency (sys) [MHz] 123.212953

Ch.    Coil    Con.

**198.** In Figure 3.15, at what field strength was this exam performed on?

| | |
|---|---|
| **A.** 1.0T | ☐ |
| **B.** 1.5T | ☐ |
| **C.** 3.0T | ☐ |
| **D.** Cannot tell | ☐ |

**199.** You are about to scan a patient with an implant. To be safe you want to lower the level of RF delivered. This can be accomplished with all the following except:

| | |
|---|---|
| **A.** Increase TR | ☐ |
| **B.** Delete sat. pulses | ☐ |
| **C.** Lower the ETL | ☐ |
| **D.** Narrow rec. B/W | ☐ |
| **E.** Turn off drive/Fast recovery | ☐ |
| **F.** Use GRE/CSE | ☐ |
| **G.** Use T/R coils if possible | ☐ |
| **H.** Lower flip angles on refocusing pulses | ☐ |
| **I.** Use a higher matrix | ☐ |
| **J.** Use a large FOV | ☐ |

# Use the factors listed below for Questions 200–203

3D MRA Seq.: TR = 23, TE 4, partitions 40, matrix $256^2$, FOV 240, 1 nex, slices = 1.2 mm

**200.** Increasing partitions on a 3D sequence from 40 to 80 will increase the SNR by _____?

| | |
|---|---|
| **A.** 34% | ☐ |
| **B.** 41% | ☐ |
| **C.** 50% | ☐ |
| **D.** 200% | ☐ |

**201.** What is the increase in scan time from question 200?

| | |
|---|---|
| **A.** 1.5 times | ☐ |
| **B.** 2 times | ☐ |
| **C.** 3 times | ☐ |
| **D.** 4 times | ☐ |

**202.** What is the scan time in the above 3D MRA?

| | |
|---|---|
| **A.** 3:41 minutes | ☐ |
| **B.** 3: 25 minutes | ☐ |
| **C.** 3: 55 minutes | ☐ |
| **D.** 3:11 minutes | ☐ |

**203.** If the 3D sequence above is made into a 2D sequential scan, what is the new scan time?

> **A.** 2:41 minutes  ☐
> **B.** 2:25 minutes  ☐
> **C.** 3: 55 minutes  ☐
> **D.** 2:11 minutes  ☐

**204.** Identify the sequence in Figure 3.16.

> **A.** 2D GRE  ☐
> **B.** 3D GRE with FC  ☐
> **C.** 2D GRE with FC  ☐
> **D.** 3D PC with FC  ☐

Fig 3-16

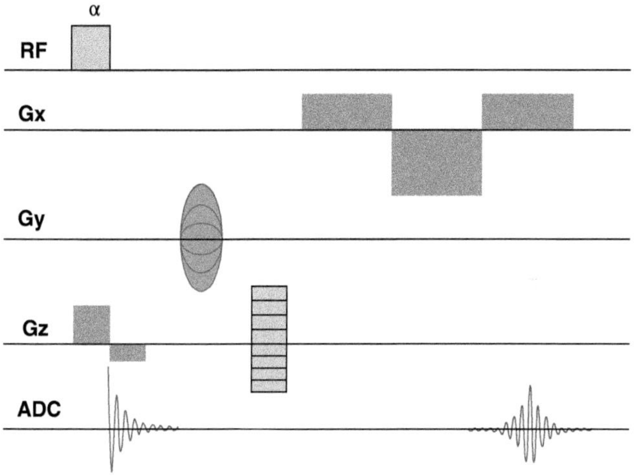

**205.** 2D and 3D TOF MRA sequences typically have _____ applied.

> **A.** Sat pulses  ☐
> **B.** F.I.D  ☐
> **C.** Flow comp.  ☐
> **D.** A and C  ☐

**206.** In 2D or 3D TOF MRA sequences, you can remove signal from unwanted vessels with the use of _____.

| | |
|---|---|
| **A.** Increased TR | ☐ |
| **B.** Sat. pulses | ☐ |
| **C.** Lower the ETL | ☐ |
| **D.** Narrow Rec. B/W | ☐ |

**207.** In 2D/3D MRA sequences, to lessen loss of signal in the voxels from flow, it is important to have _____.

| | |
|---|---|
| **A.** Small voxels | ☐ |
| **B.** Shortest possible TE | ☐ |
| **C.** Flow comp | ☐ |
| **D.** All the above | ☐ |

**208.** Normal flow in a blood vessel is known as _____.

| | |
|---|---|
| **A.** Vortex | ☐ |
| **B.** Turbulent | ☐ |
| **C.** Stagnant | ☐ |
| **D.** Laminar | ☐ |

**209.** The blood flow immediately after a stenosis is called _____.

| | |
|---|---|
| **A.** Vortex | ☐ |
| **B.** Turbulent | ☐ |
| **C.** Stagnant | ☐ |
| **D.** Laminar | ☐ |

**210.** Blood that is moving very slowly is called _____ and may appear _____ on a CSE or FSE sequences.

| | |
|---|---|
| **A.** Vortex, Bright | ☐ |
| **B.** Turbulent, Bright | ☐ |
| **C.** Stagnant, Dark | ☐ |
| **D.** Stagnant, Bright to Gray | ☐ |

**211.** Long TR sequences usually have _____ applied to decrease _____ artifact.

| | |
|---|---|
| **A.** Sat. pulses, Chemical shift | ☐ |
| **B.** Flow comp., Pulsatile | ☐ |
| **C.** Flow comp., Wrap | ☐ |
| **D.** An IR Pulse, Motion | ☐ |

**212.** A 3D MRA sequence has the advantage of _____ over a 2D MRA, but can _____ flow in smaller vessels.

| | |
|---|---|
| **A.** Higher resolution, Saturate | ☐ |
| **B.** Lower resolution, Saturate | ☐ |
| **C.** Larger coverage, Overestimate | ☐ |
| **D.** Larger coverage, Underestimate | ☐ |

**213.** A disadvantage of 2D/3D TOF MRA sequences is _____.

| | |
|---|---|
| **A.** Sensitive to Iodinated contrast | ☐ |
| **B.** Ionizing radiation | ☐ |
| **C.** Overestimation of stenosis | ☐ |
| **D.** Underestimation of stenosis | ☐ |

**214.** A minor disadvantage to using Flow comp is _____.

| | |
|---|---|
| **A.** Underexposed sequences | ☐ |
| **B.** Slight increase in TE | ☐ |
| **C.** Decreased TR | ☐ |
| **D.** A narrow Rec. B/W is required | ☐ |

**215.** PC MRA sequences have a user-selectable parameter called Venc. This factor makes the sequence sensitive to _____.

| | |
|---|---|
| **A.** Gadolinium | ☐ |
| **B.** Flow velocity | ☐ |
| **C.** Flow direction | ☐ |
| **D.** Motion | ☐ |

**216.** Advantages of a PC MRA sequence is its _____ and being _____.

- **A.** Background suppression, unaffected by IV contrast ☐
- **B.** Ultrashort scan times, sensitive to flow direction ☐
- **C.** Ultrahigh resolution, Fat-Sat ☐
- **D.** All the above ☐

**217.** A dynamic perfusion in the brain is sensitive to the _____ of the tissue.

- **A.** T2 ☐
- **B.** T1 ☐
- **C.** P.D. ☐
- **D.** Relaxation ☐

**218.** In a dynamic perfusion seq., tissues _____ in signal when the IV contrast arrives.

- **A.** Increase ☐
- **B.** Decrease ☐
- **C.** Does not change ☐

**219.** Parallel imaging decreases the scan time as well as the _____.

- **A.** SAR ☐
- **B.** PNS ☐
- **C.** TR ☐
- **D.** ETL ☐

**220.** Lowering the TR to shorter than the T1 relaxation of a tissue will _____.

- **A.** Cause saturation ☐
- **B.** Lower the SNR ☐
- **C.** Make the weighting T2* ☐
- **D.** A and B ☐

**221.** In MRI, it Is axiomatic that TR controls _____ while TE controls _____.

- **A.** T1, PD ☐
- **B.** T2, T1 ☐
- **C.** T1, T2 ☐
- **D.** T1, T2* ☐

**222.** If you double the slice thickness, the SNR will _____.

> **A.** Not be affected ☐
> **B.** Double ☐
> **C.** Triple ☐
> **D.** Quadruple ☐

**223.** If you double the FOV, the SNR will _____.

> **A.** Not be affected ☐
> **B.** Double ☐
> **C.** Triple ☐
> **D.** Quadruple ☐

**224.** If you double the frequency matrix, the SNR will _____ and the TE will _____.

> **A.** Not be affected, increase ☐
> **B.** Double, decrease ☐
> **C.** Decrease, lengthen ☐
> **D.** Decrease, not change ☐

**225.** For any given tissue, keeping the TR constant while increasing the flip angle will cause that tissue to lose signal. This is an example of _____.

> **A.** Faraday's law ☐
> **B.** Ohm's law ☐
> **C.** Tissue mitigation ☐
> **D.** Ernst angle ☐

**226.** What is the scan time formula for an inversion recovery sequence?

> **A.** $TR \times Phase \times nex \div TI \div 60\,000 = $ Scan time in ms ☐
> **B.** $TR \times Phase \times nex + TI \div 60\,000 = $ Scan time in ms ☐
> **C.** $TR \times Phase \times nex - TI \div 60\,000 = $ Scan time in ms ☐
> **D.** $TR \times Phase \times nex \div 60\,000 = $ Scan time in ms ☐

**227.** A radiologist calls and wants the GRE axials in the cervical spine more T2* weighted. You should:

| | |
|---|---|
| **A.** Increase the TR and TE | ☐ |
| **B.** Increase the TR and flip angle | ☐ |
| **C.** Increase the TE and lower the flip angle | ☐ |
| **D.** Tell him "No" it cannot be done | ☐ |

**228.** A radiologist calls and wants the GRE axials in the cervical spine more T1 weighted. You should:

| | |
|---|---|
| **A.** Decrease the TR and TE | ☐ |
| **B.** Increase the TR and flip angle | ☐ |
| **C.** decrease the TE and increase the flip angle | ☐ |
| **D.** Tell him "No" it cannot be done | ☐ |

**229.** Parallel imaging decreases the scan time as well as the _____.

| | |
|---|---|
| **A.** SAR | ☐ |
| **B.** PNS | ☐ |
| **C.** TR | ☐ |
| **D.** ETL | ☐ |

**230.** Where should the saturation pulse be placed on a 2D or 3D TOF MRA?

| | |
|---|---|
| **A.** Above the stack | ☐ |
| **B.** Below the stack | ☐ |
| **C.** Parallel to the left and right | ☐ |
| **D.** Depends on whether you are imaging above or below the heart | ☐ |

**231.** Gadolinium shortens the _____ and _____ or a tissue.

| | |
|---|---|
| **A.** T1, Transverse relaxation | ☐ |
| **B.** Proton density, T1 | ☐ |
| **C.** T2, P.D. | ☐ |
| **D.** Longitudinal, P.D. | ☐ |

**232.** When performing a 2D oblique sagittal TOF MRV of the brain, place the sat pulse _____ the slices.

| | |
|---|---|
| **A.** Lateral to the slab | ☐ |
| **B.** Above | ☐ |
| **C.** Below | ☐ |
| **D.** Do not need one | ☐ |

**233.** A single shot FSE is when the:

| | |
|---|---|
| **A.** Number of Phase encodes ÷ the ETL = 1 | ☐ |
| **B.** Number of Phase encodes × the ETL = 256 | ☐ |
| **C.** TR × Number of Phase encodes = 256 | ☐ |
| **D.** TR ÷ Number of Phase encodes = 1 | ☐ |

**234.** Image contrast in a DWI comes from the _____ and _____.

| | |
|---|---|
| **A.** TR, TE | ☐ |
| **B.** TR, b-Value | ☐ |
| **C.** TI, TE | ☐ |
| **D.** TE, b-Value | ☐ |

**235.** k-Space represents what two directions?

| | |
|---|---|
| **A.** Slice and Phase | ☐ |
| **B.** Frequency and Slice | ☐ |
| **C.** Phase and Frequency | ☐ |
| **D.** Right to Left and Anterior to Posterior | ☐ |

**236.** Decreasing the Fourier from 100% to 75% will _____.

| | |
|---|---|
| **A.** Decrease scan time and SNR | ☐ |
| **B.** Increase the scan time and SNR | ☐ |
| **C.** Increase resolution and increase SNR | ☐ |
| **D.** Lower SAR and increase resolution | ☐ |

**237.** Being able to use one half of k-Space to replicate the other half in order to decrease scan time is called _____.

| | |
|---|---|
| **A.** Half Fourier | ☐ |
| **B.** Conjugate synthesis | ☐ |
| **C.** Parallel imaging | ☐ |
| **D.** A and B | ☐ |

**238.** Acquiring just over half (60%) of the raw data and using it to synthesis the unfilled lines of k-Space is called:

A. Half Fourier ☐
B. Conjugate synthesis ☐
C. Parallel imaging ☐
D. A and B ☐

**239.** Half Fourier's disadvantage is a decrease in both _____ and _____.

A. Contrast, T1 ☐
B. SNR, Resolution ☐
C. T2, SNRD) T1, Resolution ☐

**240.** In a STIR sequence, the TR needs to be at least as long as 1 T1 of water, otherwise it will start to _____.

A. Lose signal ☐
B. Saturate ☐
C. Be T2* weighted ☐
D. Both A and B ☐

**241.** Another name or term for time of flight MRA is _____?

A. Flow relative encoding ☐
B. Flow-related enhancement ☐
C. Fast relative enhancement ☐
D. Fourier-related enhancement ☐

**242.** A technique to better see IV contrast on pre and post contrast data sets is called?

A. MPR ☐
B. MIP ☐
C. Subtraction ☐
D. Surface rendering ☐

**243.** Where is the Fourier transform performed?

A. The array processor ☐
B. The RFPA ☐
C. The Phase/Frequency time domain ☐
D. The CPU ☐

**244.** What is it called when a time domain is converted into a frequency domain?

- **A.** Faraday's domain law ☐
- **B.** Creutzfeldt–Jakob conversion ☐
- **C.** Fourier transform ☐
- **D.** Ohm's conversion ☐

**245.** When looking at the various peaks in a single-voxel spectroscopy, what you are really looking at is _____.

- **A.** Half Fourier's raw data ☐
- **B.** Conjugate synthesis of data ☐
- **C.** Chemical shift imaging ☐
- **D.** the F.I.D. curve ☐

**246.** Some parallel imaging techniques require a _____ for Fourier transform to be performed.

- **A.** Shim ☐
- **B.** Scout ☐
- **C.** Calibration/Reference ☐
- **D.** A and C ☐

**247.** Usually the saturation pulse(s) are applied _____.

- **A.** Before the 180° ☐
- **B.** After the 90° ☐
- **C.** Before TE ☐
- **D.** Before the excitation pulse ☐

**248.** In a long TR/TE sequence with low SNR, but you cannot change the nex, Matrix, Slice thickness or FOV what factor can you alter to get more signal?

- **A.** Increase slice gap ☐
- **B.** Shorten the TR ☐
- **C.** Narrow the Rec. B/W ☐
- **D.** Widen the Transmitter B/W ☐

**249.** A short tau sequence is used to suppress?

A. Long T1 relaxing tissue ☐
B. Short T1 relaxing tissue ☐
C. High proton density tissues ☐
D. Long T2 relaxing tissue ☐

**250.** Widening the transmitter bandwidth results in _____?

A. Higher resolution ☐
B. Thinner slices ☐
C. Thicker slices ☐
D. Longer TE's ☐

**251.** Widening the receiver B/W results in all the following except _____?

A. Higher SNR ☐
B. Shorter TE ☐
C. Less chemical shift ☐
D. Small echo spacing ☐

**252.** Enlarging the FOV results in all the following except _____?

A. Higher SAR ☐
B. Lower possible TE ☐
C. Lower resolution ☐
D. Larger coverage ☐

**253.** In a 3D sequence, the gap in between slices is _____?

A. A percentage of the slice thickness ☐
B. Equal to the slice thickness ☐
C. Zero ☐
D. Greater than in a 2D ☐

**254.** The time that the Readout gradient is applied changes with _____.

A. FOV ☐
B. Frequency matrix ☐
C. Receiver B/W ☐
D. A, B, and C ☐

**255.** A STIR sequence's contrast is based on the _____ of the tissues.

| | |
|---|---|
| **A.** T1 | ☐ |
| **B.** T2 | ☐ |
| **C.** P.D. | ☐ |

**256.** Spectral tissue suppression sequences decrease signal from a tissue because of _____.

| | |
|---|---|
| **A.** The precessional frequency of fat | ☐ |
| **B.** The T1 of the tissue | ☐ |
| **C.** The T2 of the tissue | ☐ |
| **D.** Precessional frequency of the tissue to be suppressed | ☐ |

**257.** In turbo spin echo, the number of slices allowed _____ with a decrease in TR.

| | |
|---|---|
| **A.** Does not change | ☐ |
| **B.** Increases | ☐ |
| **C.** Decreases | ☐ |
| **D.** Changes with TR ÷ ETL | ☐ |

**258.** Increasing the number of nex from 1 to 3 increases the SNR by a factor of?

| | |
|---|---|
| **A.** 3 | ☐ |
| **B.** 1.4 | ☐ |
| **C.** 1.7 | ☐ |
| **D.** 4 | ☐ |

**259.** If T2 Fat Sat IQ is poor for any number of reasons, a _____ is a good alternative?

| | |
|---|---|
| **A.** FLAIR | ☐ |
| **B.** STIR | ☐ |
| **C.** T1 F/S Post gad | ☐ |
| **D.** Proton density with T1 FLAIR | ☐ |

**260.** What is the precessional frequency difference between fat and water at 1.5T?

| | |
|---|---|
| **A.** 3.55 ppm | ☐ |
| **B.** 220 Hz | ☐ |
| **C.** 440 Hz | ☐ |
| **D.** A and B | ☐ |

**261.** The precessional frequency difference between fat and water is _____?

| | |
|---|---|
| **A.** 2/3 of Planck's constant | ☐ |
| **B.** Directly proportion to field strength | ☐ |
| **C.** Inversely proportional to field strength | ☐ |
| **D.** ½ of the Larmor frequency | ☐ |

**262.** How is the precessional frequency difference of fat and water determined?

| | |
|---|---|
| **A.** Field Strength × 3.5 | ☐ |
| **B.** Larmor Freq. × 3.5 | ☐ |
| **C.** Larmor Freq. × 220 | ☐ |
| **D.** Field Strength × 220 | ☐ |
| **Use Figure 3.17 as a reference*** | ☐ |

**263.** Cardiac gating a sequence, with a heart rate is 60 bpm, the R-R interval is:

| | |
|---|---|
| **A.** 60 ms | ☐ |
| **B.** 600 ms | ☐ |
| **C.** 1000 ms | ☐ |
| **D.** 100 ms | ☐ |

**264.** What if the patient's heart rate increases 75 bpm, then the R-R interval is:

| | |
|---|---|
| **A.** 80 ms | ☐ |
| **B.** 80 ms | ☐ |
| **C.** 800 ms | ☐ |
| **D.** 750 ms | ☐ |

**265.** The effective TR is the R-R interval time in ms minus the _____ and the _____.

A. Trigger delay, Trigger amplitude ☐
B. Trigger window, Trigger amplitude ☐
C. Trigger window, Trigger delay ☐
D. Trigger time, Systolic heart rate ☐

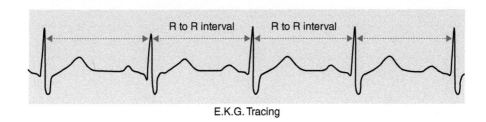

E.K.G. Tracing

**266.** In Figure 3.18, "A" points to what part of the cardiac trace?

A. S ☐
B. R ☐
C. Q ☐
D. P ☐

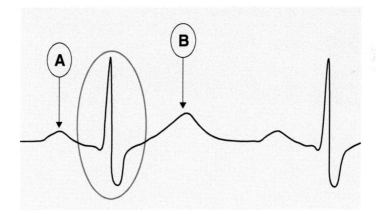

**267.** In Figure 3.18, circled is the?

A. L ☐
B. QRS ☐
C. Q ☐
D. T ☐

**268.** In Figure 3.18, "B" points to the?

A. T  ☐
B. QRS  ☐
C. Q  ☐
D. S  ☐

**269.** In Figure 3.19, the time labeled as "A" is?

A. Half the TE  ☐
B. 1 TAU  ☐
C. TE  ☐
D. A and B  ☐

**270.** In Figure 3.19, the time labeled as "B" is?

A. Half the TE  ☐
B. 1 TAU  ☐
C. TE  ☐
D. TR  ☐

**271.** In Figure 3.19, the time labeled as "C" is?

A. Half the TE  ☐
B. 1 TAU  ☐
C. TE  ☐
D. TR  ☐

**272.** In Figure 3.19, which gradient is the frequency gradient?

A. X  ☐
B. Y  ☐
C. Z  ☐

**273.** In Figure 3.19, which gradient is the phase gradient?

A. X  ☐
B. Y  ☐
C. Z  ☐

**274.** In Figure 3.19, which gradient is the slice select gradient?

**A.** X   ☐
**B.** Y   ☐
**C.** Z   ☐

**275.** The rise time of a gradient is _____?

**A.** Time to get to Max. Strength   ☐
**B.** Time to get to Max. Strength/2   ☐
**C.** Max. Gradient Amplitude $\div\ \pi$   ☐
**D.** Time/ $\pi r^2$   ☐

**276.** The slew rate of a gradient is _____?

**A.** Peak Gradient Amplitude $\div$ Rise Time   ☐
**B.** Time/ $\pi r^2$   ☐
**C.** Rise Time $\div\ \pi$   ☐
**D.** Measured in mT/mm   ☐

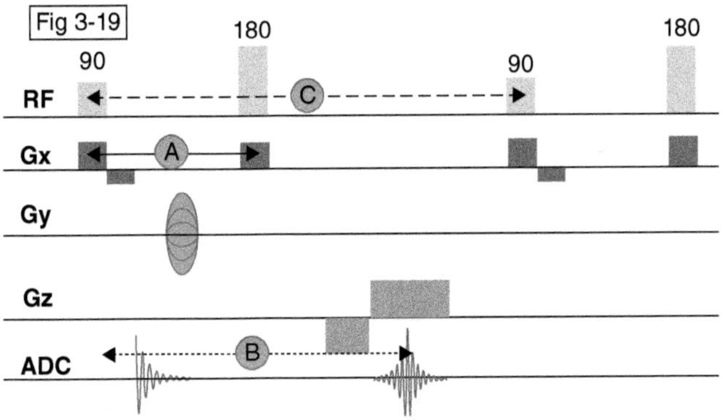

Fig 3-19

**277.** Identify the weighting in Figure 3.20:

**A.** T2   ☐
**B.** T2FLAIR   ☐
**C.** GRE   ☐
**D.** T1 FLAIR   ☐

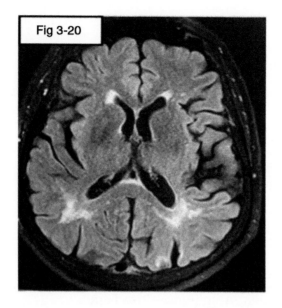

Fig 3-20

**278.** Identify the weighting in Figure 3.21:

A. T2 ☐
B. STIR ☐
C. GRE ☐
D. T1 FLAIR ☐

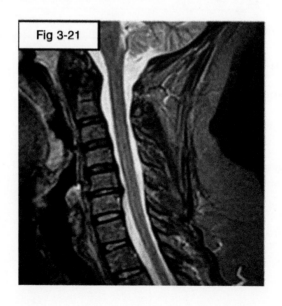

Fig 3-21

**279.** Identify the weighting in Figure 3.22:

| | |
|---|---|
| **A.** T2 | ☐ |
| **B.** T2FLAIR | ☐ |
| **C.** GRE | ☐ |
| **D.** T1 | ☐ |

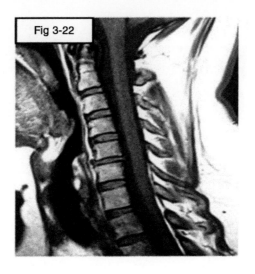

Fig 3-22

**280.** Identify the weighting in Figure 3.23:

| | |
|---|---|
| **A.** T2 | ☐ |
| **B.** T2FLAIR | ☐ |
| **C.** GRE | ☐ |
| **D.** T1 FLAIR | ☐ |

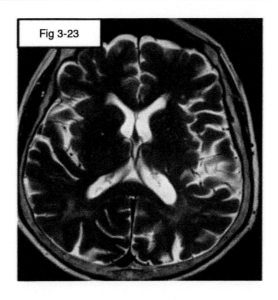

Fig 3-23

**281.** Identify the weighting in Figure 3.24:

A. T2 ☐
B. T1 ☐
C. GRE ☐
D. T1 FLAIR ☐

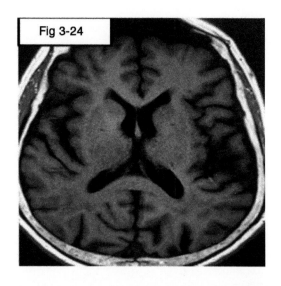

Fig 3-24

**282.** Identify the weighting in Figure 3.25:

A. T2 ☐
B. T2FLAIR ☐
C. GRE ☐
D. T1 FLAIR ☐

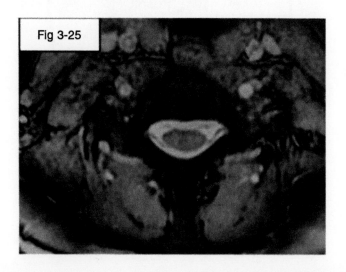

Fig 3-25

**283.** Identify the weighting in Figure 3.26:

A. T2 ☐
B. DWI ☐
C. GRE ☐
D. T2 FLAIR ☐

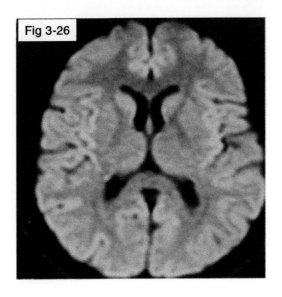

Fig 3-26

**284.** Identify the weighting in Figure 3.27:

A. T2 ☐
B. T2FLAIR ☐
C. PD ☐
D. T1 ☐

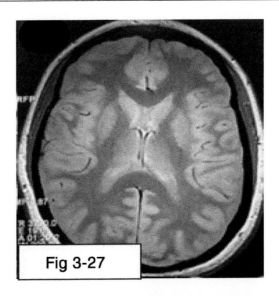

Fig 3-27

**285.** Identify the weighting in Figure 3.28:

| | |
|---|---|
| **A.** GRE | ☐ |
| **B.** T2* | ☐ |
| **C.** T2 | ☐ |
| **D.** A and B | ☐ |

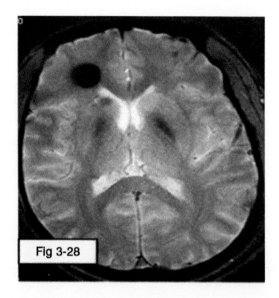

Fig 3-28

Let us do a review of the basic Spin-echo, Fast spin-echo, and Gradient echo PSDs.

**Spin-echo:** It always starts off with a 90–180 RF pulse set. If you do not see a 180 after excitation, it is a GRE. The slice select gradient (SSG) is always applied during both the 90 and 180 RFs. As you know the SSG can be in any plane, so the SSG from the Gx is a Sagittal, Gy a Coronal and Gz an Axial. Here, a picture using my LEFT-HAND (Figure 3.16) for gradient identification is helpful. The LEFT HAND is the direction the gradients encodes in real life in your conventional bore scanners. Also remember that the order that the gradients are applied is SLICE, PHASE, then FREQUENCY (SPF like sun tan lotion). After, we find the SSG that leaves the Phase and Frequency gradients and their directions. The phase encoding gradient (PEG) comes next. In SE/FSE, the PEG is always in between the 90 and the 180.

Ideally or usually the PEG is applied in the shortest axis of the body. A sagittal spine often has the phase direction A/P so you can save time by applying some amount of "Phase FOV." So, the Gy is applied for PEG. Phase is A/P. Next, frequency is a long word so that is the longest axis of the body which in the case is S/I or Gz. The frequency gradient is applied during echo formation and sometimes called the "Readout" or RO.

This is the exact scenario as shown in Figure 3.1. It is a Sagittal slice (Gx) (my middle finger) with phase running A/P (Gy) (my index finger), and frequency is S/I (Gz) (my thumb).

Let us try a coronal brain: Gy is SSG (A/P), the short axis is R/L so Gx, leaving Gz for frequency in the S/I direction.

This takes a few times to get it but practice it. You will be asked these directions.

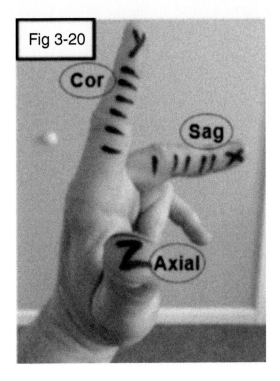

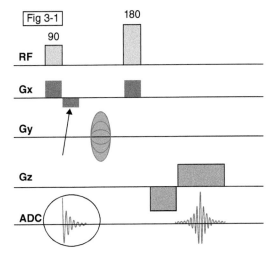

**Fast spin-echo:** Again, always starts off with a 90–180 RF pulse set but has a series of 180's, the Echo train. The same sets of rules apply to FSE as in a CSE. The difference is the series of 180's each with its own PEG to encode the different echoes into a different line of k-Space. See how the amplitude of the PEG is changed for the next echo (Figure 3.3). Also note that the amplitude of each successive echo decreases due to true T2 relaxation and imperfections in the 180 RF pulses. This is another example of a sagittal slice. If you wanted an **Axial,** which gradient would be applied during the 90 and 180's? Answer Figure 3.3.

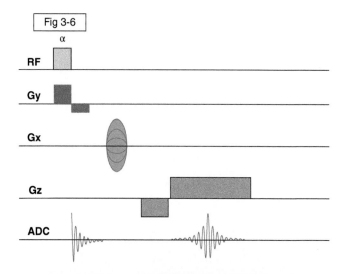

*Answer:* Gz would be applied during the RFs to get an Axial.

**Gradient echo: It** is displayed in Figure 3.6. There is an excitation pulse but *no 180.* Ding, ding, ding! no 180 = a GRE.

What imaging plane is this?
**Axial, Coronal, or Sagittal? Phase runs?** _____, **so, Frequency is**

_____.

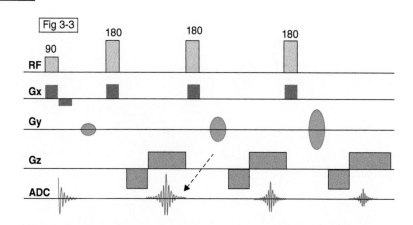

# Section 3 MR Pulse Sequences and MR Math Answers

1. **D.** A SE **always** starts off with a 90–180° RF complex. With no Echo train, it is a conventional spin-echo. If there is a 90° *but no 180°*, it is a GRE.

2. **A.** The SSG is applied during RF excitation.

3. **B.**

4. **D.** The FID, free induction decay, curve is a small amount of signal caused by the initial 90°. Its signal is very small and fades out very quickly. Too quick to get any real useful signal from. TE's would need to be less than 1 ms which is not achievable in normal everyday scanning. Maybe in a laboratory but not in routine scanning.

5. **A.**

6. **A.**

7. **A.**

8. **D.**

9. **C.**

10. **C.**

11. **A.**

12. **C.** The PEG is said to drive k-Space. Changing the amplitude of the PEG places each echo in a different line of k-Space.

13. **C.**

14. **B.**

15. **B.**

16. **B.**

17. **C.**

18. **C.** SE has 2 RF pulses, GRE has 1. In GRE it is usually less than a 90° but it can be a 90°.

19. **C.**

20. **C.** Yes, a dual echo SE. The TR is long 2000+ms, the 1st TE is a usually a short TE so is PD weighted, the 2nd Echo is a longer TE so is T2. This sequence is seldom used anymore, but was a staple years ago in Neuro imaging. It was used in the brain for M.S. and sagittals in the spine.

21. **C.** Single amplitude decrease as the TE lengthens.

22. **C.** Sagittal.

23. **C.**

24. **B.**

25. **C.**

26. **C.**

27. **C.** The ETL is what turns a SE into a FSE.

28. **B.** The 180's increase the SAR.

29. **C.**

30. **B.** Three echoes fills in three lines of Phase per TR

31. **C.**

32. **A.**

33. **B.**

34. **D.**

35. **D.** The extra RF's in an ETL equals more work for the scanner. More work a need for a longer TR. Everything the scanner needs to do to a slice needs to fit into the TR.

36. **D.**

37. **C.**

38. **C.**

39. **C.**

40. **A.** The 180s clean up the effects of metal in the FOV.

41. **C.**

42. **C.**

**43. B.** False

**44. C.** Pixel size is the FOV ÷ by the Matrix. You may have to do that math twice, once for phase and again for frequency.

**45. B.**

**46. B.**

**47. C.**

**48. A.**

**49. B.**

**50. B.**

**51. B.** 2.05 minutes = 123 seconds. Depending on the answers given, you may have to convert minutes to seconds.

**52. D.**

**53. C.**

**54. C.** Cannot determine as no scan factors are/were given.

**55. D.** The time from the 90 to the 180 = 1 TAU, 180 to the TE = 1 TAU. 90 to the TE = 2 TAU.

**56. B.** The time for the 180 to the 90 is the TI. TI is sometimes referred to as TAU as in the sequence **STIR** which is **S**hort **TAU I**nversion **R**ecovery or Short **Time** Inversion Recovery.

**57. C.** The math comes out to 3.46 minutes. 3.46 minutes = 207 seconds. (60×3 = 180, then add 0.46 of a minute or 27 seconds, so 180+27 = 207 seconds.

**58. B.**

**59. A.**

**60. B.**

**61. D.**

**62. D.** The pixel size math needs to equal the slice thickness in order to get ISOTROPIC VOXELS.

**63. A.** Looking at the answers given, there are two with unequal matrices. Those are out right off the bat. Then do the math for the other 2.

64. **B.**

65. **A.** In a STIR, the TR needs to be long enough for water to relax (2000+ms) or it will begin to saturate and lose signal.

66. **B.**

67. **A.**

68. **C.** The 3 RF pulses immediately prior to the 90° are RF pulses tuned to the PF of fat. This series of RFs puts fat into an almost steady state and makes it unable to give signal.

69. **A.**

70. **C.** As ELT goes up, there can be increased blurring of the image. Please see Figure 5.9 in Chapter 5 of MRI Physics: Tech to Tech Explanations.

71. **A.** Sort of a trick question. The basic and or FSE scan time formula applies to a Fat Sat. No special or different formula. The F/S pulses will cause the TR to be lengthened.

72. **D.** A Narrow Rec. B/W is the cause of chemical shift artifact. A narrow B/W forces to many frequencies into a pixel. These extra frequencies "ooze" out of the pixel in the frequency direction causing the artifact.

73. **C.**

74. **B.** Coronal. The RF and Gy are applied simultaneously.

75. **A.** Right to Left.

76. **C.** The 1st lobe de-phases and the 2nd re-phases to create the echo.

77. **D.** Analog to Digital Converter. The Echo is an ANALOG or Sine wave. Fourier transform cannot work on Sine waves, it needs numbers. The echo is **converted** into numbers by the ADC so Fourier transform to do its job.

78. **C.** GREs have no 180°. When you look at a PSD, number 1: is there a 180 after excitation? NO, it is GRE, if YES, it is SE, Multiple 180s, its FSE. number 2. Does it start off with a 180? Yes, it is an IR.

79. **A.** The basic scan time formula applies to a 2D GRE.

80. **D.**

81. **A.**

82. **A.**

**83. C.**

**84. C.** A narrow Rec. B/W is actually a slower sampling rate so, the Min TE will increase. SNR increases as your sampling the sweet spot of the echo where signal is highest, and with a narrow Rec. B/W, lots of frequencies are put into a pixel. If the pixel is over full, they spill out in the frequency direction causing a chemical shift artifact.

**85. C.** As the F/A increases, there is more T1'ing the NMV has to do to recover. If an excitation pulse is applied before full recovery, tissues saturate. So, for a given TR, as F/A increases there will be a point where saturation begins.

**86. A.** Weighting in a GRE is not actually T2 but T2*. It is a long TE so fluids get bright, but it is never a "T2" weighted GRE. True T2 weighting is only produced by a spin echo. You could say a GRE is T2 like as fluids get bright but it is not a true T2.

**87. C.** As the TR increases, there is more time for full T1 relaxation so less chance of saturation. This is especially true in STIR sequences where if the TR is to short, fluids like edema and CSF lose signal due to saturation. See Chapter 6: Tissue Suppression for more.

**88. C.** Note the extra SSG.

**89. B.** Coronal.

**90. B.**

**91. A.** The F/A is how far into the X/Y plane the NMV is placed. The further over, the more T1'ing the transverse NMV has to do. Think of the flip angle as how much T1 you r putting into the system. Put in T1, expect to get T1 back in the echo.

**92. B.** SNR changes with the $\sqrt{}$ of the number of Locs.

**93. C.** The number of Locs is how many times the extra SSG is applied.

**94. A.** True. 3D, in general, has thinner slices than a 2D.

**95. A.** 8:24.

**96. C.** Anisotropic.

**97. C.** $0.72 \times 1.02$ is the pixel size. FOV ÷ Matrix = Pixel size.

**98. A.** $0.72 \times 1.02 \times 2 = 1.45 \, mm^3$.

**99. C.**

**100. C.** As the blood (Flow) is in the slab longer, it gets more RF's and begins to saturate.

**101. D.** Ideally, blood flow should be at 90° (⊥) to the flow. You may/should angle the slab/slice to be perpendicular (⊥) to the flow in the target vessel(s).

**102. D.**

**103. B.** SNR is a function of the √ of the number of nex/Acq or NSA. The √ of $1 = 1$, $\sqrt{2} = 1.4$, $\sqrt{3} = 1.7$, $\sqrt{4} = 2$. It is not until you scan the data 4 times will you get a doubling in SNR.

**104. B.** TE controls T2 not T1.

**105. B.**

**106. D.**

**107. True.** An increased F/A means the RF ($B_1$) is turned on longer.

**108. D.**

**109. B.**

**110. C.**

**111. B.** False. The late echoes in any Echo train inherently have a low SNR compared to the 1st echo due to True T2 relaxation (Spin–Spin relaxation) and inhomogeneities in the 180° refocusing pulse(s).

**112. C.** Partitions in a 3D are akin to the number of phase encodes in the matrix. It is how many TRs are needed to image the slab vs. making the TR longer. Both affect scan time.

**113. A.** This is a dual echo GRE. IN-OOP Phase, Opposed Phase, or a Dixon.

**114. A.** Axial.

**115. C.** Right/Left as it comes from the Gx gradient.

**116. True.** Flow comp. is extra gradient applications in either the SSG or frequency directions.

**117. D.** All.

**118. D.** A GRE. An OOP echo can only happen/occur in a GRE sequence. **The 180° in a SE/FSE makes the protons to ALWAYS to be INPHASE at the TE.** Even if you select an OOP TE in a SE sequence, you would not get the OOP effect. Cannot happen.

**119. B.** True.

**120. A.**

**121. B.** The OOP echo is also called chemical shift of the 2nd kind. Note that the black outline is in two directions: Phase and Frequency. **2** directions chem shift of the **2nd** kind.

**122. D.** A Dixon sequence is a dual echo GRE. Simply put, the four different contrasts come from adding and subtracting the In and Out of phase echoes. In a Dixon, you acquire 2 echoes, the In and Out (1 and 2), then add them together gives a water only (3), subtract them to get the fat only (4).

**123. C.** Dixon technique is used to get Fat Sat on low fields.

**124. D.**

**125. D.** Very commonly used to evaluate adrenals.

**126. A.**

**127. A.**

**128. D.**

**129. C.**

**130. C.**

**131. C.**

**132.** True, think "T" (Temporal) is for **T**ime, and **S**patial is over **S**pace (distance).

**133. C.**

**134.** K and M do not apply.

**135. D.**

**136. C.**

**137. C.**

**138. C.**

**139. D.** *Segmentation* is cutting out the background tissue. We all call it a MIP, but a MIP is an image of all the slices piled on top of each other giving you quick look to check the I.Q. MIP stands for Maximum Intensity Projection.

**140. A.**

141. C.

142. C.

143. A. This describes Fourier transform (FT). There are several ways to say, ask or describe it.

144. B.

145. D. There are of course multiple ways to describe "Partial Fourier."

146. B.

147. C.

148. B.

149. A.

150. D.

151. B. The ETL is how many lines of k-Space are filled per slice per TR.

152. D. This is how many lines of k-Space are filled per TR, so $19 \times 12 = 228$.

153. C.

154. B.

155. B.

156. B.

157. B.

158. C.

159. B.

160. C.

161. C.

162. D.

163. B.

164. B.

165. B.

166. C.

167. B.

168. C.

169. B.

170. D.

171. B.

172. B.

173. D.

174. D.

175. B.

176. **A.** True. EPI sequences can start off a number of ways: SE, STIR, or GRE. This one starts of as a SE. SE usually for DWI, STIR for Fat suppression, GRE for Perfusion.

177. **B.** All EPI's have lots of gradient reversals, so PNS is a real concern.

178. **D.** DWI's have extra gradients pulses in three or more directions. The PSD in Figure 3.13 shows the diffusion gradients in the SLICE direction ONLY. A DWI would run the sequence diffusing in the Slice, then runs again diffusing in the Phase direction and then the Frequency direction.

179. A.

180. B.

181. B.

182. D.

183. D.

184. B.

185. A.

186. C.

187. B.

188. **A.** At 0 ms after excitation, the protons are all In-phase.

189. **B.** When doing either Fat Saturation or Water Excitation images, you are using or taking advantage of the "Chemical Shift" between these two "chemicals".

190. C.

191. D.

192. D.

193. A.

194. D.

195. B.

196. A.

197. B.

198. C.

199. D, I, J.

200. B.

201. B.

202. C.

203. C.

204. **D.** Note that there is an extra positive and double negative gradient complex applied just before the echo. The extra positive and double neg. is Flow comp.

205. **D.** Sat pulse is used to remove signal from the unwanted vessels, and Flow comp to make the vessels as bright as possible.

206. B.

207. D.

208. D.

209. A.

210. D.

211. B.

212. A.

213. C.

214. B.

**215. B.**

**216. A.** Remember to give the most correct answer. Yes, PC can give flow direction information. PC sequences are not often "Ultrashort" in scan times so **B** is out, and with good back ground suppression, in **C**, Fat sat on a PC is both overkill and makes the sequence even longer.

**217. A.** Gado, being a metal, causes perfused tissue to drop in signal on arrival.

**218. B.**

**219. A.**

**220. D.**

**221. C.**

**222. B.** This would double the number of protons in the voxel so doubling the signal.

**223. D.** Doubling the FOV increases the voxel size in 2 directions. $2 \times 2 = 4$.

**224. C.**

**225. D.**

**226. D.**

**227. C.** TE always affects the T2 (T2* in the case of a GRE). Here, the Rad. wants brighter fluid. He may not know how this is achieved. That is your job not his. An increase in the TE allows for more T2* to happen so fluid gets brighter, and a decrease in Flip angle lessens the T1 contrast in the image. All told, both these adjustments will make fluid brighter.

**228. C.**

**229. A.** Filling less lines of phase will mean fewer RF pulses which = a lower SAR.

**230. D.**

**231. A.**

**232. C.**

**233. A.** If dividing the phase lines by the ETL does not come out to 1 then the sequence in a "Multi-shot." A multi-shot of say 2 uses 2 TR's to acquire the data.

**234. D.**

235. **C.**

236. **A.**

237. **D.** Same concept just different terminology.

238. **D.** Same concept just different terminology.

239. **B.**

240. **A.**

241. **B.** FRE or Flow-related enhancement is a new way of describing T.O.F MRA. When I stated MR, it was called T.O.F. What FRE means: is the **Enhancement** (bright vessels) is **Related to Flow.**

242. **C.**

243. **A.**

244. **C.**

245. **C.**

246. **C.**

247. **D.**

248. **C.**

249. **B.**

250. **C.**

251. **A.**

252. **A.**

253. **C.** There is no gap in 3D seqs. Partitions are made by variations in amplitude of the SGG like the PEG. Slabs are excited by a single RF pulse and divided into "Locs" by the SSG.

254. **D.**

255. **A.**

256. **D.**

257. **C.**

**258. C.**

**259. B.** STIRs and T2 Fat-Sats have the same "contrast profile" meaning that fat is dark and fluid is bright.

**260. D.** Either A or B is applicable here. Answer "A" is the Precessional Frequency difference between Fat and water at any field strength when no specific field strength is stated. And "B" is the difference at 1.5T. Note: It is not "C" as this is the Precessional Frequency difference at 3T.

**261. B.**

**262. B.**

**263. C.** With a heart rate of 60bpm, the R-R interval is 1000ms: 1 minute = 60 seconds, and 1 second = 1000ms, so 60 heartbeats per minute = 1 beat every 1000ms. So, divide 60000 by the BPM (60) to find out the R-R interval. $60\,000 \div 60 = 1000$.

**264. C.** $60\,000\,\text{ms} \div 75 = 800\,\text{ms}$. The scanner will do this for you, but you may be asked.

**265. C.** See Figure 3.18b. The **Trigger Delay** is a user selectable time you tell the scanner to **wait** after it sees the QRS complex to not image during maximum heart movement. The **Trigger Window** is also a user selectable time you put in as sort of like a margin for error **so you are not imaging into the next QRS**. Basically, in case the patient's rate increases or an Arrhythmia during the sequence. The effective TR is the time left over to image and get the least amount of motion.

**266. D.**

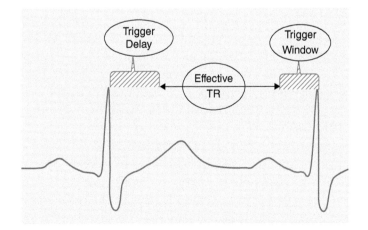

267. **B.**

268. **A.**

269. **D.**

270. **C.**

271. **D.**

272. **C.** Z Gradient.

273. **B.** Y Gradient.

274. **A.** × gradient.

275. **A.** The time it takes for the gradient to come up to required strength.

276. **A.** The Slew Rate is the Peak Gradient Strength ÷ Rise time. The Slew Rate is a very important number when purchasing a scanner. The shorter the Slew Rate, the faster you can scan.

277. **B.**

278. **B.**

279. **B.**

280. **A.**

281. **B.**

282. **C.**

283. **B.**

284. **C.** If this one has or had you confused, it was meant to. Remember, pick the best answer. Let us work the answers: Is it "A" a T2? Maybe. Is it T2 FLAIR? No, the CSF is bright so it cannot be T2 FLAIR, Is it a PD? Maybe, CSF and Fat are both bright. Is it T1? No, the CSF is too bright to be a T1. So now we are down to two possibilities. T2 or PD. Use another question to answer this one. Go back to question 280's image. That a T2 no question. The image for number 284 is PD weighted.

   I threw this image in because few places do PD in the brain anymore. They used to be included routinely in a brain study and used for M.S. but with the advent of T2 FLAIR, the PD axial in the brain has been replaced. Not that PD weighting is no longer valid, it is just that T2 FLAIR contrasts show M.S. plaques better.

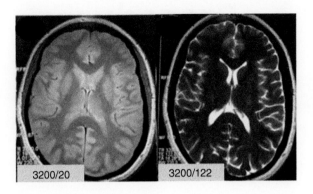

**285. D.** GRE or T2* apply to this image.

# 4 Procedures

This section will concentrate on Procedures or Anatomy. The last portion will be identifying and steps to reduce them. Imaging procedures/protocols vary greatly from department to department. There are/will be approximately 50 questions concerning procedures. The breakdown is listed below. Your general knowledge of anatomy is being tested here in this section. That is not our job. The **approximate** breakdown for the different anatomical regions is listed. Note where questions are "light": The Thorax/Mediastinum.

- Head/neck ≈ 16
- Spine ≈ 12
- Thorax ≈ 5
- Abdomen/pelvis ≈14
- Musculoskeletal ≈15

Besides just giving the answers, there will be some discussion or explanations as to the how/why/what's. Lastly, I will also give you some ways to remember certain anatomies in a section called Mnemonics. Some will be corny, others not so. Some you will know; others you will not. **Remember: Select the most correct answer for each question.**

*MRI Registry Review: Tech to Tech Questions and Answers*, First Edition. Stephen J. Powers.
© 2021 John Wiley & Sons Ltd. Published 2021 by John Wiley & Sons Ltd.

1. What anatomical area would you image for a patient with bowel and bladder dysfunction?

   **A.** Brachial plexus ☐
   **B.** Thoraco-lumbar junction ☐
   **C.** Sacral plexus ☐
   **D.** Cerebral pontine angle ☐

2. When placed into the static magnetic field, what part of the patient's EKG trace can increase?

   **A.** P wave ☐
   **B.** T wave ☐
   **C.** Q wave ☐
   **D.** QRS complex ☐

3. What condition is the result of decreased blood supply to bone?

   **A.** Septic necrosis ☐
   **B.** Hemangioma ☐
   **C.** Avascular necrosis ☐
   **D.** Hemosiderin ☐

4. What part of the femur is most often affected by avascular necrosis?

   **A.** Femoral head ☐
   **B.** Lesser trochanter ☐
   **C.** Surgical neck ☐
   **D.** Mid shaft ☐

5. The Achilles tendon is best seen in what plane?

   **A.** Axial ☐
   **B.** Coronal ☐
   **C.** Sagittal ☐
   **D.** Oblique sagittal ☐

**6.** The prostate is located where in relation to the bladder?

> **A.** Anterior and Superior ☐
> **B.** Inferior and Anterior ☐
> **C.** Inferior and Posterior ☐
> **D.** Superior and Posterior ☐

**7.** What sequence is most sensitive to M.S. plaques?

> **A.** GRE ☐
> **B.** FSE/TSE ☐
> **C.** T2 FLAIR ☐
> **D.** T1 FLAIR ☐

**8.** What blood vessel has the greatest pressure?

> **A.** Aortic arch ☐
> **B.** Pulmonary veins ☐
> **C.** Renal arteries ☐
> **D.** Coronary artery ☐

**9.** T wave elevation during an MRI is an example of _____.

> **A.** Patient anxiety ☐
> **B.** Magneto-Hemodynamic effect ☐
> **C.** Equipment failure ☐
> **D.** Loose skin contacts ☐

**10.** The sciatic nerve originates from the _____.

> **A.** Sacral plexus ☐
> **B.** L2/3 ☐
> **C.** Upper thigh ☐
> **D.** Medulla oblongata ☐

**11.** What is the first branch off the abdominal aorta?

> **A.** Renal ☐
> **B.** Celiac ☐
> **C.** Superior mesenteric ☐
> **D.** Inferior mesenteric ☐

**12.** What is the mnemonic to remember the muscles of the rotator cuff?

A. F.I.T.S ☐
B. T.I.S.T ☐
C. S.I.T.S ☐
D. C.I.S.T ☐

**13.** What structure in the brain is responsible for CSF production?

A. The ventricles ☐
B. Corpus collosum ☐
C. Arachnoid mater ☐
D. Choroid plexus ☐

**14.** The nerve affected by carpal tunnel syndrome is the _____.

A. Median ☐
B. Carpal ☐
C. Ulna ☐
D. Brachialis longus ☐

**15.** The pituitary stalk is also known as the _____.

A. Infrundibulum ☐
B. Infundibulum ☐
C. Peduncle ☐
D. Falx cerebri ☐

**16.** The venous drainage of the liver in through what major vessel?

A. Portal vein ☐
B. IVC ☐
C. Hepatic vein ☐
D. Superior mesenteric vein ☐

**17.** What is the first branch major branch off the aortic arch?

A. Brachiocephalic ☐
B. Left common carotid ☐
C. Subclavian ☐
D. Tertiary ☐

**18.** There are two ligamentum teres in the body. One each in the liver and hip.

| | |
|---|---|
| **A.** True | ☐ |
| **B.** False | ☐ |

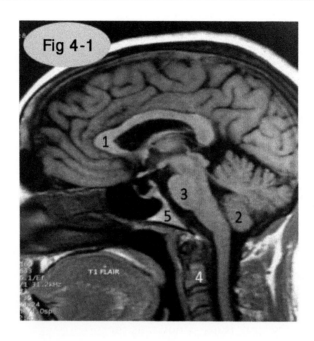

**19.** In Figure 4.1, what structure is labeled 1?

| | |
|---|---|
| **A.** Sella turcica | ☐ |
| **B.** Genu of corpus callosum | ☐ |
| **C.** Body of lateral ventricle | ☐ |
| **D.** Splenium | ☐ |

**20.** In Figure 4.1, what structure is labeled 2?

| | |
|---|---|
| **A.** Cerebellum | ☐ |
| **B.** Cerebellar tonsils | ☐ |
| **C.** Cervical cord | ☐ |
| **D.** Sphenoid sinus | ☐ |

**21.** In Figure 4.1, what structure is labeled 3?

| | |
|---|---|
| **A.** Pons | ☐ |
| **B.** Medulla oblongata | ☐ |
| **C.** Genu of corpus callosum | ☐ |
| **D.** Ethmoid sinus | ☐ |

**22.** In Figure 4.1, what structure is labeled 4?

| | |
|---|---|
| **A.** Odontoid | ☐ |
| **B.** C-2 | ☐ |
| **C.** Dens | ☐ |
| **D.** A, B, and C | ☐ |

**23.** In Figure 4.1, what portion of the sphenoid bone is labeled 5?

| | |
|---|---|
| **A.** Ala | ☐ |
| **B.** Clivus | ☐ |
| **C.** Optic clivus | ☐ |
| **D.** Sphenoid sinus | ☐ |

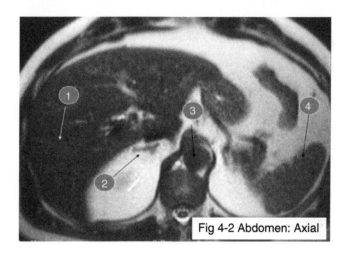

Fig 4-2 Abdomen: Axial

**24.** Number 1 in Figure 4.2 points to the:

| | |
|---|---|
| **A.** Liver | ☐ |
| **B.** Spleen | ☐ |
| **C.** Aorta | ☐ |
| **D.** Kidney | ☐ |

**25.** Number 2 in Figure 4.2 points to the:

| | |
|---|---|
| **A.** Adrenal gland | ☐ |
| **B.** Spinal cord | ☐ |
| **C.** Stomach | ☐ |
| **D.** Liver | ☐ |

**26.** Number 3 in Figure 4.2 points to the:

A. Liver ☐
B. Aorta ☐
C. Adrenal ☐
D. Spleen ☐

**27.** In Figure 4.2, number 4 points to the _____.

A. Stomach ☐
B. Left kidney ☐
C. Splenic flexure ☐
D. Spleen ☐

**28.** In Figure 4.3, number 4 points to the _____.

A. Stomach ☐
B. Left kidney ☐
C. IVC ☐
D. Aorta ☐

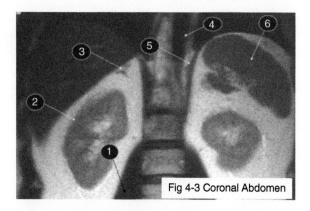

Fig 4-3 Coronal Abdomen

**29.** In Figure 4.3, number 5 points to the _____.

A. Adrenal ☐
B. Crura of diaphragm ☐
C. Splenic ligament ☐
D. Spleen ☐

**30.** In Figure 4.3, number 2 points to the _____.

|  |  |
|---|---|
| **A.** Stomach | ☐ |
| **B.** Kidney | ☐ |
| **C.** Adrenal gland | ☐ |
| **D.** Porta hepatis | ☐ |

**31.** In Figure 4.3, number 1 points to the _____.

|  |  |
|---|---|
| **A.** Psoas muscle | ☐ |
| **B.** Medulla oblongata | ☐ |
| **C.** Transverse ligament | ☐ |
| **D.** Ureter | ☐ |

**32.** In Figure 4.3, number 3 points to the _____.

|  |  |
|---|---|
| **A.** Adrenal | ☐ |
| **B.** Left lobe of liver | ☐ |
| **C.** Hepatic artery | ☐ |
| **D.** Mesenteric vein | ☐ |

**33.** In Figure 4.3, number 6 points to the _____.

|  |  |
|---|---|
| **A.** Ala of pelvic bone | ☐ |
| **B.** Fundus of stomach | ☐ |
| **C.** Corpus selenium | ☐ |
| **D.** Spleen | ☐ |

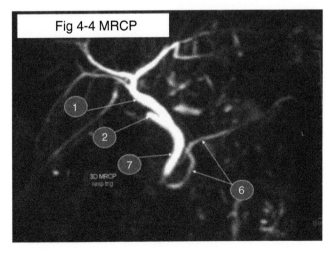

Fig 4-4 MRCP

**34.** In Figure 4.4, number 1 points to the _____.

| | |
|---|---|
| **A.** CBD | ☐ |
| **B.** Hepatic duct | ☐ |
| **C.** Cystic duct | ☐ |
| **D.** Pancreatic duct | ☐ |

**35.** In Figure 4.4, number 2 points to the _____.

| | |
|---|---|
| **A.** CBD | ☐ |
| **B.** Hepatic duct | ☐ |
| **C.** Cystic duct | ☐ |
| **D.** Pancreatic duct | ☐ |

**36.** In Figure 4.4, number 7 points to the _____.

| | |
|---|---|
| **A.** CBD | ☐ |
| **B.** Hepatic duct | ☐ |
| **C.** Cystic duct | ☐ |
| **D.** Pancreatic duct | ☐ |

**37.** In Figure 4.4, number 6 points to the _____.

| | |
|---|---|
| **A.** CBD | ☐ |
| **B.** Hepatic duct | ☐ |
| **C.** Cystic duct | ☐ |
| **D.** Pancreatic duct | ☐ |

**38.** In Figure 4.5, number 3 points to the _____.

| | |
|---|---|
| **A.** Lumbar vessels | ☐ |
| **B.** Celiac axis | ☐ |
| **C.** IMA | ☐ |
| **D.** SMA | ☐ |

**39.** In Figure 4.5, number 1 points to the _____.

| | |
|---|---|
| **A.** Lumbar vessels | ☐ |
| **B.** Celiac axis | ☐ |
| **C.** IMA | ☐ |
| **D.** SMA | ☐ |

**40.** In Figure 4.5, number 2 points to the _____.

A. Lumbar vessels ☐
B. Celiac axis ☐
C. IMA ☐
D. SMA ☐

**41.** The branches of the celiac axis are the hepatic splenic and the

_____.

A. Left gastric ☐
B. Duodenal ☐
C. Minor adrenal ☐
D. Major adrenal ☐

**42.** In the coronal plane, the IVC is seen _____ of the aorta.

A. Right ☐
B. Posterior ☐
C. Left ☐
D. Anterior ☐

**43.** In Figure 4.6, number 1 points to the _____.

A. Symphysis pubis ☐
B. Prostate ☐
C. Urinary bladder ☐
D. Rectum ☐

**44.** In Figure 4.6, number 2 points to the _____.

A. Symphysis pubis ☐
B. Obturator ☐
C. Urinary bladder ☐
D. Rectum ☐

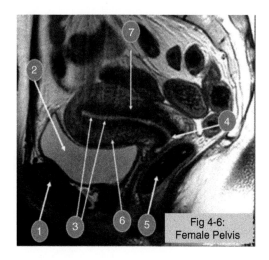

Fig 4-6:
Female Pelvis

**45.** In Figure 4.6, number 7 points to the _____.

| | |
|---|---|
| **A.** Endometrium | ☐ |
| **B.** Myometrium | ☐ |
| **C.** Junctional zone | ☐ |
| **D.** Cervix | ☐ |

**46.** In Figure 4.6, number 3 points to the _____.

| | |
|---|---|
| **A.** Junctional zone | ☐ |
| **B.** Myometrium | ☐ |
| **C.** Endometrium | ☐ |
| **D.** Cervix | ☐ |

**47.** In Figure 4.6, number 6 points to the _____.

| | |
|---|---|
| **A.** Endometrium | ☐ |
| **B.** Myometrium | ☐ |
| **C.** Junctional zone | ☐ |
| **D.** Cervix | ☐ |

**48.** In Figure 4.6, number 5 points to the _____.

| | |
|---|---|
| **A.** Cecum | ☐ |
| **B.** Rectum | ☐ |
| **C.** Junctional zone | ☐ |
| **D.** Cervix | ☐ |

**49.** In Figure 4.6, number 4 points to the _____.

| | |
|---|---|
| **A.** Endometrium | ☐ |
| **B.** Myometrium | ☐ |
| **C.** Junctional zone | ☐ |
| **D.** Cervix | ☐ |

**50.** The image in Figure 4.6 is an example of _____ weighting.

| | |
|---|---|
| **A.** T1 | ☐ |
| **B.** GRE | ☐ |
| **C.** T2 | ☐ |
| **D.** PG | ☐ |

**51.** In Figure 4.6, the prostate is not well seen because it is_____.

| | |
|---|---|
| **A.** Full of urine | ☐ |
| **B.** Saturated | ☐ |
| **C.** Surgically absent | ☐ |
| **D.** A female Pelvis | ☐ |

**52.** The uterus's position can change during scan as the bladder fills with urine. True or False.

**53.** In Figure 4.7, number 1 points to the _____.

| | |
|---|---|
| **A.** Caudate nucleus | ☐ |
| **B.** Infundibulum | ☐ |
| **C.** Ventricular septum | ☐ |
| **D.** Corpus collosum | ☐ |

**54.** In Figure 4.7, number 2 points to the _____.

| | |
|---|---|
| **A.** Temporal lobe | ☐ |
| **B.** Lateral ventricle | ☐ |
| **C.** Temporal horn | ☐ |
| **D.** Sylvian fissure | ☐ |

**55.** In Figure 4.7, number 7 points to the _____.

A. Pituitary stalk ☐
B. Infundibulum ☐
C. Choroid plexus ☐
D. A or B ☐

**56.** In Figure 4.7, number 3 points to the _____.

A. Frontal lobe ☐
B. Parietal lobe ☐
C. Temporal lobe ☐
D. Occipital lobe ☐

**57.** In Figure 4.7, number 6 points to the _____.

A. Mandibular tuberosity ☐
B. TMJ ☐
C. Mandibular symphysis ☐
D. Medial condyle ☐

**58.** In Figure 4.7, number 4 points to the _____.

A. Carotid ☐
B. Cavernous sinus ☐
C. Carotid syphon ☐
D. Basilar artery ☐

**59.** In Figure 4.7, number 5 points to the _____.

A. Optic nerve ☐
B. Infundibulum ☐
C. Optic chiasm ☐
D. Carotid syphon ☐

**60.** In Figure 4.7, number 8 points to the _____.

A. Basilar arteriosus ☐
B. Carotid ☐
C. Anterior communicating artery ☐
D. Middle cerebral ☐

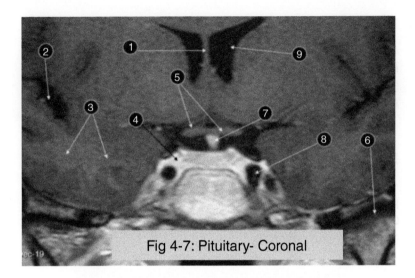

Fig 4-7: Pituitary- Coronal

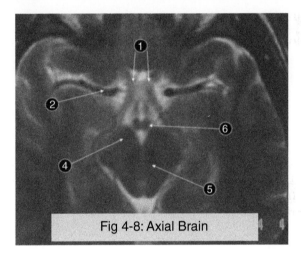

Fig 4-8: Axial Brain

**61.** In Figure 4.8, number 1 points to the _____.

| | |
|---|---|
| **A.** Optic chiasm | ☐ |
| **B.** Pituitary gland | ☐ |
| **C.** Optic retinaculum | ☐ |
| **D.** Choroid plexus | ☐ |

**62.** In Figure 4.8, number 2 points to the _____.

| | |
|---|---|
| **A.** Transverse ligament | ☐ |
| **B.** Medial rectus | ☐ |
| **C.** Middle cerebellar artery | ☐ |
| **D.** Basilar artery | ☐ |

**63.** In Figure 4.8, number 4 points to the _____.

> **A.** Cerebral peduncle ☐
> **B.** Cerebellar tonsil ☐
> **C.** Medulla ☐
> **D.** Corpus callosum ☐

**64.** In Figure 4.8, number 5 points to the _____.

> **A.** Medulla ☐
> **B.** Cerebellar tonsil ☐
> **C.** Pons ☐
> **D.** Forth ventricle ☐

**65.** In Figure 4.8, number 6 points to the _____.

> **A.** Endometrium ☐
> **B.** Mammary bodies ☐
> **C.** Mamillary glands ☐
> **D.** Cervix ☐

**66.** In Figure 4.9, number 1 points to the _____.

> **A.** Lateral ventricle ☐
> **B.** Forth ventricle ☐
> **C.** Third ventricle ☐
> **D.** Mid brain ☐

**67.** In Figure 4.9, number 2 points to the _____.

> **A.** Lateral ventricle ☐
> **B.** Forth ventricle ☐
> **C.** Ventricular septum ☐
> **D.** Mid brain ☐

**68.** In Figure 4.9, number 3 points to the _____.

> **A.** Temporal lobe ☐
> **B.** Frontal lobe ☐
> **C.** Occipital lobe ☐
> **D.** Mid brain ☐

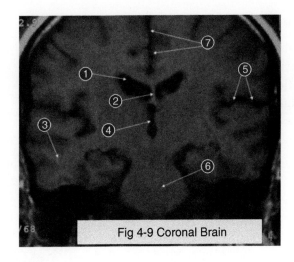

Fig 4-9 Coronal Brain

**69.** In Figure 4.9, number 4 points to the _____.

| | |
|---|---|
| **A.** Lateral ventricle | ☐ |
| **B.** Forth ventricle | ☐ |
| **C.** Third ventricle | ☐ |
| **D.** Mid brain | ☐ |

**70.** In Figure 4.9, number 5 points to the _____.

| | |
|---|---|
| **A.** Lateral ventricle | ☐ |
| **B.** Forth ventricle | ☐ |
| **C.** Sylvian fissure | ☐ |
| **D.** Mid brain | ☐ |

**71.** In Figure 4.9, number 6 points to the _____.

| | |
|---|---|
| **A.** Pons | ☐ |
| **B.** Forth ventricle | ☐ |
| **C.** Occipital lobe | ☐ |
| **D.** Mid brain | ☐ |

**72.** In Figure 4.9, number 7 points to the _____.

| | |
|---|---|
| **A.** Optic chiasm | ☐ |
| **B.** Ventricular septum | ☐ |
| **C.** Inter-Hemispheric fissure | ☐ |
| **D.** Choroid plexus | ☐ |

**73.** In Figure 4.10, number 1 points to the _____.

| | |
|---|---|
| **A.** Posterior cerebral | ☐ |
| **B.** Anterior cerebral artery | ☐ |
| **C.** Middle cerebellar artery | ☐ |
| **D.** Basilar artery | ☐ |

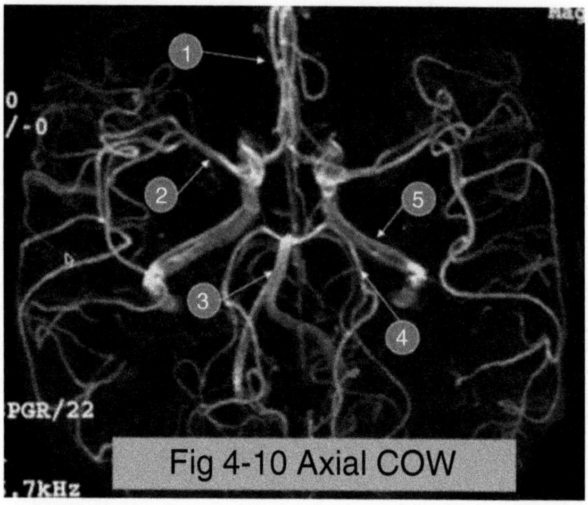

Fig 4-10 Axial COW

**74.** In Figure 4.10, number 2 points to the _____.

| | |
|---|---|
| **A.** Posterior cerebral | ☐ |
| **B.** Anterior cerebral artery | ☐ |
| **C.** Middle cerebellar artery | ☐ |
| **D.** Basilar artery | ☐ |

**75.** In Figure 4.10, number 3 points to the _____.

| | |
|---|---|
| **A.** Posterior cerebral | ☐ |
| **B.** Anterior cerebral artery | ☐ |
| **C.** Middle cerebellar artery | ☐ |
| **D.** Basilar artery | ☐ |

**76.** In Figure 4.10, number 4 points to the _____.

| | |
|---|---|
| **A.** Posterior cerebral | ☐ |
| **B.** Anterior cerebral artery | ☐ |
| **C.** Middle cerebellar artery | ☐ |
| **D.** Basilar artery | ☐ |

**77.** In Figure 4.10, number 5 points to the _____.

| | |
|---|---|
| **A.** Posterior cerebral | ☐ |
| **B.** Carotid artery | ☐ |
| **C.** Middle cerebellar artery | ☐ |
| **D.** Basilar artery | ☐ |

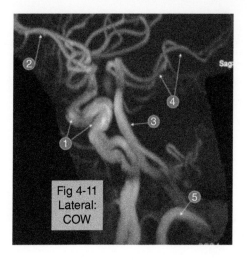

Fig 4-11
Lateral:
COW

**78.** In Figure 4.11, number 1 points to the _____.

| | |
|---|---|
| **A.** Posterior cerebral | ☐ |
| **B.** Anterior cerebral artery | ☐ |
| **C.** Carotid siphon | ☐ |
| **D.** Basilar artery | ☐ |

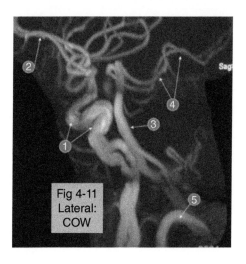

Fig 4-11
Lateral:
COW

**79.** In Figure 4.11, number 2 points to the _____.

> **A.** Posterior cerebral ☐
> **B.** Anterior cerebral artery ☐
> **C.** Middle cerebellar artery ☐
> **D.** Basilar artery ☐

**80.** In Figure 4.11, number 3 points to the _____.

> **A.** Posterior cerebral ☐
> **B.** Anterior cerebral artery ☐
> **C.** Middle cerebellar artery ☐
> **D.** Basilar artery ☐

**81.** In Figure 4.11, number 4 points to the _____.

> **A.** Posterior cerebral ☐
> **B.** Anterior cerebral artery ☐
> **C.** Middle cerebellar artery ☐
> **D.** Basilar artery ☐

**82.** In Figure 4.11, number 5 points to the _____.

> **A.** Vertebral artery ☐
> **B.** Anterior cerebral artery ☐
> **C.** Middle cerebellar artery ☐
> **D.** Carotid ☐

**83.** In Figure 4.12, number 1 points to the _____.

> **A.** Axis ☐
> **B.** Atlas ☐
> **C.** C-2 ☐
> **D.** A and C ☐

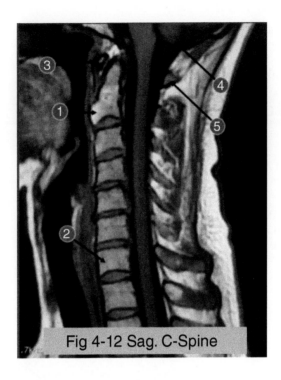

Fig 4-12 Sag. C-Spine

**84.** In Figure 4.12, number 2 points to the _____.

| | |
|---|---|
| **A.** C-6 | ☐ |
| **B.** C-7 | ☐ |
| **C.** T-1 | ☐ |
| **D.** C-9 | ☐ |

**85.** In Figure 4.12, number 3 points to the _____.

| | |
|---|---|
| **A.** C-1 | ☐ |
| **B.** Cerebellar tonsil | ☐ |
| **C.** Atlas | ☐ |
| **D.** A and C | ☐ |

**86.** In Figure 4.12, number 5 points to the _____.

| | |
|---|---|
| **A.** C-1 | ☐ |
| **B.** Cerebellar tonsil | ☐ |
| **C.** Atlas | ☐ |
| **D.** A and C | ☐ |

**87.** In Figure 4.12, number 4 points to the _____.

| | |
|---|---|
| **A.** C-1 | ☐ |
| **B.** Cerebellar tonsil | ☐ |
| **C.** Atlas | ☐ |
| **D.** A and C | ☐ |

**88.** Figure 4.12 demonstrates what kind of weighting?

| | |
|---|---|
| **A.** T2 | ☐ |
| **B.** T1 FLAIR | ☐ |
| **C.** Proton density | ☐ |
| **D.** Proton density fat sat | ☐ |

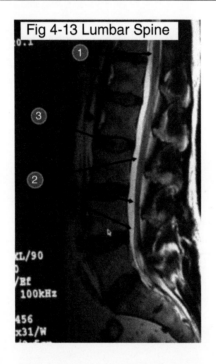

Fig 4-13 Lumbar Spine

**89.** In Figure 4.13, number 1 points to the _____.

| | |
|---|---|
| **A.** Filum terminally | ☐ |
| **B.** Cervical cord | ☐ |
| **C.** Conus medullaris | ☐ |
| **D.** Cauda equina | ☐ |

**90.** In Figure 4.13, number 2 points to the _____.

| | |
|---|---|
| **A.** Filum terminally | ☐ |
| **B.** Cervical cord | ☐ |
| **C.** Conus medullaris | ☐ |
| **D.** Cauda equina | ☐ |

**91.** In Figure 4.13, number 3 points to the _____.

| | |
|---|---|
| **A.** Filum terminally | ☐ |
| **B.** Intervertebral disc | ☐ |
| **C.** Conus medullaris | ☐ |
| **D.** Cauda equina | ☐ |

**92.** In Figure 4.13, demonstrates what weighting?

| | |
|---|---|
| **A.** Proton density | ☐ |
| **B.** T1 | ☐ |
| **C.** STIR | ☐ |
| **D.** T2 | ☐ |

**93.** In Figure 4.14, number 1 points to the _____.

| | |
|---|---|
| **A.** Supraspinatus tendon | ☐ |
| **B.** Teres minor | ☐ |
| **C.** Deltoid muscle | ☐ |
| **D.** Biceps muscle | ☐ |

**94.** In Figure 4.14, number 2 sits on the _____.

| | |
|---|---|
| **A.** Supraspinatus muscle | ☐ |
| **B.** Teres minor | ☐ |
| **C.** Deltoid muscle | ☐ |
| **D.** Biceps muscle | ☐ |

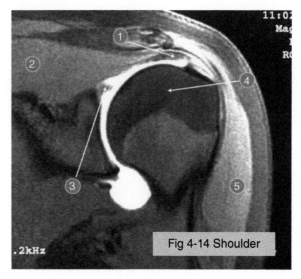

Fig 4-14 Shoulder

**95.** In Figure 4.14, number 3 points to the _____.

| | |
|---|---|
| **A.** Supraspinatus tendon | ☐ |
| **B.** Teres minor | ☐ |
| **C.** Deltoid muscle | ☐ |
| **D.** Labrum | ☐ |

**96.** In Figure 4.14, number 5 sits on the _____.

| | |
|---|---|
| **A.** Supraspinatus muscle | ☐ |
| **B.** Teres minor | ☐ |
| **C.** Deltoid muscle | ☐ |
| **D.** Biceps muscle | ☐ |

**97.** In Figure 4.14, number 4 points to the _____.

| | |
|---|---|
| **A.** A/C joint | ☐ |
| **B.** Humeral groove | ☐ |
| **C.** Humeral biceps | ☐ |
| **D.** Humeral head | ☐ |

**98.** Figure 4.14 demonstrates what kind of weighting?

| | |
|---|---|
| **A.** T2 | ☐ |
| **B.** T1 FLAIR | ☐ |
| **C.** Proton density | ☐ |
| **D.** T1 Fat sat | ☐ |

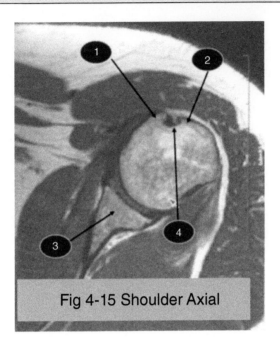

Fig 4-15 Shoulder Axial

**99.** In Figure 4.15, number 1 points to the _____.

| | |
|---|---|
| **A.** Bicipital groove | ☐ |
| **B.** Greater tubercle | ☐ |
| **C.** Lesser tubercle | ☐ |
| **D.** Radial head | ☐ |

**100.** In Figure 4.15, number 2 points to the _____.

| | |
|---|---|
| **A.** Bicipital groove | ☐ |
| **B.** Greater tubercle | ☐ |
| **C.** Lesser tubercle | ☐ |
| **D.** Radial head | ☐ |

**101.** In Figure 4.15, number 3 points to the _____.

|  |  |
|---|---|
| **A.** Scaphoid | ☐ |
| **B.** Scapular | ☐ |
| **C.** Scrupulous | ☐ |
| **D.** Sub scrupulous | ☐ |

**102.** In Figure 4.15, number 4 points to the _____.

|  |  |
|---|---|
| **A.** Biceps femora | ☐ |
| **B.** Deltoid insertion | ☐ |
| **C.** Subscapularis | ☐ |
| **D.** Bicipital groove | ☐ |

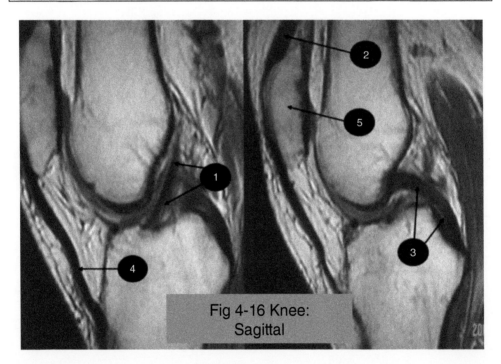

Fig 4-16 Knee: Sagittal

**103.** In Figure 4.16, number 1 points to the _____.

|  |  |
|---|---|
| **A.** Patella tendon | ☐ |
| **B.** ACL | ☐ |
| **C.** PCL | ☐ |
| **D.** Quadriceps tendon | ☐ |

**104.** In Figure 4.16, number 2 sits on the _____.

> **A.** Patella tendon ☐
> **B.** ACL ☐
> **C.** PCL ☐
> **D.** Quadriceps tendon ☐

**105.** In Figure 4.16, number 3 points to the _____.

> **A.** Patella tendon ☐
> **B.** ACL ☐
> **C.** PCL ☐
> **D.** Quadriceps tendon ☐

**106.** In Figure 4.16, number 5 points to the _____.

> **A.** Patella ☐
> **B.** ACL ☐
> **C.** PCL ☐
> **D.** Quadriceps tendon ☐

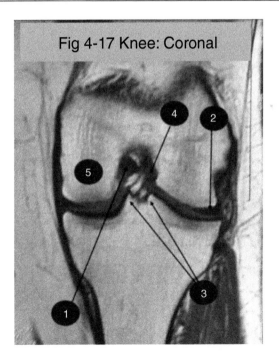

Fig 4-17 Knee: Coronal

**107.** In Figure 4.16, number 4 points to the _____.

> **A.** Patella tendon ☐
> **B.** ACL ☐
> **C.** PCL ☐
> **D.** Quadriceps tendon ☐

**108.** In Figure 4.17, number 1 points to the _____.

> **A.** ACL ☐
> **B.** PCL ☐
> **C.** Patellar lig. ☐
> **D.** Inter meniscal lig. ☐

**109.** In Figure 4.17, number 2 points to the _____.

> **A.** ACL ☐
> **B.** PCL ☐
> **C.** Meniscus ☐
> **D.** Inter meniscal lig. ☐

**110.** In Figure 4.17, number 3 points to the _____.

> **A.** Tibial plateau ☐
> **B.** Tibial eminences ☐
> **C.** Lesser trochanter ☐
> **D.** Radial head ☐

**111.** In Figure 4.17, number 4 points to the _____.

> **A.** ACL ☐
> **B.** PCL ☐
> **C.** Patellar lig. ☐
> **D.** Inter meniscal lig. ☐

**112.** In Figure 4.17, number 5 sits on the _____.

> **A.** Femoral condyle ☐
> **B.** Deltoid insertion ☐
> **C.** Femoral head ☐
> **D.** Bicipital groove ☐

**113.** Figure 4.17 demonstrates what weighting?

    **A.** STIR ☐
    **B.** T2 ☐
    **C.** FLAIR ☐
    **D.** T1 ☐

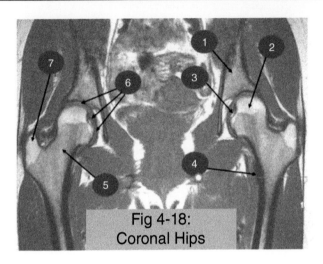

Fig 4-18:
Coronal Hips

**114.** In Figure 4.18, number 1 points to the _____.

    **A.** Iliac crest ☐
    **B.** Ilium ☐
    **C.** Ileum ☐
    **D.** Renal pelvis ☐

**115.** In Figure 4.18, number 2 points to the _____.

    **A.** Femoral plateau ☐
    **B.** Femoral head ☐
    **C.** Teres lig. ☐
    **D.** Greater trochanter ☐

**116.** In Figure 4.18, number 3 points to the _____.

    **A.** Femoral plateau ☐
    **B.** Femoral head ☐
    **C.** Fovea capitis ☐
    **D.** Lesser trochanter ☐

**117.** In Figure 4.18, number 4 points to the _____.

A. Fovea capitis ☐
B. Femoral head ☐
C. Greater trochanter ☐
D. Lesser trochanter ☐

**118.** In Figure 4.18, number 5 points to the _____.

A. Neck of the femur ☐
B. Body of the femur ☐
C. Os calcis ☐
D. Quadriceps tendon ☐

**119.** In Figure 4.18, number 6 points to the _____.

A. Fovea capitis ☐
B. Femoral head ☐
C. Greater trochanter ☐
D. Acetabulum ☐

**120.** In Figure 4.18, number 7 points to the _____.

A. Fovea capitis ☐
B. Femoral head ☐
C. Greater trochanter ☐
D. Acetabulum ☐

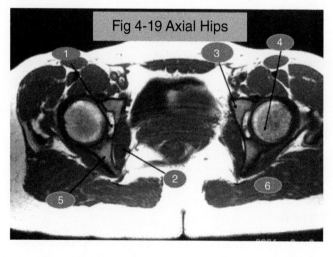

Fig 4-19 Axial Hips

**121.** In Figure 4.19, number 1 points to the _____.

| | |
|---|---|
| **A.** Acetabulum | ☐ |
| **B.** Femoral head | ☐ |
| **C.** Hamate | ☐ |
| **D.** Greater trochanter | ☐ |

**122.** In Figure 4.19, number 4 points to the _____.

| | |
|---|---|
| **A.** Acetabulum | ☐ |
| **B.** Femoral head | ☐ |
| **C.** Hamate | ☐ |
| **D.** Greater trochanter | ☐ |

**123.** In Figure 4.19, number 3 points to the _____.

| | |
|---|---|
| **A.** Ischium | ☐ |
| **B.** Ilium | ☐ |
| **C.** Pubis | ☐ |
| **D.** Bicipital groove | ☐ |

**124.** In Figure 4.19, number 6 sits on the _____?

| | |
|---|---|
| **A.** Obturator muscle | ☐ |
| **B.** Gluteus muscle | ☐ |
| **C.** Quadriceps | ☐ |
| **D.** Teres minor | ☐ |

**125.** In Figure 4.19, number 2 points to the _____.

| | |
|---|---|
| **A.** Obturator muscle | ☐ |
| **B.** Gluteus muscle | ☐ |
| **C.** Quadriceps | ☐ |
| **D.** Teres minor | ☐ |

**126.** In Figure 4.19, number 5 points to the _____.

| | |
|---|---|
| **A.** Ischium | ☐ |
| **B.** Ilium | ☐ |
| **C.** Pubis | ☐ |
| **D.** Bicipital groove | ☐ |

**127.** In Figure 4.20, number 3 points to the _____.

| | |
|---|---|
| **A.** Capitulum | ☐ |
| **B.** Trochlea | ☐ |
| **C.** Olecranon | ☐ |
| **D.** Coronoid | ☐ |

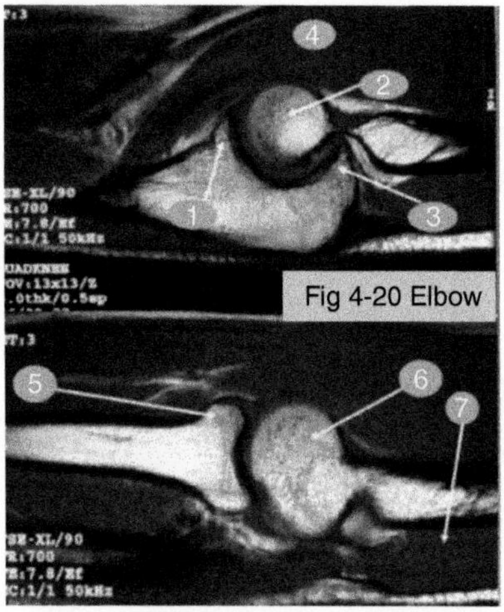

Fig 4-20 Elbow

**128.** In Figure 4.20, number 1 points to the _____.

| | |
|---|---|
| **A.** Capitulum | ☐ |
| **B.** Trochlea | ☐ |
| **C.** Olecranon | ☐ |
| **D.** Coronoid | ☐ |

**129.** In Figure 4.20, number 2 points to the _____.

| | |
|---|---|
| **A.** Capitulum | ☐ |
| **B.** Trochlea | ☐ |
| **C.** Olecranon | ☐ |
| **D.** Coronoid | ☐ |

**130.** In Figure 4.20, number 4 sits on the _____.

| | |
|---|---|
| **A.** Capitulum | ☐ |
| **B.** Triceps | ☐ |
| **C.** Olecranon | ☐ |
| **D.** Brachialis muscle | ☐ |

**131.** In Figure 4.20, number 7 points to the _____.

A. Capitulum ☐
B. Biceps muscle ☐
C. Greater trochanter ☐
D. Triceps muscle ☐

**132.** In Figure 4.20, number 5 points to the _____.

A. Capitulum ☐
B. Triceps muscle ☐
C. Greater multangular ☐
D. Radial head ☐

**133.** In Figure 4.20, number 6 points to the _____.

A. Capitulum ☐
B. Trochlea ☐
C. Olecranon ☐
D. Coronoid ☐

**134.** In Figure 4.20, number 8 points to the _____?

A. Olecranon ☐
B. Coronoid ☐
C. Radial head ☐
D. Capitulum ☐

**135.** In Figure 4.20, number 9 points to the _____.

A. Olecranon ☐
B. Coronoid ☐
C. Radial head ☐
D. Capitulum ☐

**136.** In Figure 4.21, number 1 points to the _____.

A. Lunate ☐
B. Capitate ☐
C. Hamate ☐
D. Scaphoid ☐

**137.** In Figure 4.21, number 2 points to the _____.

> **A.** Lunate ☐
> **B.** Capitate ☐
> **C.** Hamate ☐
> **D.** Trapezoid ☐

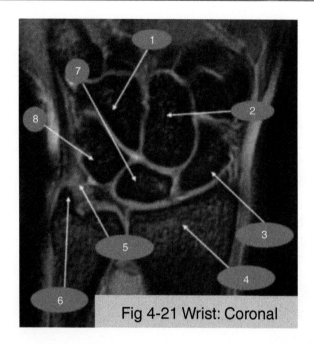

Fig 4-21 Wrist: Coronal

**138.** In Figure 4.21, number 3 points to the _____.

> **A.** Lunate ☐
> **B.** Capitate ☐
> **C.** Hamate ☐
> **D.** Scaphoid ☐

**139.** In Figure 4.21, number 4 points to the _____.

> **A.** Ulna ☐
> **B.** Radius ☐
> **C.** Capitate ☐
> **D.** Lunate ☐

**140.** In Figure 4.21, number 5 points to the _____.

> **A.** Trapezoid ☐
> **B.** Triquetrum ☐
> **C.** TFCC ☐
> **D.** Coronoid ☐

**141.** In Figure 4.21, number 6 points to the _____.

> **A.** Ulna styloid process ☐
> **B.** Ulna trunk ☐
> **C.** Olecranon ☐
> **D.** Biceps muscle ☐

**142.** In Figure 4.21, number 7 points to the _____.

> **A.** Trapezoid ☐
> **B.** Triquetrum ☐
> **C.** TFCC ☐
> **D.** Lunate ☐

**143.** In Figure 4.21, number 8 points to the _____.

> **A.** Trapezoid ☐
> **B.** Triquetrum ☐
> **C.** TFCC ☐
> **D.** Coronoid ☐

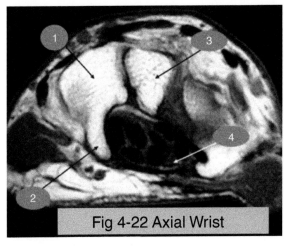

Fig 4-22 Axial Wrist

**144.** In Figure 4.22, number 1 points to the _____.

A. Lunate ☐
B. Capitate ☐
C. Hamate ☐
D. Scaphoid ☐

**145.** In Figure 4.22, number 2 points to the _____.

A. Lunate ☐
B. Capitate ☐
C. Hook of the hamate ☐
D. Scaphoid ☐

**146.** In Figure 4.22, number 3 points to the _____.

A. Lunate ☐
B. Capitate ☐
C. Hamate ☐
D. Scaphoid ☐

**147.** In Figure 4.22, number 4 points to the _____.

A. Peroneus longus ☐
B. Peroneus brevis ☐
C. Ulna nerve ☐
D. Median nerve ☐

**148.** In Figure 4.23, number 1 points to the _____.

A. Fibula ☐
B. Tibia ☐
C. Talus ☐
D. Calcaneus ☐

**149.** Figure 4.23 was scanned with a _____ TR and a _____ TE.

A. Short, Long ☐
B. Long, Long ☐
C. Long, Short ☐
D. Short, Short ☐

**150.** In Figure 4.23, number 2 points to the _____.

| | |
|---|---|
| **A.** Fibula | ☐ |
| **B.** Tibia | ☐ |
| **C.** Talus | ☐ |
| **D.** Calcaneus | ☐ |

**151.** In Figure 4.23, number 3 points to the _____.

| | |
|---|---|
| **A.** Fibula | ☐ |
| **B.** Cuboid | ☐ |
| **C.** Talus | ☐ |
| **D.** Navicular | ☐ |

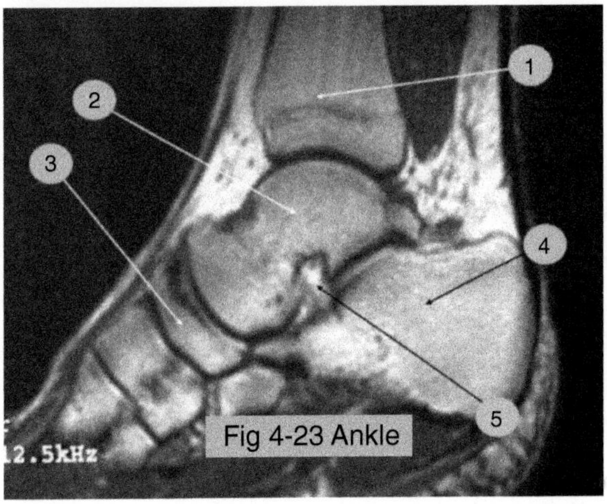

Fig 4-23 Ankle

**152.** In Figure 4.23, number 4 points to the _____.

| | |
|---|---|
| **A.** Fibula | ☐ |
| **B.** Tibia | ☐ |
| **C.** Talus | ☐ |
| **D.** Calcaneus | ☐ |

**153.** In Figure 4.23, number 5 points to the _____.

| | |
|---|---|
| **A.** Sinus tarsi | ☐ |
| **B.** Sub-Talar joint | ☐ |
| **C.** Posterior tibialis | ☐ |
| **D.** Calcaneal flexure | ☐ |

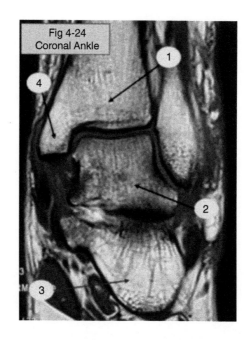

Fig 4-24
Coronal Ankle

**154.** In Figure 4.24, number 1 points to the _____.

| | |
|---|---|
| **A.** Fibula | ☐ |
| **B.** Tibia | ☐ |
| **C.** Talus | ☐ |
| **D.** Calcaneus | ☐ |

**155.** In Figure 4.24, number 2 points to the _____.

| | |
|---|---|
| **A.** Fibula | ☐ |
| **B.** Tibia | ☐ |
| **C.** Talus | ☐ |
| **D.** Calcaneus | ☐ |

**156.** In Figure 4.24, number 3 points to the _____.

| | |
|---|---|
| **A.** Fibula | ☐ |
| **B.** Tibia | ☐ |
| **C.** Talus | ☐ |
| **D.** Calcaneus | ☐ |

**157.** In Figure 4.24, number 4 points to the _____.

| | |
|---|---|
| **A.** Medial malleolus | ☐ |
| **B.** Tibia | ☐ |
| **C.** Talus | ☐ |
| **D.** Lateral malleolus | ☐ |

**158.** Figure 4.24 is an_____ image.

| | |
|---|---|
| **A.** Axial | ☐ |
| **B.** Coronal | ☐ |
| **C.** Sagittal | ☐ |

**159.** Figure 4.24 is a _____ weighted image.

| | |
|---|---|
| **A.** T1 | ☐ |
| **B.** T2 | ☐ |
| **C.** STIR | ☐ |
| **D.** FLAIR | ☐ |

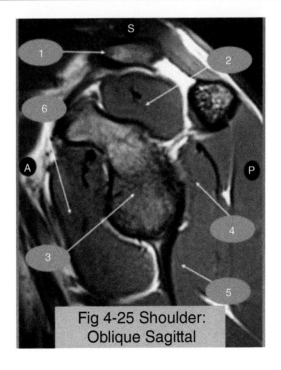

Fig 4-25 Shoulder:
Oblique Sagittal

**160.** In Figure 4.25, number 1 points to the _____.

| | |
|---|---|
| **A.** Humerus | ☐ |
| **B.** Clavicle | ☐ |
| **C.** Teres minor | ☐ |
| **D.** Subscapularis | ☐ |

**161.** In Figure 4.25, number 2 points to the _____.

| | |
|---|---|
| **A.** Supraspinatus mus. | ☐ |
| **B.** Infraspinatus mus. | ☐ |
| **C.** Teres minor | ☐ |
| **D.** Subscapularis | ☐ |

**162.** In Figure 4.25, number 3 points to the _____.

| | |
|---|---|
| **A.** Genus | ☐ |
| **B.** Glenoid | ☐ |
| **C.** Scapula | ☐ |
| **D.** Navicular | ☐ |

**163.** In Figure 4.25, number 4 points to the _____.

| | |
|---|---|
| **A.** Supraspinatus mus. | ☐ |
| **B.** Infraspinatus mus. | ☐ |
| **C.** Teres minor | ☐ |
| **D.** Subscapularis | ☐ |

**164.** In Figure 4.25, number 5 points to the _____.

| | |
|---|---|
| **A.** Supraspinatus mus. | ☐ |
| **B.** Infraspinatus mus. | ☐ |
| **C.** Teres minor | ☐ |
| **D.** Subscapularis | ☐ |

**165.** In Figure 4.25, number 6 points to the _____.

| | |
|---|---|
| **A.** Supraspinatus mus. | ☐ |
| **B.** Infraspinatus mus. | ☐ |
| **C.** Teres minor | ☐ |
| **D.** Subscapularis | ☐ |

**166.** In Figure 4.26, angling your slices to line number ________ would give you images as seen in Figure 4.25.

**A.** Number 1 ☐
**B.** Number 2 ☐

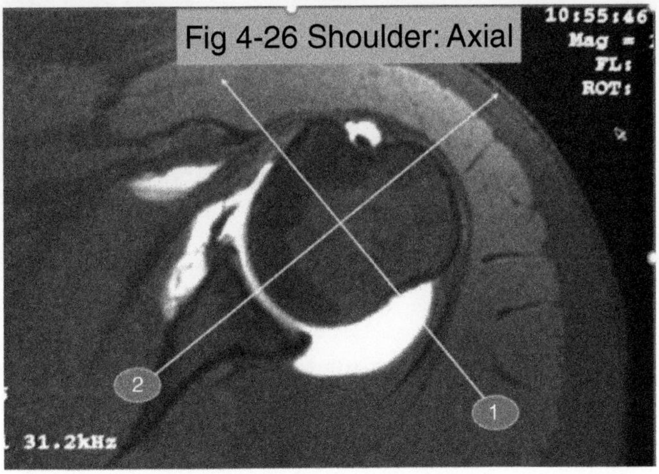
Fig 4-26 Shoulder: Axial
10:55:46
Mag =
FL:
ROT:
2
1
31.2kHz

**167.** Figure 4.26 is ________ weighted.

**A.** T2 ☐
**B.** STIR ☐
**C.** T1 Fat Sat ☐
**D.** Proton density ☐

**168.** Figure 4.26 is an example of an ________ exam.

**A.** Arteriogram ☐
**B.** Arthrogram ☐
**C.** Capsulogram ☐
**D.** Post IV contrast ☐

**169.** Imaging a patient for "Anosmia," you would concentrate on the ________.

**A.** First cranial nerve ☐
**B.** Mandible ☐
**C.** Fifth cranial nerve ☐
**D.** Soft tissue neck ☐

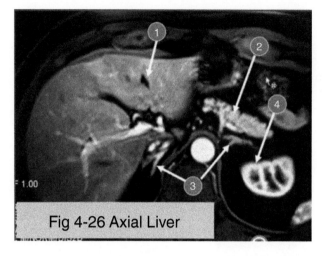

F 1.00

Fig 4-26 Axial Liver

**170.** In Figure 4.26, number 1 points to the _____.

| | |
|---|---|
| **A.** Ligament of tries | ☐ |
| **B.** Ligament of teres | ☐ |
| **C.** Teres minor | ☐ |
| **D.** Sub-Diaphragmatic fissure | ☐ |

**171.** In Figure 4.26, number 2 points to the _____.

| | |
|---|---|
| **A.** Adrenals | ☐ |
| **B.** Ligament of teres | ☐ |
| **C.** Pancreas | ☐ |
| **D.** Sub-Diaphragmatic fissure | ☐ |

**172.** In Figure 4.26, number 3 points to the _____.

| | |
|---|---|
| **A.** Pancreas | ☐ |
| **B.** Adrenals | ☐ |
| **C.** Left kidney | ☐ |
| **D.** Sub-Diaphragmatic fissure | ☐ |

**173.** In Figure 4.26, number 4 points to the _____.

| | |
|---|---|
| **A.** Pancreas | ☐ |
| **B.** Adrenals | ☐ |
| **C.** Left kidney | ☐ |
| **D.** Sub-Diaphragmatic fissure | ☐ |

**174.** On delayed contrast images, the renal pelvises may become as black because?

| | |
|---|---|
| **A.** Staghorn calculi | ☐ |
| **B.** Tumor | ☐ |
| **C.** Gadolinium reconstituting | ☐ |
| **D.** Renal failure | ☐ |

**175.** What are the three layers of meninges?

| | |
|---|---|
| **A.** Cortex, Medulla, and Pia | ☐ |
| **B.** Pia, Dura, and Arachnoid | ☐ |
| **C.** Pia, Dura, and Scleral | ☐ |
| **D.** Plea, Dura, and Subarachnoid | ☐ |

**176.** Of the 3 meninges, the inner most is _____ and the outer is the

_____.

| | |
|---|---|
| **A.** Dura, Pia | ☐ |
| **B.** Arachnoid, Dura | ☐ |
| **C.** Pia, Arachnoid | ☐ |
| **D.** Pia, Dura | ☐ |

**177.** A tangled collection of blood vessels is called a _____.

| | |
|---|---|
| **A.** Hematoma | ☐ |
| **B.** Hemangioma | ☐ |
| **C.** Hemorrhoid | ☐ |
| **D.** Hyoid | ☐ |

**178.** What nerve is affected by Bell's palsy?

| | |
|---|---|
| **A.** 5th | ☐ |
| **B.** 6th | ☐ |
| **C.** 7th | ☐ |
| **D.** 8th | ☐ |

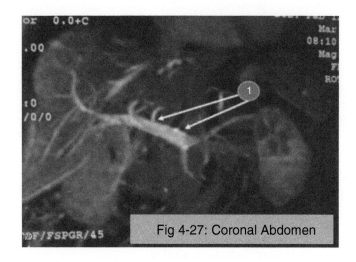

Fig 4-27: Coronal Abdomen

**179.** In Figure 4.27, arrows point to the _____?

| | |
|---|---|
| **A.** Teres ligament | ☐ |
| **B.** I.V.C | ☐ |
| **C.** Portal vein | ☐ |
| **D.** Celiac axis | ☐ |

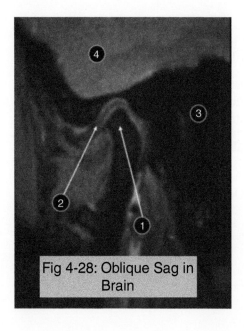

Fig 4-28: Oblique Sag in Brain

**180.** In Figure 4.28, number 1 points the _____.

|  |  |
|---|---|
| **A.** Inter condylar meniscus | ☐ |
| **B.** TMJ | ☐ |
| **C.** Lateral meniscus | ☐ |
| **D.** Splenium | ☐ |

**181.** In Figure 4.28, number 2 points the _____.

|  |  |
|---|---|
| **A.** Inter condylar meniscus | ☐ |
| **B.** TMJ | ☐ |
| **C.** Meniscus | ☐ |
| **D.** Splenium | ☐ |

**182.** In Figure 4.28, number 3 sits on the _____.

|  |  |
|---|---|
| **A.** Sphenoid sinus | ☐ |
| **B.** Mastoid air cells | ☐ |
| **C.** Temporal ridge | ☐ |
| **D.** Occipital lobe | ☐ |

**183.** In Figure 4.28, number 4 sits on the _____.

|  |  |
|---|---|
| **A.** Clivus | ☐ |
| **B.** Frontal lobe | ☐ |
| **C.** Temporal lobe | ☐ |
| **D.** Occipital lobe | ☐ |

**184.** Imaging for a suspected Arnold Chiari malformation should concentrate on the _____?

|  |  |
|---|---|
| **A.** Ventricles | ☐ |
| **B.** Frontal lobe | ☐ |
| **C.** Temporal lobe | ☐ |
| **D.** Cerebellum | ☐ |

**185.** An infectious process will cause an increased _____ count.

|  |  |
|---|---|
| **A.** RBC | ☐ |
| **B.** Platelets | ☐ |
| **C.** WBC | ☐ |
| **D.** Hemoglobin | ☐ |

**186.** A serum creatinine level is used to evaluate a patients' _____.

- **A.** Liver ☐
- **B.** Adrenals ☐
- **C.** Kidneys ☐
- **D.** Thyroid ☐

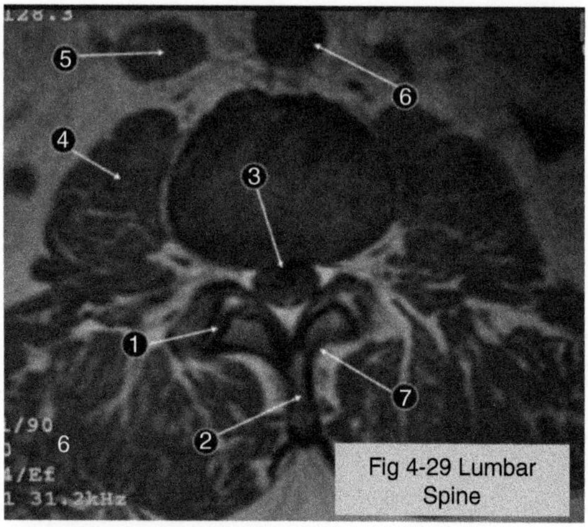

Fig 4-29 Lumbar Spine

**187.** In Figure 4.29, number 1 points to what structure?

- **A.** Facet joint ☐
- **B.** I.V.C ☐
- **C.** Lamina ☐
- **D.** Spinous process ☐

**188.** In Figure 4.29, number 2 points to the _____.

- **A.** Facet joint ☐
- **B.** I.V.C ☐
- **C.** Lamina ☐
- **D.** Spinous process ☐

**189.** In Figure 4.29, number 3 points to the _____.

- **A.** Aorta ☐
- **B.** IVC ☐
- **C.** Thecal sac ☐
- **D.** Lamina ☐

**190.** In Figure 4.29, number 4 points to the _____.

| | |
|---|---|
| **A.** Iliacus | ☐ |
| **B.** Ilio-Sacral muscle | ☐ |
| **C.** Quadratum lumborum | ☐ |
| **D.** Psoas muscle | ☐ |

**191.** In Figure 4.29, number 5 points to the _____.

| | |
|---|---|
| **A.** Aorta | ☐ |
| **B.** IVC | ☐ |
| **C.** Portal vein | ☐ |
| **D.** Azygous vein | ☐ |

**192.** In Figure 4.29, number 6 points to the _____.

| | |
|---|---|
| **A.** Aorta | ☐ |
| **B.** IVC | ☐ |
| **C.** Portal vein | ☐ |
| **D.** Azygous vein | ☐ |

**193.** In Figure 4.29, number 7 points to the _____.

| | |
|---|---|
| **A.** Vertebral body | ☐ |
| **B.** Spinous process | ☐ |
| **C.** Lamina | ☐ |
| **D.** Transverse process | ☐ |

**194.** What plane is useful for visualizing scoliosis in the spine?

| | |
|---|---|
| **A.** Axial | ☐ |
| **B.** Sagittal | ☐ |
| **C.** Oblique | ☐ |
| **D.** Coronal | ☐ |

**195.** Dyspnea is used to describe?

| | |
|---|---|
| **A.** Difficulty urinating | ☐ |
| **B.** Unable to swallow | ☐ |
| **C.** Difficulty breathing | ☐ |
| **D.** Unable to smell | ☐ |

**196.** Difficulty swallowing is known as?

> **A.** Dysphagia ☐
> **B.** Disnuclear ☐
> **C.** Dysarthria ☐
> **D.** Decarbonate ☐

**197.** Difficulty speaking is known as?

> **A.** Dystonia ☐
> **B.** Disassociation ☐
> **C.** Dysarthria ☐
> **D.** Disarticulate ☐

**198.** The vertebral arteries originate off of the _____ ?

> **A.** Aorta ☐
> **B.** Carotids ☐
> **C.** Subclavian's ☐
> **D.** Jugular's ☐

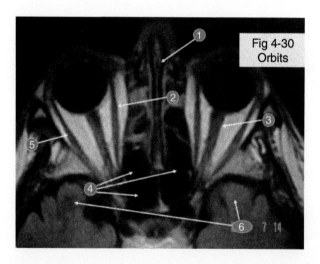

Fig 4-30
Orbits

**199.** In Figure 4.30, number 1 points to?

> **A.** Nasal bone ☐
> **B.** Nasal hyoid ☐
> **C.** Nasal septum ☐
> **D.** Ethmoid sinuses ☐

**200.** In Figure 4.30, number 2 points to?

   **A.** Nasal bone ☐
   **B.** Rectus muscle ☐
   **C.** Nasal septum ☐
   **D.** Medial rectus muscle ☐

**201.** In Figure 4.30, number 3 points to?

   **A.** Temporal lobes ☐
   **B.** Left globe ☐
   **C.** Optic nerve ☐
   **D.** Ethmoid sinuses ☐

**202.** In Figure 4.30, number 4 points to?

   **A.** Nasal bone ☐
   **B.** Nasal hyoid ☐
   **C.** Nasal septum ☐
   **D.** Ethmoid sinuses ☐

**203.** In Figure 4.30, number 5 points to?

   **A.** Temporal lobe ☐
   **B.** Nasal hyoid ☐
   **C.** Lateral rectus muscle ☐
   **D.** Ethmoid sinuses ☐

**204.** In Figure 4.30, number 6 points to?

   **A.** Temporal lobe ☐
   **B.** Nasal hyoid ☐
   **C.** Lateral rectus muscle ☐
   **D.** Ethmoid sinuses ☐

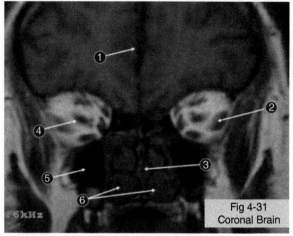

Fig 4-31
Coronal Brain

**205.** In Figure 4.31, number 1 points to the _____?

|   |   |
|---|---|
| **A.** Falx cerebri | ☐ |
| **B.** Inter-Hemispheric fissure | ☐ |
| **C.** Corpus callosum | ☐ |
| **D.** A and B | ☐ |

**206.** In Figure 4.31, number 2 points to the _____?

|   |   |
|---|---|
| **A.** Optic nerve | ☐ |
| **B.** Optic sheath | ☐ |
| **C.** Rectus muscle | ☐ |
| **D.** Lateral rectus muscle | ☐ |

**207.** In Figure 4.31, number 3 points to the _____?

|   |   |
|---|---|
| **A.** Turbinates | ☐ |
| **B.** Nasal bone | ☐ |
| **C.** Nasal septum | ☐ |
| **D.** Maxillary sinus | ☐ |

**208.** In Figure 4.31, number 4 points to the _____.

|   |   |
|---|---|
| **A.** Optic nerve | ☐ |
| **B.** Optic sheath | ☐ |
| **C.** Rectus muscle | ☐ |
| **D.** Lateral rectus muscle | ☐ |

**209.** In Figure 4.31, number 5 points to the _____.

| | |
|---|---|
| **A.** Optic nerve | ☐ |
| **B.** Sphenoid sinus | ☐ |
| **C.** Maxillary sinus | ☐ |
| **D.** Lateral rectus muscle | ☐ |

**210.** In Figure 4.31, number 6 points to the _____.

| | |
|---|---|
| **A.** Nasal turbinates | ☐ |
| **B.** Optic sheath | ☐ |
| **C.** Rectus muscle | ☐ |
| **D.** Lateral rectus muscle | ☐ |

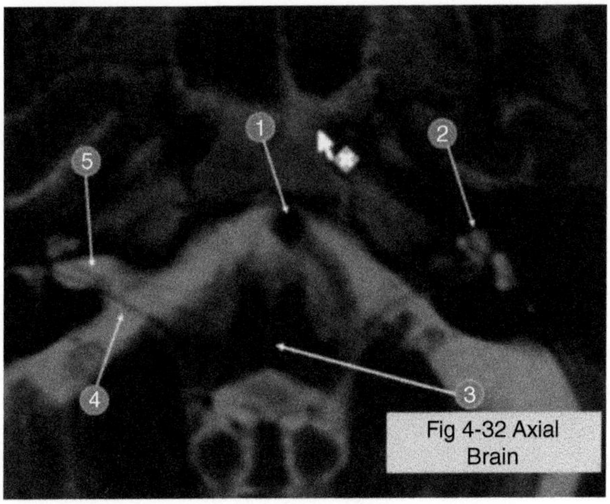

Fig 4-32 Axial Brain

**211.** In Figure 4.32, number 1 points to the _____.

| | |
|---|---|
| **A.** Carotid | ☐ |
| **B.** Middle cerebral | ☐ |
| **C.** Pupilar | ☐ |
| **D.** Basilar artery | ☐ |

**212.** In Figure 4.32, number 2 points to the _____.

| | |
|---|---|
| **A.** IAC | ☐ |
| **B.** Incus | ☐ |
| **C.** Semi-Circular canals | ☐ |
| **D.** Mastoid | ☐ |

**213.** In Figure 4.32, number 3 points to the _____.

| | |
|---|---|
| **A.** Carotid | ☐ |
| **B.** Brain stem | ☐ |
| **C.** Tonsils | ☐ |
| **D.** Basilar artery | ☐ |

**214.** Figure 4.32, number 4 points to the _____.

| | |
|---|---|
| **A.** Acoustic nerve | ☐ |
| **B.** Trigeminal nerve | ☐ |
| **C.** Facial nerve | ☐ |
| **D.** Optic nerve | ☐ |

**215.** Figure 4.32, number 5 points to the _____.

| | |
|---|---|
| **A.** Acoustic nerve | ☐ |
| **B.** Trigeminal nerve | ☐ |
| **C.** Facial nerve | ☐ |
| **D.** Optic nerve | ☐ |

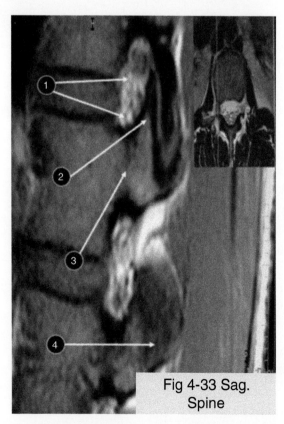

Fig 4-33 Sag.
Spine

**216.** In Figure 4.33, number 1 points to the _____.

| | |
|---|---|
| **A.** Foramen ovalle | ☐ |
| **B.** Neural foramen | ☐ |
| **C.** Facet joint | ☐ |
| **D.** Pedicle | ☐ |

**217.** In Figure 4.33, number 2 points to the _____.

| | |
|---|---|
| **A.** Foramen ovalle | ☐ |
| **B.** Neural foramen | ☐ |
| **C.** Facet joint | ☐ |
| **D.** Pedicle | ☐ |

**218.** In Figure 4.33, number 3 points to the _____.

| | |
|---|---|
| **A.** Foramen ovalle | ☐ |
| **B.** Neural foramen | ☐ |
| **C.** Facet joint | ☐ |
| **D.** Pedicle | ☐ |

**219.** In Figure 4.33, number 4 points to the _____.

| | |
|---|---|
| **A.** Foramen ovalle | ☐ |
| **B.** Spinous process | ☐ |
| **C.** Facet joint | ☐ |
| **D.** Pedicle | ☐ |

**220.** The 3 ossicles of the inner ear consist of the Stapes, _____ and _____.

| | |
|---|---|
| **A.** Malleus, Ictal | ☐ |
| **B.** Incus, Malleus | ☐ |
| **C.** Malleolar, Incus | ☐ |
| **D.** Tympani, Incus | ☐ |

**221.** The 5th cranial nerve is the _____.

| | |
|---|---|
| **A.** Trochlear | ☐ |
| **B.** Trigeminal | ☐ |
| **C.** Abducens | ☐ |
| **D.** Glossal-Pharyngeal | ☐ |

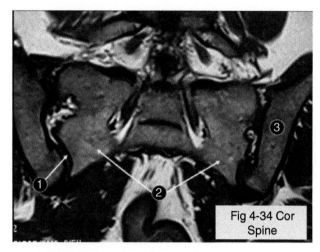

Fig 4-34 Cor Spine

**222.** In Figure 4.34, number 1 points to the _____.

| | |
|---|---|
| **A.** Sacrum | ☐ |
| **B.** Ala | ☐ |
| **C.** SI Joint | ☐ |
| **D.** Iliac wing | ☐ |

**223.** In Figure 4.34, number 2 points to the _____.

| | |
|---|---|
| **A.** Sacrum | ☐ |
| **B.** Ala | ☐ |
| **C.** SI joint | ☐ |
| **D.** Iliac wing | ☐ |

**224.** In Figure 4.34, number 3 points to the _____.

| | |
|---|---|
| **A.** Sacrum | ☐ |
| **B.** Ischium | ☐ |
| **C.** SI joint | ☐ |
| **D.** Iliac wing | ☐ |

**225.** Figure 4.34 is what weighting _____?

| | |
|---|---|
| **A.** PD | ☐ |
| **B.** STIR | ☐ |
| **C.** T2 Fat Sat | ☐ |
| **D.** T1 | ☐ |

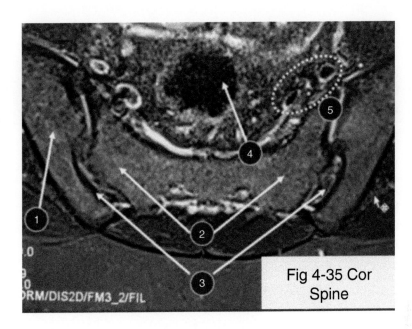

Fig 4-35 Cor Spine

ORM/DIS2D/FM3_2/FIL

**226.** In Figure 4.35, number 5 (circled) shows blood vessels which demonstrate what phenomenon _____.

| | |
|---|---|
| **A.** Pulsatile artifact | ☐ |
| **B.** High velocity signal loss | ☐ |
| **C.** Flow void | ☐ |
| **D.** B or C | ☐ |

**227.** In Figure 4.35, number 1 points to the _____.

| | |
|---|---|
| **A.** Sacrum | ☐ |
| **B.** Ischium | ☐ |
| **C.** SI joints | ☐ |
| **D.** Iliac wing | ☐ |

**228.** In Figure 4.35, number 2 points to the _____.

| | |
|---|---|
| **A.** Sacrum | ☐ |
| **B.** Ischium | ☐ |
| **C.** SI joints | ☐ |
| **D.** Iliac wing | ☐ |

**229.** In Figure 4.35, number 3 points to the _____.

| | |
|---|---|
| **A.** Sacrum | ☐ |
| **B.** Ischium | ☐ |
| **C.** SI joints | ☐ |
| **D.** Iliac wing | ☐ |

**230.** In Figure 4.35, number 4 points to the _____.

| | |
|---|---|
| **A.** Bladder | ☐ |
| **B.** Uterus | ☐ |
| **C.** Prostate | ☐ |
| **D.** Rectum | ☐ |

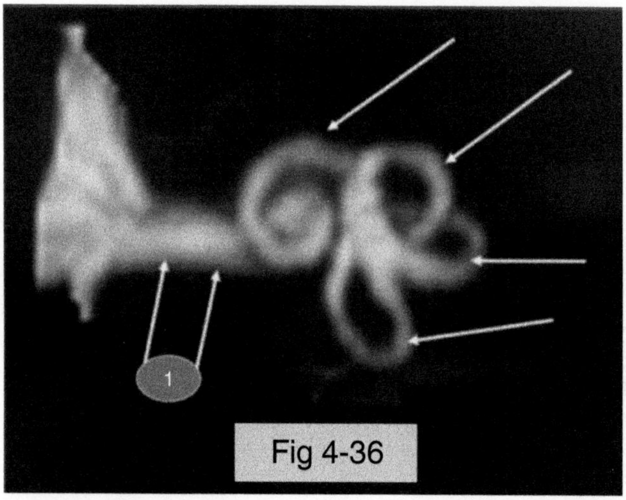

Fig 4-36

**231.** Figure 4.36 is a 3D T2 weighted image. Number 1 points to:

| | |
|---|---|
| **A.** Meckel's cave | ☐ |
| **B.** Internal auditory canal | ☐ |
| **C.** Foramen ovalle | ☐ |
| **D.** 3rd ventricle | ☐ |

**232.** In Figure 4.36, the arrows point to the _____?

| | |
|---|---|
| **A.** Semi-Circular canals | ☐ |
| **B.** Rami of the inner ears | ☐ |
| **C.** Ear worm | ☐ |
| **D.** Circular volvulus | ☐ |

**233.** Figure 4.36: The 2 cranial nerves that run through the region labeled number 1 are the:

| | |
|---|---|
| **A.** 3rd and 4th | ☐ |
| **B.** 5th and 6th | ☐ |
| **C.** 4th and 5th | ☐ |
| **D.** 7th and 8th | ☐ |

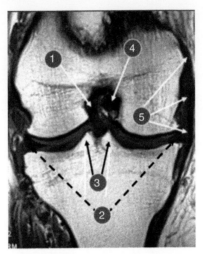

Fig 4-37 Cor. Knee

**234.** In Figure 4.37, number 1 points to the _____.

| | |
|---|---|
| **A.** PCL | ☐ |
| **B.** ACL | ☐ |
| **C.** Medial collateral | ☐ |
| **D.** Ilio-Tibial band | ☐ |

**235.** In Figure 4.37, number 2 points to the _____.

| | |
|---|---|
| **A.** Menisci | ☐ |
| **B.** Chondral bone | ☐ |
| **C.** Tibial plateaus | ☐ |
| **D.** Condyles | ☐ |

**236.** In Figure 4.37, number 3 points to the _____.

| | |
|---|---|
| **A.** Menisci | ☐ |
| **B.** Chondral bone | ☐ |
| **C.** Tibial eminences | ☐ |
| **D.** Condyles | ☐ |

**237.** In Figure 4.37, number 4 points to the _____.

A. PCL ☐
B. ACL ☐
C. Medial collateral ☐
D. Ilio-Tibial band ☐

**238.** In Figure 4.37, number 5 points to the _____.

A. PCL ☐
B. ACL ☐
C. Collateral ligament ☐
D. Ilio-Tibial band ☐

**239.** True or False: Ligaments attach bone to bone and Tendons connect muscles to bone.

**240.** When scanning a knee and the patient relates a twisting injury with pain and swelling afterward, attention should be paid to the_____.

A. PCL ☐
B. ACL ☐
C. Patella collaterals ☐
D. Ilio-Tibial band ☐

**241.** What structure in the brain is responsible for CSF production?

A. Foramen ovalle ☐
B. Neural foramen ☐
C. Forth ventricle ☐
D. Choroid plexus ☐

**242.** Meningitis is an indication for post gado study of the brain.

A. False ☐
B. True ☐

**243.** Brain exams with a trauma history should always include _____.

A. IV contrast ☐
B. FSE axials ☐
C. GRE axials ☐
D. MRA ☐

**244.** The vertebral arteries originate off of the _____.

A. Aorta ☐
B. Carotids ☐
C. Subclavian' s ☐
D. Jugular's ☐

**245.** Imaging of the adrenal glands commonly includes a _____ sequence.

A. T2 FLAIR ☐
B. In and Out of phase ☐
C. Coronal DWI ☐
D. Oral contrast ☐

**246.** What drug can be administered to slow a patient's peristalsis?

A. Glucose ☐
B. Glucagon ☐
C. Gluten ☐
D. Gluteal ☐

**247.** What structure connects the right and left hemispheres in the brain?

A. Pars Intra-Articularus ☐
B. Pituitary ☐
C. Cerebellum ☐
D. Corpus callosum ☐

**248.** The corpus callosum has three parts, the middle is called the?

| | |
|---|---|
| **A.** Pars Intra-Articularus | ☐ |
| **B.** Body | ☐ |
| **C.** Cerebellum | ☐ |
| **D.** Center corpus | ☐ |

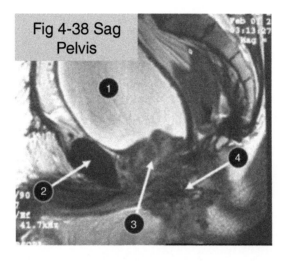

Fig 4-38 Sag Pelvis

**249.** In Figure 4.38, number 1 sits on the _____.

| | |
|---|---|
| **A.** Bladder | ☐ |
| **B.** Symphysis | ☐ |
| **C.** Rectum | ☐ |
| **D.** Prostate | ☐ |

**250.** In Figure 4.38, number 2 points to the _____.

| | |
|---|---|
| **A.** Bladder | ☐ |
| **B.** Symphysis | ☐ |
| **C.** Rectum | ☐ |
| **D.** Prostate | ☐ |

**251.** In Figure 4.38, number 3 points to the _____.

| | |
|---|---|
| **A.** Bladder | ☐ |
| **B.** Symphysis | ☐ |
| **C.** Rectum | ☐ |
| **D.** Prostate | ☐ |

**252.** In Figure 4.38, number 4 points to the _____.

|  |  |
|---|---|
| **A.** Bladder | ☐ |
| **B.** Symphysis | ☐ |
| **C.** Rectum | ☐ |
| **D.** Prostate | ☐ |

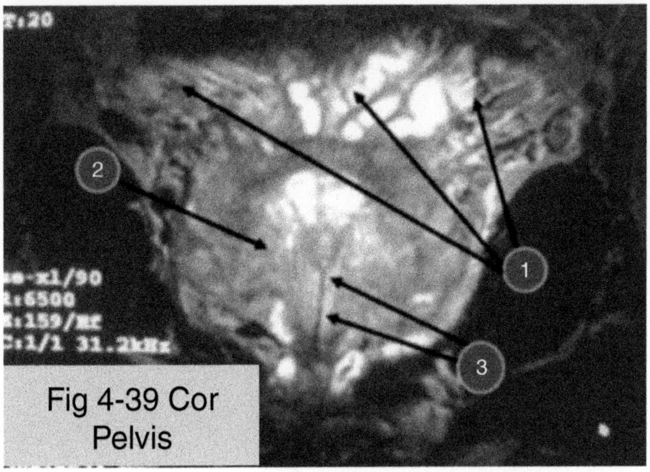

Fig 4-39 Cor Pelvis

**253.** In Figure 4.39, number 1 points to the _____.

|  |  |
|---|---|
| **A.** Symphysis | ☐ |
| **B.** Rectum | ☐ |
| **C.** Seminal vesicles | ☐ |
| **D.** Prostate | ☐ |

**254.** In Figure 4.39, number 2 points to the _____.

|  |  |
|---|---|
| **A.** Symphysis | ☐ |
| **B.** Rectum | ☐ |
| **C.** Seminal vesicles | ☐ |
| **D.** Prostate | ☐ |

**255.** In Figure 4.39, number 3 points to the _____.

|  |  |
|---|---|
| **A.** Urethra | ☐ |
| **B.** Blood vessel | ☐ |
| **C.** Seminal vesicles | ☐ |
| **D.** Prostate | ☐ |

**256.** What structure does number 4 sit on in Figure 4.40?

| | |
|---|---|
| **A.** Obturator muscle | ☐ |
| **B.** Symphysis | ☐ |
| **C.** Ureter | ☐ |
| **D.** Prostate | ☐ |

**257.** In Figure 4.40, number 2 sits in/on the _____.

| | |
|---|---|
| **A.** Rectum | ☐ |
| **B.** Bladder | ☐ |
| **C.** Sigmoid | ☐ |
| **D.** Uterus | ☐ |

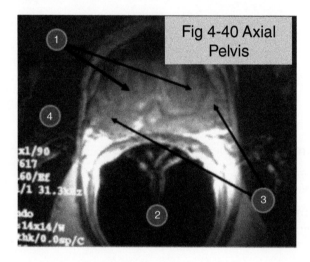

Fig 4-40 Axial Pelvis

**258.** In Figure 4.40, number 3 points to the _____?

| | |
|---|---|
| **A.** Peripheral zone | ☐ |
| **B.** Rectum | ☐ |
| **C.** Seminal vesicles | ☐ |
| **D.** Prostate | ☐ |

**259.** In Figure 4.40, number 1 points to the _____?

| | |
|---|---|
| **A.** Peripheral zone | ☐ |
| **B.** Rectum | ☐ |
| **C.** Seminal vesicles | ☐ |
| **D.** Prostate | ☐ |

**260.** Figure 4.40 was acquired with what kind of coil?

| | |
|---|---|
| **A.** No coil | ☐ |
| **B.** Surface | ☐ |
| **C.** Body | ☐ |
| **D.** Endo-Coil | ☐ |

**261.** Figures 4.39 and 4.40 is what weighting?

| | |
|---|---|
| **A.** T1 | ☐ |
| **B.** DWI | ☐ |
| **C.** T2 | ☐ |
| **D.** P.D. | ☐ |

**262.** Figure 4.40 was acquired in what plane?

| | |
|---|---|
| **A.** Axial | ☐ |
| **B.** Coronal | ☐ |
| **C.** Sagittal | ☐ |

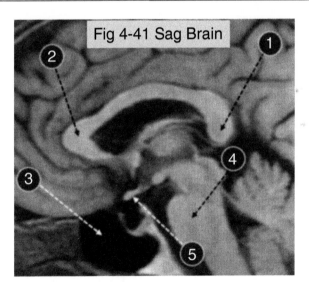

Fig 4-41 Sag Brain

**263.** In Figure 4.41, number 1 points to the _____.

| | |
|---|---|
| **A.** Genu | ☐ |
| **B.** Body | ☐ |
| **C.** Splenium | ☐ |
| **D.** Corpus | ☐ |

**264.** In Figure 4.41, number 2 points to the _____.

> **A.** Genu ☐
> **B.** Protonimus ☐
> **C.** Splenium ☐
> **D.** Corpus ☐

**265.** In Figure 4.41, number 3 points to the _____.

> **A.** Ethmoid sinus ☐
> **B.** Sphenoid sinus ☐
> **C.** Dural sinus ☐
> **D.** Mastoid sinus ☐

**266.** In Figure 4.41, number 4 points to the _____.

> **A.** Pons ☐
> **B.** Medulla oblongata ☐
> **C.** 4th ventricle ☐
> **D.** Optic nerve ☐

**267.** In Figure 4.41, number 5 points to the _____.

> **A.** Pituitary ☐
> **B.** Pituitary stalk ☐
> **C.** Infundibulum ☐
> **D.** Optic chiasm ☐

**268.** Gadolinium is best seen on a _____ weighted image?

> **A.** T2 Fat-Sat ☐
> **B.** STIR ☐
> **C.** PD Fat-Sat ☐
> **D.** T1 and T1 Fat-Sat ☐

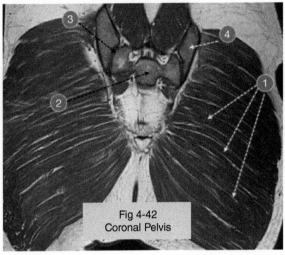

Fig 4-42
Coronal Pelvis

**269.** In Figure 4.42, number 3 points to the _____.

| | |
|---|---|
| **A.** S/I Jt. | ☐ |
| **B.** Iliac crest | ☐ |
| **C.** Ischium | ☐ |
| **D.** Coccyx | ☐ |

**270.** What structure does number 1 point to on Figure 4.42?

| | |
|---|---|
| **A.** Obturator muscle | ☐ |
| **B.** Gluteal muscle | ☐ |
| **C.** Quadriceps | ☐ |
| **D.** Psoas muscle | ☐ |

**271.** In Figure 4.42, number 2 points to the _____.

| | |
|---|---|
| **A.** Peri anal muscle | ☐ |
| **B.** Sacrum | ☐ |
| **C.** Seminal vesicles | ☐ |
| **D.** Uterus | ☐ |

**272.** In Figure 4.42, number 4 points to the _____?

| | |
|---|---|
| **A.** Iliac bone | ☐ |
| **B.** Rectum | ☐ |
| **C.** Iliac crest | ☐ |
| **D.** Quadriceps femoris | ☐ |

**273.** The brain stem is made up of the _____?

   **A.** Pons, Medulla, and Hind Brain ☐
   **B.** Mid Brain, Pons, and Medulla ☐
   **C.** Thalamus, Pons, and Hind Brain ☐
   **D.** Thalamus, Hind Brain, and Pons ☐

**274.** Figure 4.42 was acquired with what scan factors?

   **A.** Short TR/TE ☐
   **B.** Long TR/TE ☐
   **C.** Long TR/TE, Short TI ☐
   **D.** Short TR, Long TE ☐

**275.** How many pairs of gluteal muscles are there?

   **A.** 1 ☐
   **B.** 2 ☐
   **C.** 3 ☐
   **D.** 4 ☐

**276.** What enzyme is usually elevated in a patient with pancreatitis?

   **A.** BUN ☐
   **B.** Creatinine ☐
   **C.** Amylase ☐
   **D.** GFR ☐

**277.** There is multiple form of Hepatitis A, B, and C. They are caused by _____.

   **A.** Bacteria ☐
   **B.** Protozoa ☐
   **C.** Flagella ☐
   **D.** a Virus ☐

**278.** There are several factors used to calculate a patient's eGFR. They include the patient's creatinine, age, race, and _____.

   **A.** Sex ☐
   **B.** Weight ☐
   **C.** Body mass ☐
   **D.** BUN ☐

**279.** What is the standard dose of gadolinium for neurologic exams according to the package inserts?

    **A.** 1.0 cc/kg ☐
    **B.** 0.2 ml/kg ☐
    **C.** 0.1 mmol/kg ☐
    **D.** Either B or C. ☐

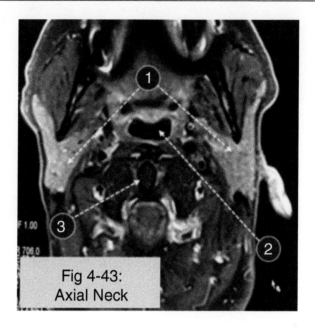

Fig 4-43:
Axial Neck

**280.** In Figure 4.43, number 1 points to the _____.

    **A.** Mastoids ☐
    **B.** Lingula ☐
    **C.** Parotids ☐
    **D.** Masticator ☐

**281.** In Figure 4.43, number 2 points to the _____.

    **A.** Nasion ☐
    **B.** Lingula ☐
    **C.** Oro-Pharynx ☐
    **D.** Masticator ☐

**282.** In Figure 4.43, number 3 points to the _____.

| | |
|---|---|
| **A.** Dens | ☐ |
| **B.** Tonsils | ☐ |
| **C.** C-1 | ☐ |
| **D.** Parotid | ☐ |

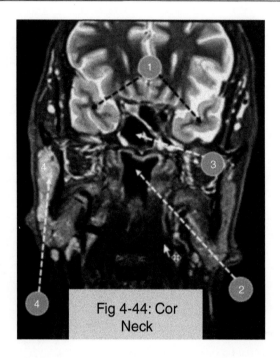

Fig 4-44: Cor Neck

**283.** What structure does number 1 point to on Figure 4.44?

| | |
|---|---|
| **A.** Frontal lobes | ☐ |
| **B.** Parietal lobes | ☐ |
| **C.** Temporal lobes | ☐ |
| **D.** Occipital lobes | ☐ |

**284.** In Figure 4.44, number 2 points to the _____.

| | |
|---|---|
| **A.** Nasal pharynx | ☐ |
| **B.** Sphenoid sinus | ☐ |
| **C.** Glottis | ☐ |
| **D.** Nasal septum | ☐ |

**285.** In Figure 4.42, number 3 points to the _____?

| | |
|---|---|
| **A.** Nasal pharynx | ☐ |
| **B.** Sphenoid sinus | ☐ |
| **C.** Glottis | ☐ |
| **D.** Nasal septum | ☐ |

**286.** In Figure 4.42, number 4 points to the _____?

| | |
|---|---|
| **A.** Nasal gland | ☐ |
| **B.** Sphenoid sinus | ☐ |
| **C.** Glottis | ☐ |
| **D.** Parotid gland | ☐ |

**287.** Figure 4.42 was acquired with what scan factors?

| | |
|---|---|
| **A.** Short TR and TE | ☐ |
| **B.** Long TR and TE | ☐ |
| **C.** Long TR and TE, Short TI | ☐ |
| **D.** Short TR, Long TE | ☐ |

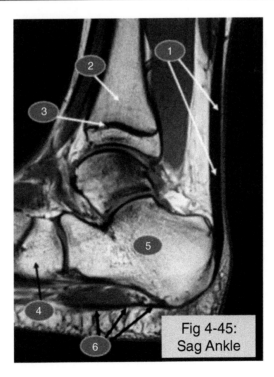

Fig 4-45:
Sag Ankle

**288.** In Figure 4.45, number 1 points to:

|   |   |
|---|---|
| **A.** Semi-Membranoid tendon | ☐ |
| **B.** Talus ligament | ☐ |
| **C.** Achilles tendon | ☐ |
| **D.** Saphenous tendon | ☐ |

**289.** In Figure 4.45, number 2 points to the _____.

|   |   |
|---|---|
| **A.** Tibia | ☐ |
| **B.** Fibula | ☐ |
| **C.** Talus | ☐ |
| **D.** Femur | ☐ |

**290.** In Figure 4.45, number 3 points to the _____.

|   |   |
|---|---|
| **A.** Distal tibia | ☐ |
| **B.** Tibial fracture | ☐ |
| **C.** Epiphyseal plate | ☐ |
| **D.** Femur | ☐ |

**291.** In Figure 4.45, number 4 points to the _____.

|   |   |
|---|---|
| **A.** Navicular | ☐ |
| **B.** Cuboid | ☐ |
| **C.** Calcaneus | ☐ |
| **D.** Hamate | ☐ |

**292.** In Figure 4.45, number 5 sits on the _____.

|   |   |
|---|---|
| **A.** Navicular | ☐ |
| **B.** Cuboid | ☐ |
| **C.** Calcaneus | ☐ |
| **D.** Hamate | ☐ |

**293.** In Figure 4.45, number 6 (red arrows) points to the _____.

|   |   |
|---|---|
| **A.** Achilles | ☐ |
| **B.** Plantar fascia | ☐ |
| **C.** Plantar aponeurosis | ☐ |
| **D.** B or C | ☐ |

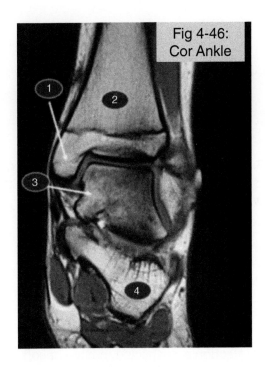

Fig 4-46: Cor Ankle

**294.** In Figure 4.46, number 1 points to the _____.

    **A.** Lateral condyle  ☐
    **B.** Lateral malleolus  ☐
    **C.** Medial condyle  ☐
    **D.** Medial malleolus  ☐

**295.** What structure does number 2 sit on Figure 4.46?

    **A.** Tibia  ☐
    **B.** Fibula  ☐
    **C.** Talus  ☐
    **D.** Femur  ☐

**296.** In Figure 4.46, number 3 points to the _____.

    **A.** Tibia  ☐
    **B.** Fibula  ☐
    **C.** Talus  ☐
    **D.** Femur  ☐

**297.** In Figure 4.46, number 4 sits on the _____?

| | |
|---|---|
| **A.** Tibia | ☐ |
| **B.** Calcaneus | ☐ |
| **C.** Talus | ☐ |
| **D.** Fibula | ☐ |

**298.** In Figure 4.46, number 3 does not look like the rest of the cortical bones. The lower signal on this T1 weighted image may suggest _____ in the marrow and depending on the patient's history this may suggest

_____.

| | |
|---|---|
| **A.** Edema, Fracture | ☐ |
| **B.** Edema, Infection | ☐ |
| **C.** Either A or B | ☐ |
| **D.** None of these | ☐ |

**299.** If edema or infection is suspected in bone or soft tissue, which of the weightings listed below will show it best?

| | |
|---|---|
| **A.** Short TR/TE | ☐ |
| **B.** Long TR, Short TE | ☐ |
| **C.** Long TR/TE, Short TI | ☐ |
| **D.** Short TR, Long TE | ☐ |

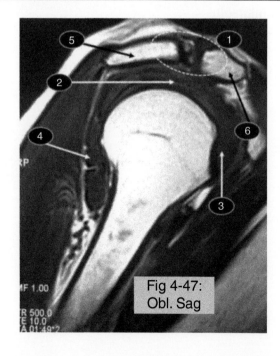

Fig 4-47:
Obl. Sag

**300.** In Figure 4.47, number 1 circled is the _____.

| | |
|---|---|
| **A.** S/C Jt. | ☐ |
| **B.** A/C Jt. | ☐ |
| **C.** MC/PH Jt. | ☐ |
| **D.** Glenohumeral Jt. | ☐ |

**301.** In Figure 4.47, number 2 points to the _____.

| | |
|---|---|
| **A.** Supraspinatus | ☐ |
| **B.** Infraspinatus | ☐ |
| **C.** Subscapularis | ☐ |
| **D.** Teres minor | ☐ |

**302.** In Figure 4.47, number 3 points to the _____.

| | |
|---|---|
| **A.** Supraspinatus | ☐ |
| **B.** Infraspinatus | ☐ |
| **C.** Subscapularis | ☐ |
| **D.** Teres minor | ☐ |

**303.** In Figure 4.47, number 4 points to the _____.

| | |
|---|---|
| **A.** Supraspinatus | ☐ |
| **B.** Infraspinatus | ☐ |
| **C.** Subscapularis | ☐ |
| **D.** Teres minor | ☐ |

**304.** In Figure 4.47, number 5 points to the _____.

| | |
|---|---|
| **A.** Acromion | ☐ |
| **B.** Coracoid | ☐ |
| **C.** Capitate | ☐ |
| **D.** Scapula | ☐ |

**305.** In Figure 4.47, number 6 points to the _____.

| | |
|---|---|
| **A.** Acromion | ☐ |
| **B.** Coracoid | ☐ |
| **C.** Capitate | ☐ |
| **D.** Clavicle | ☐ |

**306.** The salivary glands include the Parotid, Submandibular, and the
_____.

| | |
|---|---|
| **A.** Sub-oral | ☐ |
| **B.** Infra-Glottis | ☐ |
| **C.** Sublingual | ☐ |
| **D.** Minor parotid | ☐ |

**307.** In Figure 4.48, number 1 points to _____.

| | |
|---|---|
| **A.** Superior sagittal sinus | ☐ |
| **B.** Inferior sagittal sinus | ☐ |
| **C.** Sigmoid sinus | ☐ |
| **D.** Transverse sinus | ☐ |

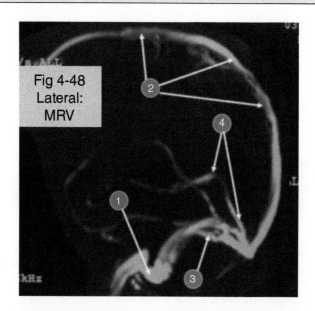

Fig 4-48
Lateral:
MRV

**308.** In Figure 4.48, number 3 points to the _____.

| | |
|---|---|
| **A.** Superior sagittal sinus | ☐ |
| **B.** Inferior sagittal sinus | ☐ |
| **C.** Sigmoid sinus | ☐ |
| **D.** Transverse sinus | ☐ |

**309.** In Figure 4.46, number 2 points to the _____.

| | |
|---|---|
| **A.** Superior sagittal sinus | ☐ |
| **B.** Inferior sagittal sinus | ☐ |
| **C.** Sigmoid sinus | ☐ |
| **D.** Transverse sinus | ☐ |

**310.** In Figure 4.48, number 4 points to the _____.

| | |
|---|---|
| **A.** Superior sagittal sinus | ☐ |
| **B.** Inferior sagittal sinus | ☐ |
| **C.** Sigmoid sinus | ☐ |
| **D.** Transverse sinus | ☐ |

**311.** All the above-mentioned sinuses eventually drain into what two vessels?

| | |
|---|---|
| **A.** Internal carotids | ☐ |
| **B.** Internal jugulars | ☐ |
| **C.** Outer cavernous | ☐ |
| **D.** Major azygous | ☐ |

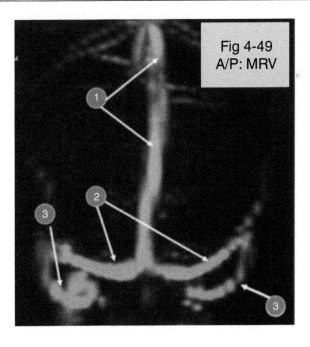

Fig 4-49
A/P: MRV

**312.** In Figure 4.49, number 1 points to the _____.

| | |
|---|---|
| **A.** Superior sagittal sinus | ☐ |
| **B.** Inferior sagittal sinus | ☐ |
| **C.** Sigmoid sinus | ☐ |
| **D.** Transverse sinus | ☐ |

**313.** In Figure 4.49, number 2 points to the _____.

| | |
|---|---|
| **A.** Superior sagittal sinus | ☐ |
| **B.** Inferior sagittal sinus | ☐ |
| **C.** Sigmoid sinus | ☐ |
| **D.** Transverse sinus | ☐ |

**314.** In Figure 4.49, number 3 points to the _____.

| | |
|---|---|
| **A.** Superior sagittal sinus | ☐ |
| **B.** Inferior sagittal sinus | ☐ |
| **C.** Sigmoid sinus | ☐ |
| **D.** Transverse sinus | ☐ |

**315.** A subclavian steal results from the occlusion or narrowing of what blood vessel?

| | |
|---|---|
| **A.** Basilar artery | ☐ |
| **B.** Subclavian artery | ☐ |
| **C.** Radial artery | ☐ |
| **D.** Vertebral artery | ☐ |

**316.** Which heart chamber has the thickest wall?

| | |
|---|---|
| **A.** Rt. ventricle | ☐ |
| **B.** Lt. atrium | ☐ |
| **C.** Lt. ventricle | ☐ |
| **D.** Rt. atrium | ☐ |

**317.** Which heart chamber is the most anterior?

| | |
|---|---|
| **A.** Rt. ventricle | ☐ |
| **B.** Lt. atrium | ☐ |
| **C.** Lt. ventricle | ☐ |
| **D.** Rt. atrium | ☐ |

**318.** What bone is located in the soft tissue of the neck just anterior to the larynx?

A. Infra-oral ☐
B. Infra-Glottis ☐
C. Hyoid ☐
D. Lingula ☐

**319.** The _____ valve sits between the Rt. ventricle and Rt. atrium.

A. Mitral ☐
B. Pulmonary ☐
C. Tricuspid ☐
D. Aortic ☐

**320.** The _____ valve sits between the Lt. ventricle and atrium.

A. Mitral ☐
B. Pulmonary ☐
C. Tricuspid ☐
D. Aortic ☐

**321.** When one structure is said to be "Medial" to another it means it is:

A. Above ☐
B. Below ☐
C. Closer to the mid-line ☐
D. Outside of ☐

**322.** Something that is said to be "Superior" to another structure is:

A. Above ☐
B. Below ☐
C. Closer to the middle ☐
D. Behind ☐

**323.** When something is "Anterior" to another structure it is:

A. In front of something ☐
B. Behind something ☐
C. Under another ☐
D. Inside another ☐

**324.** "Intra" means to be:

> **A.** Inside ☐
> **B.** Outside ☐
> **C.** Through ☐
> **D.** Around ☐

**325.** "Trans" means:

> **A.** Through or Across ☐
> **B.** Around ☐
> **C.** Mesial ☐
> **D.** Radial ☐

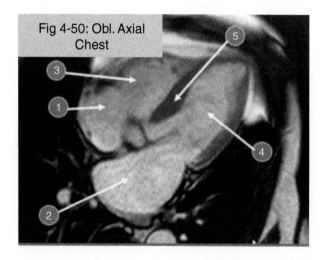

Fig 4-50: Obl. Axial Chest

**326.** In Figure 4.50, number 1 points to:

> **A.** Aorta ☐
> **B.** Subclavian artery ☐
> **C.** Left ventricle ☐
> **D.** Right auricle ☐

**327.** In Figure 4.50, number 2 points to:

> **A.** Pulmonary root ☐
> **B.** Subclavian vein ☐
> **C.** Left ventricle ☐
> **D.** Left atrium ☐

**328.** In Figure 4.50, number 3 points to:

| | |
|---|---|
| **A.** Aorta | ☐ |
| **B.** Right auricle | ☐ |
| **C.** Lt. ventricle | ☐ |
| **D.** Rt. ventricle | ☐ |

**329.** In Figure 4.50, number 4 points to:

| | |
|---|---|
| **A.** Left ventricle | ☐ |
| **B.** Pulmonary root | ☐ |
| **C.** Ventricular septum | ☐ |
| **D.** Atrial septum | ☐ |

**330.** In Figure 4.50, number 5 points to:

| | |
|---|---|
| **A.** Atrial septum | ☐ |
| **B.** Pulmonary root | ☐ |
| **C.** Ventricular septum | ☐ |
| **D.** Atrial septum | ☐ |

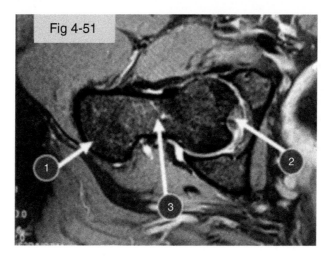

Fig 4-51

**331.** In Figure 4.51, number 1 points to:

| | |
|---|---|
| **A.** Acetabulum | ☐ |
| **B.** Greater trochanter | ☐ |
| **C.** Surgical neck | ☐ |
| **D.** Fovea capitus | ☐ |

**332.** In Figure 4.51, number 2 points to:

A. Fovea capitus ☐
B. Greater trochanter ☐
C. Lesser trochanter ☐
D. Femoral neck ☐

**333.** In Figure 4.51, number 3 points to:

A. Labrum ☐
B. Greater trochanter ☐
C. Lesser trochanter ☐
D. Femoral neck ☐

**334.** "Para" means:

A. Through or Across ☐
B. Around ☐
C. Mesial ☐
D. Radial ☐

**335.** In Figure 4.52, number 1 points to the _____.

A. Aorta ☐
B. Rt. pulmonary artery ☐
C. SVC ☐
D. Main pulmonary artery ☐

**336.** In Figure 4.52, number 2 points to the _____.

A. Ascending aorta ☐
B. Rt. pulmonary artery ☐
C. SVC ☐
D. Main pulmonary artery ☐

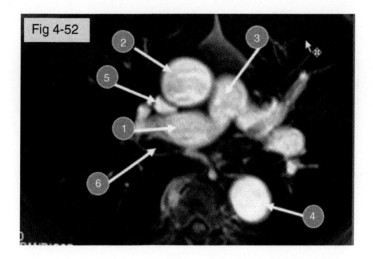

Fig 4-52

**337.** In Figure 4.52, number 3 points to the _____.

| | |
|---|---|
| **A.** Aorta | ☐ |
| **B.** Rt. pulmonary artery | ☐ |
| **C.** SVC | ☐ |
| **D.** Main pulmonary artery | ☐ |

**338.** In Figure 4.52, number 4 points to:

| | |
|---|---|
| **A.** Descending aorta | ☐ |
| **B.** Right auricle | ☐ |
| **C.** Lt. ventricle | ☐ |
| **D.** Rt. ventricle | ☐ |

**339.** In Figure 4.52, number 5 points to:

| | |
|---|---|
| **A.** IVC | ☐ |
| **B.** Rt. pulmonary vein | ☐ |
| **C.** Ascending aorta | ☐ |
| **D.** SVC | ☐ |

**340.** In Figure 4.52, number 6 points to:

| | |
|---|---|
| **A.** Atrial appendage | ☐ |
| **B.** RT. bronchus | ☐ |
| **C.** Azygous vein | ☐ |
| **D.** Esophagus | ☐ |

**341.** The _____ angle or "line" typically used for angling axial slices in the brain is?

| | |
|---|---|
| **A.** Orbital-Meatal line | ☐ |
| **B.** Inter-Trochanteric | ☐ |
| **C.** AC/PC line | ☐ |
| **D.** Submental-Vertical | ☐ |

**342.** When placing coronal slices in the brain in a patient with a seizure disorder, you should angle _____ to the _____.

| | |
|---|---|
| **A.** Parallel, Occipital Lobes | ☐ |
| **B.** Parallel, Temporal Lobes | ☐ |
| **C.** Perpendicular, Temporal Lobes | ☐ |
| **D.** Perpendicular, Parietal | ☐ |

**343.** There are normal curves in the human spine. The cervical and lumbar have _____ while the thoracic has a _____.

| | |
|---|---|
| **A.** Complex, Concave | ☐ |
| **B.** Concave, Complex | ☐ |
| **C.** Lordotic, Kyphotic | ☐ |
| **D.** Kyphotic, Lordotic | ☐ |

**344.** Buccal refers to the_____.

| | |
|---|---|
| **A.** Tonsils | ☐ |
| **B.** Mouth and or Cheeks | ☐ |
| **C.** Teeth | ☐ |
| **D.** Esophagus | ☐ |

**345.** Peri-Ocular refers to _____.

| | |
|---|---|
| **A.** Near or around the eye | ☐ |
| **B.** Around the nasion | ☐ |
| **C.** Near or around the occiput | ☐ |
| **D.** Around or near the occipital lobe | ☐ |

**346.** The auricle or auricular refers to the _____.

> **A.** Mouth ☐
> **B.** Ear ☐
> **C.** Heart ☐
> **D.** B and C ☐

**347.** The cauda equina is seen best in the coronal and sagittal plane in the _____.

> **A.** Cervical ☐
> **B.** Lumbar ☐
> **C.** Thoracic ☐
> **D.** Either B or C ☐

**348.** Due to lack of myelination in the pediatric population, Gray/White matter differentiation in the brain can best be seen with _____.

> **A.** T1 Weighting ☐
> **B.** STIR ☐
> **C.** Gradient echo ☐
> **D.** Post IV contrast ☐

**349.** In a perfusion study of the brain, normal tissue will _____ in signal intensity while less perfused tissue will _____ in signal intensity.

> **A.** Increase, decrease ☐
> **B.** Decrease, not change ☐
> **C.** Decrease, not change ☐
> **D.** Not change, decrease ☐

**350.** Positioning for a shoulder exam, the arm usually has a/an_____ rotation of the arm.

> **A.** Internal ☐
> **B.** External ☐
> **C.** Neutral ☐

**351.** "Supra Renal Gland" refers to the _____.

A. Adnexa ☐
B. Areola ☐
C. Adrenal ☐
D. Arm pit ☐

**352.** Tic douloureux is a painful condition affecting the _____.

A. Eyes ☐
B. Ears ☐
C. Face ☐
D. Scalp ☐

**353.** Douloureux affects/originates from the _____ cranial nerve.

A. 3rd ☐
B. 4th ☐
C. 5th ☐
D. 6th ☐

**354.** The 5th cranial nerve is the _____.

A. Trochlea ☐
B. Trigeminal ☐
C. Abducens ☐
D. Facial ☐

**355.** Evaluating a patient with a complaint tinnitus, the _____ should be imaged.

A. Pituitary ☐
B. Orbits ☐
C. IAC's ☐
D. Temporal lobes ☐

**356.** When imaging a patient with asymmetric sensorineural hearing loss (ASNHL), the _____ should be imaged.

A. Pituitary ☐
B. Orbits ☐
C. IAC's ☐
D. Temporal lobes ☐

# Image Artifacts

This portion of will cover artifacts commonly seen in MRI. Please go to Chapter 12 in *MRI Physics: Tech to Tech to Tech Explanations* for additional information and more detailed explanations.

In this series of questions, you will be asked to identify the artifact (s), their cause, how to fix and how to avoid/minimize the artifact.

## Remember, Choose the Answer Most Correct

**357.** What artifact is seen in Figure 4.53?

| | |
|---|---|
| **A.** Wrap | ☐ |
| **B.** Truncation | ☐ |
| **C.** Under-sampling | ☐ |
| **D.** Motion | ☐ |

**358.** What is the best way to fix or minimize the artifact seen in Figure 4.53?

| | |
|---|---|
| **A.** Immobilization | ☐ |
| **B.** Increase FOV | ☐ |
| **C.** Shorten the TE | ☐ |
| **D.** Increase the TR | ☐ |

**359.** Phase direction in Figure 4.53 is in the_____?

| | |
|---|---|
| **A.** Axial | ☐ |
| **B.** A/P | ☐ |
| **C.** S/I | ☐ |
| **D.** RT./LT. | ☐ |

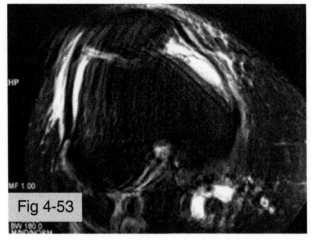

Fig 4-53

**360.** Shortening the scan time, for Figure 4.53 can affect the _____.

|   |   |
|---|---|
| **A.** SNR | ☐ |
| **B.** Resolution | ☐ |
| **C.** Contrast | ☐ |
| **D.** All the above | ☐ |

**361.** Figure 4.54 shows what artifact?

|   |   |
|---|---|
| **A.** Motion | ☐ |
| **B.** Pulsatile | ☐ |
| **C.** Aliasing | ☐ |
| **D.** Gibbs | ☐ |

**362.** What scan factor might best reduce or eliminate the artifact seen in Figure 4.54?

|   |   |
|---|---|
| **A.** Sat pulses | ☐ |
| **B.** Flow comp/GMR | ☐ |
| **C.** Anti-Aliasing | ☐ |
| **D.** A and B | ☐ |

**363.** Figure 4.54, In this image the artifact could be caused by?

> **A.** A long Echo train ☐
> **B.** A long TR/TE/TI ☐
> **C.** IV contrast ☐
> **D.** B and C ☐

**364.** In Figure 4.54, swapping phase and frequency will_____.

> **A.** Eliminate the artifact ☐
> **B.** Put it in a different direction ☐
> **C.** Cause the artifact to get worse ☐
> **D.** Increase patient's SAR ☐

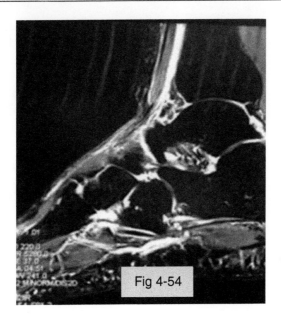

Fig 4-54

**365.** What artifact is seen in Figure 4.55?

> **A.** Wrap ☐
> **B.** RF leak ☐
> **C.** Truncation ☐
> **D.** Motion ☐

**366.** What is the best way to fix or minimize the artifact seen in Figure 4.55?

| | |
|---|---|
| **A.** Repeat scan | ☐ |
| **B.** Close the scan room door | ☐ |
| **C.** Check for bad light bulb | ☐ |
| **D.** All the above | ☐ |

**367.** Swapping phase and frequency in Figure 4.55 will relocate this artifact.

| | |
|---|---|
| **A.** False | ☐ |
| **B.** True | ☐ |

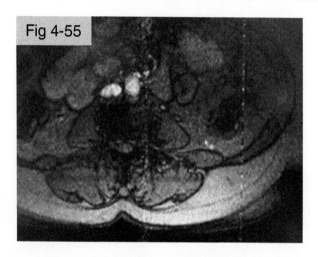

Fig 4-55

**368.** Another name for the artifact in Figure 4.55 is _____.

| | |
|---|---|
| **A.** White pixel artifact | ☐ |
| **B.** Zipper | ☐ |
| **C.** Mourier | ☐ |
| **D.** A or B | ☐ |

**369.** Figure 4.56 shows what artifact?

| | |
|---|---|
| **A.** Motion | ☐ |
| **B.** Pulsatile | ☐ |
| **C.** Aliasing | ☐ |
| **D.** Gibbs | ☐ |

**370.** What scan factor might best reduce or eliminate the artifact seen in Figure 4.56?

|  |  |
|---|---|
| **A.** A superior sat pulse | ☐ |
| **B.** Increase phase matrix | ☐ |
| **C.** Increase the FOV | ☐ |
| **D.** A and B | ☐ |

**371.** Swapping phase and frequency on Figure 4.56 will put the artifact in the _____?

|  |  |
|---|---|
| **A.** S/I | ☐ |
| **B.** RT/LT | ☐ |
| **C.** A/P | ☐ |
| **D.** Slice select | ☐ |

**372.** In Figure 4.56, if resolution is prime concern for I.Q. and anti-aliasing is not available, then another consideration would be _____.

|  |  |
|---|---|
| **A.** Saturation pulses | ☐ |
| **B.** Increase phase and frequency matrix | ☐ |
| **C.** Decrease the FOV | ☐ |
| **D.** Increase nex/Acquisitions | ☐ |

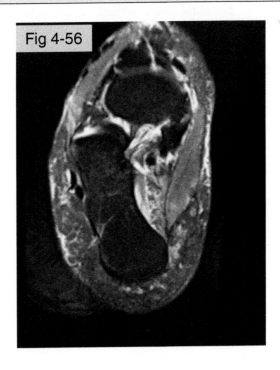

Fig 4-56

**373.** In Figure 4.56, the artifact is seen because the _____ was not met or satisfied.

    **A.** Faraday's law   ☐

    **B.** Nyquist theorem   ☐

    **C.** Larmor equation   ☐

    **D.** Basic scan time formula   ☐

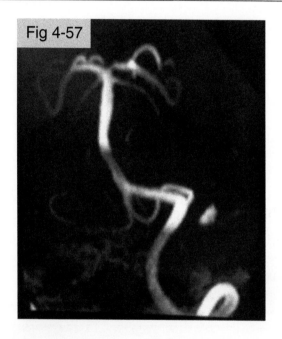

Fig 4-57

**374.** What artifact/phenomenon is seen in Figure 4.57?

    **A.** Wrap   ☐

    **B.** RF leak   ☐

    **C.** In-Plane saturation   ☐

    **D.** Motion   ☐

**375.** What is the best way to improve I.Q. in Figure 4.57?

    **A.** Give IV contrast   ☐

    **B.** Scan parallel to blood flow   ☐

    **C.** Scan perpendicular to flow   ☐

    **D.** Remove all sat. pulses   ☐

**376.** Another option to improve I.Q. in Figure 4.57 is to_____.

|  |  |
|---|---|
| **A.** Pulse gate | ☐ |
| **B.** Decrease the flip angle | ☐ |
| **C.** Use ramp pulse | ☐ |
| **D.** Inferior saturation pulse | ☐ |

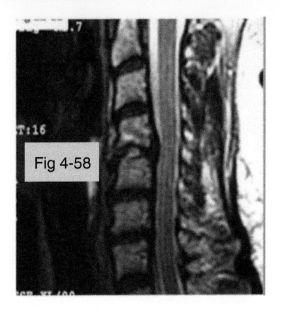

Fig 4-58

**377.** The name for the artifact in Figure 4.58 is _____.

|  |  |
|---|---|
| **A.** Motion | ☐ |
| **B.** Gibbs/truncation | ☐ |
| **C.** Mourier | ☐ |
| **D.** Zebra | ☐ |

**378.** The artifact seen in Figure 4.58 comes from _____?

|  |  |
|---|---|
| **A.** Scan matrix | ☐ |
| **B.** Short TR/TE | ☐ |
| **C.** Transmitter band width | ☐ |
| **D.** F.O.V. | ☐ |

**379.** To reduce the artifact in Figure 4.58, you could?

A. Increase scan matrix ☐
B. Lengthen the TR/TE ☐
C. Narrow the transmitter B/W ☐
D. Increase the F.O.V ☐

**380.** In Figure 4.58, the artifact may also be caused by _____.

A. Phase/Frequency direction ☐
B. Saturation pulses ☐
C. Isotropic pixels ☐
D. Anisotropic pixels ☐

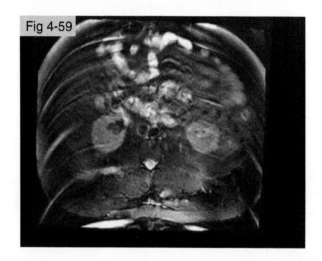

Fig 4-59

**381.** What two artifacts are seen in Figure 4.59?

A. Wrap and Aliasing ☐
B. RF leak and Motion ☐
C. Wrap and Motion ☐
D. Gibbs and Wrap ☐

**382.** In Figure 4.59, how can wrap artifact be corrected?

A. Give IV contrast ☐
B. Increase the FOV ☐
C. Free breath the patient ☐
D. Remove all sat. pulses ☐

**383.** An option to improve I.Q. in Figure 4.59 is _____.

| | |
|---|---|
| **A.** Pulse gate | ☐ |
| **B.** Respiratory triggering | ☐ |
| **C.** Put patient prone | ☐ |
| **D.** Inferior saturation pulse | ☐ |

**384.** The name for the artifact in Figure 4.60 is _____.

| | |
|---|---|
| **A.** Cross talk | ☐ |
| **B.** Gibbs/truncation | ☐ |
| **C.** Motion | ☐ |
| **D.** RF artifact | ☐ |

**385.** The artifact seen in Figure 4.60 comes from _____?

| | |
|---|---|
| **A.** Slices crossing posteriorly | ☐ |
| **B.** Long TR/TE | ☐ |
| **C.** Bad coil selection | ☐ |
| **D.** Slices crossing anteriorly | ☐ |

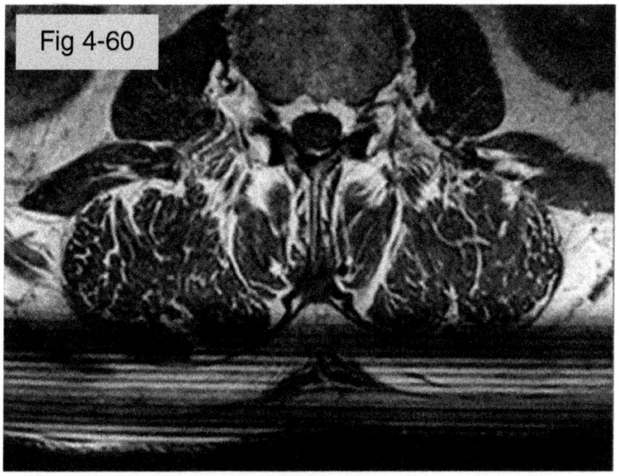

Fig 4-60

**386.** To reduce or eliminate the artifact in Figure 4.60?

| | |
|---|---|
| **A.** Change the angle of slices | ☐ |
| **B.** Shorten the TR/TE | ☐ |
| **C.** Better coil selection | ☐ |
| **D.** Increase slice thickness | ☐ |

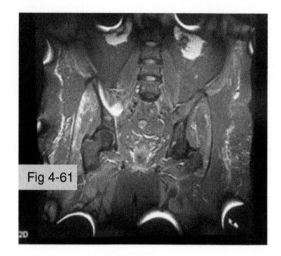

Fig 4-61

**387.** In Figure 4.61, the artifact is called.

A. Wrap ☐
B. Cross excitation ☐
C. Gradient warp ☐
D. Susceptibility ☐

**388.** In Figure 4.61, if you _____ the _____, you can decrease the artifact.

A. Increase, Slice thickness ☐
B. Decrease, Scan matrix ☐
C. Decrease, FOV ☐
D. Increase, FOV ☐

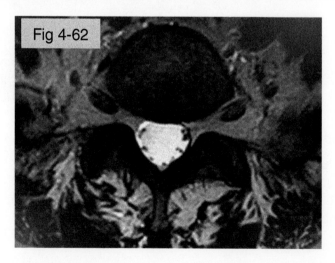

Fig 4-62

**389.** What artifact is seen in Figure 4.62?

> **A.** Aliasing ☐
> **B.** Over-Sampling ☐
> **C.** Under-Sampling ☐
> **D.** Chemical shift ☐

**390.** In Figure 4.62, how can the artifact be lessened?

> **A.** Narrow the rec. bandwidth ☐
> **B.** Increase the FOV ☐
> **C.** Narrow the transmitted B/W ☐
> **D.** Widen the rec. B/W ☐

**391.** Another option to lessen the artifact in Figure 4.62 is?

> **A.** Swap Phase/Freq. ☐
> **B.** Increase the ETL ☐
> **C.** Use Fat-Sat ☐
> **D.** Flow compensation ☐

**392.** The artifact seen in Figure 4.62 is worse at which field strength?

> **A.** 1.0T ☐
> **B.** 1.5T ☐
> **C.** 3T ☐
> **D.** .5T ☐

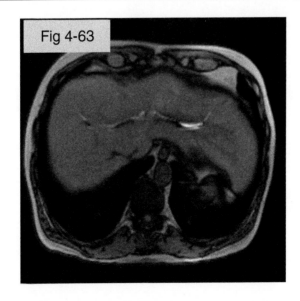

Fig 4-63

**393.** The artifact seen in Figure 4.63 comes from scan option_____?

| | |
|---|---|
| **A.** Half Fourier | ☐ |
| **B.** Re-Ordered k-Space | ☐ |
| **C.** Parallel imaging | ☐ |
| **D.** Motion | ☐ |

**394.** To eliminate the artifact in Figure 4.63, you could?

| | |
|---|---|
| **A.** Decrease the FOV | ☐ |
| **B.** Increase the FOV | ☐ |
| **C.** Decrease phase or rectangular FOV | ☐ |
| **D.** B and or C | ☐ |

**395.** The artifact seen in Figure 4.63 is _____.

| | |
|---|---|
| **A.** Wrap | ☐ |
| **B.** Cross excitation | ☐ |
| **C.** Gradient warp | ☐ |
| **D.** Susceptibility | ☐ |

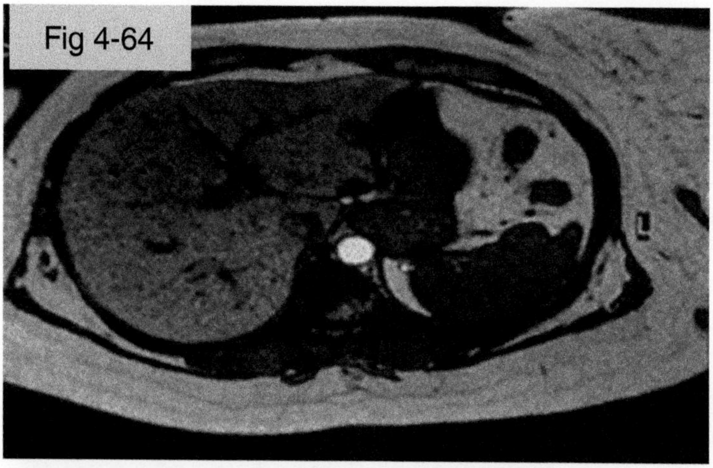

Fig 4-64

**396.** In this pre-contrast T1 weighted GRE, Figure 4.64, the aorta is bright because of the _____, _____and _____.

| | |
|---|---|
| **A.** Lg. FOV, Thin Slice, and Large Flip Angle | ☐ |
| **B.** Short TR, TE, and Flip Angle | ☐ |
| **C.** Small FOV, Short TR/Short TE | ☐ |
| **D.** Short TR, Long TE, Shallow Flip Angle | ☐ |

**397.** In Figure 4.64, the bright Aorta is bright due to what is called _____?

| | |
|---|---|
| **A.** Exit slice phenomenon | ☐ |
| **B.** Entry slice phenomenon | ☐ |
| **C.** IV Contrast | ☐ |
| **D.** No Sat Pulse | ☐ |

**398.** In Figure 4.64, in slices inferior to the shown slice, the aorta will lose signal due to_____.

| | |
|---|---|
| **A.** Saturation pulses | ☐ |
| **B.** In-Plane saturation | ☐ |
| **C.** Venous return | ☐ |
| **D.** Cardiac arrythmias | ☐ |

**399.** The artifact shown in Figure 4.65 is called or known as _____.

| | |
|---|---|
| **A.** Di-Electric | ☐ |
| **B.** Flow void | ☐ |
| **C.** Standing wave | ☐ |
| **D.** A and C | ☐ |

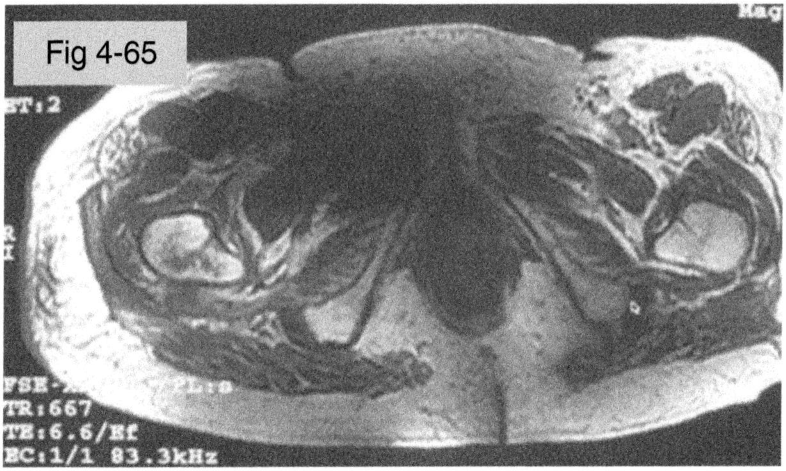

Fig 4-65

**400.** In Figure 4.65, this artifact is/can be seen at all fields strengths but is most common at?

| | |
|---|---|
| **A.** 1.5 T | ☐ |
| **B.** 0.5 T | ☐ |
| **C.** 3 T | ☐ |
| **D.** 1.0 T | ☐ |

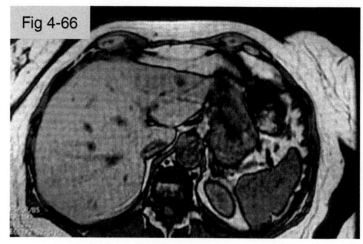

Fig 4-66

**401.** The artifact seen in Figure 4.66 is due to the _____?

| | |
|---|---|
| **A.** Flip angle | ☐ |
| **B.** Phase matrix | ☐ |
| **C.** TR | ☐ |
| **D.** TE | ☐ |

**402.** In Figure 4.66, the artifact is called?

| | |
|---|---|
| **A.** Opposed echo | ☐ |
| **B.** Chemical shift of 2nd kind | ☐ |
| **C.** Out of Phase echo | ☐ |
| **D.** A, B, and C | ☐ |

**403.** In Figure 4.66, you will only see this artifact in a _____.

| | |
|---|---|
| **A.** Fast spin-echo | ☐ |
| **B.** STIR | ☐ |
| **C.** GRE | ☐ |
| **D.** Spin-echo | ☐ |

**404.** Adding Fat Sat to a GRE sequence enhances the Out of Phase effect.

| | |
|---|---|
| **A.** True | ☐ |
| **B.** False | ☐ |

**405.** In and Out of Phase TE's do not change with field strengths.

> **A.** True ☐
> **B.** False ☐

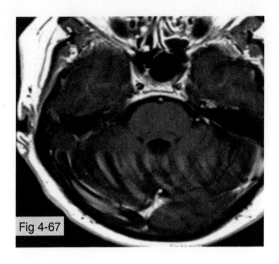

Fig 4-67

**406.** In Figure 4.67, this artifact is called _____.

> **A.** Pulsatile flow ☐
> **B.** Motion ☐
> **C.** Standing wave ☐
> **D.** Wrap ☐

**407.** In Figure 4.67, this artifact is/can be caused by:

> **A.** Pulse gating ☐
> **B.** A long TI in a FLAIR ☐
> **C.** IV contrast ☐
> **D.** Cardiac arrythmias ☐

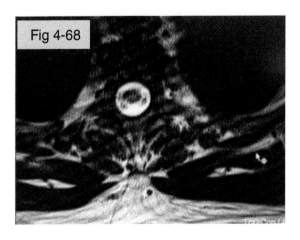

Fig 4-68

**408.** In Figure 4.68, this artifact is called:

| | |
|---|---|
| **A.** Plaid artifact | ☐ |
| **B.** Woolen artifact | ☐ |
| **C.** Corduroy artifact | ☐ |
| **D.** RF leak | ☐ |

**409.** In Figure 4.68, this artifact can be caused by:

| | |
|---|---|
| **A.** Static electricity | ☐ |
| **B.** Low humidity | ☐ |
| **C.** Bad light bulb | ☐ |
| **D.** All of these | ☐ |

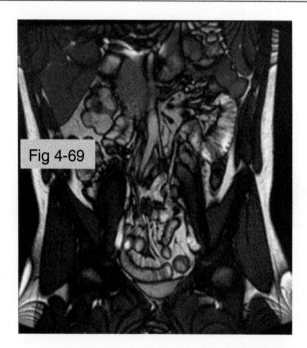

Fig 4-69

**410.** The artifact seen in Figure 4.69 is called_____?

| | |
|---|---|
| **A.** Motion | ☐ |
| **B.** Gradient warp | ☐ |
| **C.** Moiré | ☐ |
| **D.** Aliasing | ☐ |

**411.** In Figure 4.69, this artifact is seen often in which sequence?

**A.** Spin-echo ☐
**B.** Fast spin-echo ☐
**C.** STIR ☐
**D.** Gradient echo ☐

**412.** Figure 4.69, the artifact can be lessened with?

**A.** Shimming and Anti-Aliasing ☐
**B.** Fat-Sat and Shimming ☐
**C.** Decreased FOV and Shimming ☐
**D.** Fat-Sat and Anti-Aliasing ☐

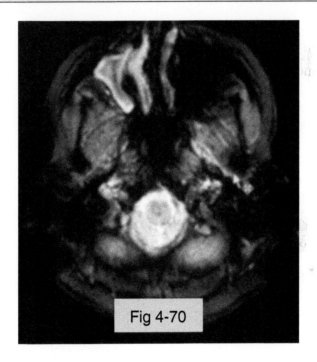

Fig 4-70

**413.** What artifact is seen in Figure 4.70?

**A.** Motion ☐
**B.** Zipper artifact ☐
**C.** Susceptibility ☐
**D.** Over-Sampling ☐

**414.** In Figure 4.70, the artifact results from_____.

> **A.** A long Echo train ☐
> **B.** Entry slice phenomenon ☐
> **C.** Lack of 180's in the sequence ☐
> **D.** Metal ☐

**415.** In Figure 4.70, the sequence is a _____.

> **A.** DWI ☐
> **B.** GRE ☐
> **C.** Spin-echo ☐
> **D.** FSE ☐

**416.** In Figure 4.70, this artifact can be lessened by:

> **A.** Removing the metal if able ☐
> **B.** Fat saturation ☐
> **C.** Use a sequence with 180's ☐
> **D.** A and C ☐

**417.** In Figure 4.71, attention to the urinary bladder. What is causing the layering effect in the bladder?

> **A.** This is a post contrast image ☐
> **B.** Gadolinium is concentrating dependently ☐
> **C.** Pure gadolinium does not produce signal ☐
> **D.** All the above ☐

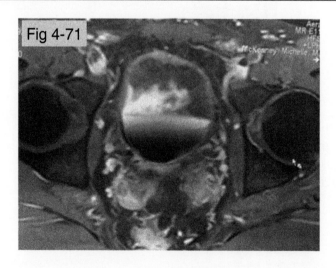

Fig 4-71

**418.** In Figure 4.71, why is the urine dark on this image?

A. Image is T2 weighted ☐
B. Image is a STIR ☐
C. Image is T1 weighted ☐
D. Image is a FLAIR ☐

## Artifacts

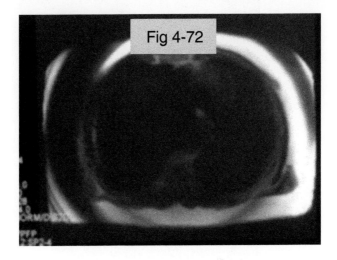

Fig 4-72

**419.** In Figure 4.72, the artifact is mostly due to _____.

A. Center frequency has drifted ☐
B. A very large stack of slices ☐
C. Magnetic field inhomogeneity ☐
D. A, B, and C ☐

**420.** It is common to see this effect in a/an _____ sequence.

A. SS-Free precession ☐
B. F/S fast spin-echo ☐
C. Inversion recovery ☐
D. CE-MRA ☐

**421.** The artifact/effect in Figure 4.72 can be avoided or lessened by
_____?

| | |
|---|---|
| **A.** Shim | ☐ |
| **B.** Splitting into two stacks | ☐ |
| **C.** Turn off F/S | ☐ |
| **D.** Thinner slices | ☐ |

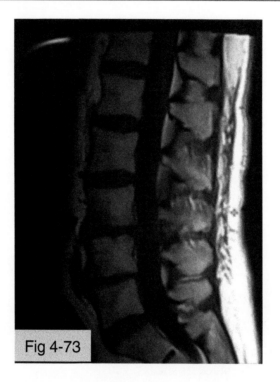

Fig 4-73

**422.** What artifact is seen in Figure 4.73?

| | |
|---|---|
| **A.** Motion | ☐ |
| **B.** Zipper artifact | ☐ |
| **C.** Annifact | ☐ |
| **D.** Over-Sampling | ☐ |

**423.** In Figure 4.73, the artifact comes from_____?

| | |
|---|---|
| **A.** To many coils turned on for the FOV | ☐ |
| **B.** To few coils turned on for the FOV | ☐ |
| **C.** Coil not plugged in | ☐ |
| **D.** Wrap | ☐ |

**424.** In Figure 4.73, a possible solution for this artifact could be? Choose all that apply.

A. Less coils ☐
B. More coils ☐
C. Sat bands above + below the FOV ☐
D. Swap phase/frequency ☐
E. Change image weighting ☐
F. Change patient orientation ☐
G. Apply full over-sampling ☐

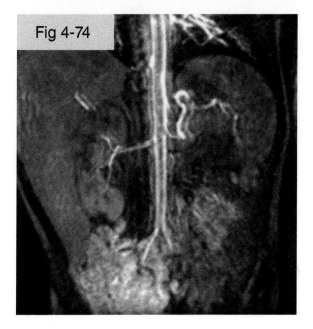

Fig 4-74

**425.** In Figure 4.74, this artifact is called?

A. Motion ☐
B. Ringing or "Maki" ☐
C. Inverted vessel ☐
D. Reversed k-Space artifact ☐

**426.** In Figure 4.74, the artifact is caused by.

A. Acquiring the center of k-Space to early ☐
B. Acquiring the center of k-Space to late ☐
C. Pure gadolinium does not give signal ☐
D. A and C ☐

**427.** In Figure 4.74, how can you avoid this artifact?

A. Double the scan time ☐
B. Halve the scan time ☐
C. Better timing of data acquisition ☐
D. Do a 2D TOF ☐

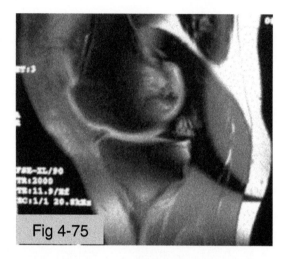

Fig 4-75

**428.** The artifact seen in Figure 4.75 comes from_____?

A. Mag. susceptibility ☐
B. Gradient warp ☐
C. Moiré ☐
D. Metal ☐

**429.** In Figure 4.75, the artifact is seen in this _____ sequence?

A. PD Fat Sat ☐
B. GRE ☐
C. STIR ☐
D. PD-FSE ☐

**430.** In Figure 4.75, the artifact can be avoided by_____.

A. Proper screening ☐
B. Change patient into hospital gowns ☐
C. Use metal detector ☐
D. A, B, and C ☐

## Miscellaneous Questions:

**431.** What two arteries joint to make the basilar?

| | |
|---|---|
| **A.** Carotids | ☐ |
| **B.** Subclavian | ☐ |
| **C.** Vertebral | ☐ |
| **D.** Posterior cerebrals | ☐ |

**432.** Another name for the brachiocephalic artery is the _____.

| | |
|---|---|
| **A.** Brachialis artery | ☐ |
| **B.** Basilar artery | ☐ |
| **C.** Innominate artery | ☐ |
| **D.** Inferior cerebral artery | ☐ |

**433.** Hepatic veins drain into the _____.

| | |
|---|---|
| **A.** Renal veins | ☐ |
| **B.** Azygous vein | ☐ |
| **C.** I.V.C | ☐ |
| **D.** Portal vein | ☐ |

**434.** Islet cells are found in which organ?

| | |
|---|---|
| **A.** Kidney | ☐ |
| **B.** Pancreas | ☐ |
| **C.** Liver | ☐ |
| **D.** Conus medullaris | ☐ |

**435.** In a "Subclavian Steal" blood flow is _____ in the _____.

| | |
|---|---|
| **A.** Retrograde, Carotid | ☐ |
| **B.** Antegrade, Subclavian | ☐ |
| **C.** Retrograde, Vertebral | ☐ |
| **D.** Antegrade, Vertebral | ☐ |

**436.** A "Subclavian Steal" can be suspected with the absence of flow in what artery on a 2D TOF.

A. Carotid ☐
B. Subclavian ☐
C. Vertebral ☐
D. Cerebral ☐

**437.** To help rule out or prove a "Subclavian Steal," in a 2D TOF of the neck, simply swap the position of the _____ from _____ to _____.

A. Sat Pulse, Anterior, Posterior ☐
B. Sat Pulse, Right, Left ☐
C. Sat Pulse, Superior, Inferior ☐
D. Slices, Superior, Inferior ☐

**438.** What are the paired openings from the lateral ventricles going into the 3rd ventricle called?

A. Aqueducts of Sylvius ☐
B. Foramen of Monroe ☐
C. Foramen of Magendie ☐
D. Lateral ventricles ☐

**439.** The connection between the 3rd ventricle and the 4th ventricle is called the _____.

A. Aqueducts of Sylvius ☐
B. Foramen of Monroe ☐
C. Foramen of Magendie ☐
D. Lateral Ventricles ☐

**440.** The aperture from the 4th ventricle to the central canal in the spinal cord is called the _____.

A. Aqueducts of Sylvius ☐
B. Foramen of Monroe ☐
C. Foramen of Magendie ☐
D. Lateral ventricles ☐

**441.** While scanning, you notice Truncation/Gibbs artifact. How can you decrease the artifact?

| | |
|---|---|
| **A.** Decrease the scan matrix | ☐ |
| **B.** Increase the scan matrix | ☐ |
| **C.** Decrease slice thickness | ☐ |
| **D.** Widen the receiver bandwidth | ☐ |

**442.** A "Tethered Cord" is considered if the conus medullaris lies below what spinal level?

| | |
|---|---|
| **A.** T11/12 | ☐ |
| **B.** T12/L1 | ☐ |
| **C.** L1/2 | ☐ |
| **D.** L5/S1 | ☐ |

**443.** On post contrast images of the spine, which structure enhanced first?

| | |
|---|---|
| **A.** Disc | ☐ |
| **B.** Nerve sheaths | ☐ |
| **C.** Scar tissue | ☐ |
| **D.** The Pars Intra-Articularus | ☐ |

**444.** Various types of blood flow include all of the following except?

| | |
|---|---|
| **A.** Vernacular | ☐ |
| **B.** Laminar | ☐ |
| **C.** Turbulent | ☐ |
| **D.** Vortex | ☐ |

**445.** What view will best visualize the co-lateral ligaments in the knee?

| | |
|---|---|
| **A.** Axial | ☐ |
| **B.** Coronal | ☐ |
| **C.** Sagittal | ☐ |
| **D.** Double oblique | ☐ |

**446.** A ligament attaches what?

| | |
|---|---|
| **A.** Bone to Bone | ☐ |
| **B.** Bone to Muscle | ☐ |
| **C.** Tendon to Bone | ☐ |
| **D.** Muscle to Muscle | ☐ |

**447.** The aorta bifurcates into the _____.

| | |
|---|---|
| **A.** Femoral arteries | ☐ |
| **B.** Iliac arteries | ☐ |
| **C.** Deep and Superficial femoral arteries | ☐ |
| **D.** Renal arteries | ☐ |

**448.** Which blood vessels feed the circle of Willis?

| | |
|---|---|
| **A.** Internal cerebral and Carotid arteries | ☐ |
| **B.** Carotid and Basilar arteries | ☐ |
| **C.** Jugular and Carotid arteries | ☐ |
| **D.** Middle Cerebral and Anterior arteries | ☐ |

**449.** What are the three parts of the pituitary gland?

| | |
|---|---|
| **A.** Anterior, Medulla, and Cortex | ☐ |
| **B.** Anterior, Cortex, and Posterior | ☐ |
| **C.** Adeno, Intermediate, and Neuro Hypophysis | ☐ |
| **D.** Superior, Middle, and Inferior | ☐ |

**450.** What gland secretes adrenalin?

| | |
|---|---|
| **A.** Spleen | ☐ |
| **B.** Pancreas | ☐ |
| **C.** Kidneys | ☐ |
| **D.** Supra-Renal glands | ☐ |

**451.** The three bones of the inner ear are called the _____?

| | |
|---|---|
| **A.** Os Calsii | ☐ |
| **B.** Ossicles | ☐ |
| **C.** Otitis | ☐ |
| **D.** Semi-Circulars | ☐ |

**452.** The three bones of the inner ear are named _____, _____ and the _____.

A. Malleus, Incus, and Staples ☐
B. Malleus, Incus, and Stapes ☐
C. Malleolus, Incus, Stapes ☐
D. Medial, Lateral, Internus ☐

**453.** The series of curved tubes medial to the inner ear are called the

_____.

A. Rounded canals ☐
B. Semi-Circular canals ☐
C. Ovalis ☐
D. Semi-Ovalis ☐

**454.** There are three portions of the sternum. They are the _____.

A. Manubrium, Body, and Xiphoid ☐
B. Gladiolus, Body, and Xiphoid ☐
C. Upper, Middle, and Tip ☐
D. A and B ☐

**455.** Another name for the Iliac Wing is the _____.

A. Mons bone ☐
B. Semi-Circular bone ☐
C. Ala ☐
D. Ovalis ☐

*Mnemonics*: Are different sayings or rhymes to help you to remember various sets/groups/names of bones, nerves, and other anatomies. Some are family friendly; others are PG or R rated. Reader discretion is advised.

#1. *Branches of the aortic arch: A, B, C, S.* **A**orta, **B**rachiocephalic, **C**arotid, **S**ubclavian.

Two images labeled #1: Artists rendition of the great vessels on the left and a CE-MRA on the right.

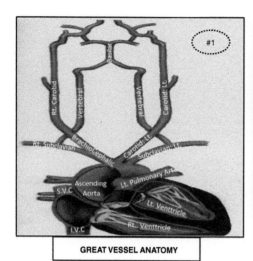

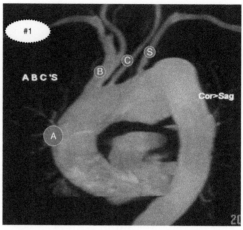

GREAT VESSEL ANATOMY

You could be asked a question such as: What is the second branch of the aortic arch? Remember your ABC'S. When learning CPR, you memorized ABC for Airway, Breathing, and Circulation correct? Yes, you did. Now add an S and it becomes the acronym for the branches off the aortic arch: Aorta, Brachiocephalic, Carotid (LEFT), and Subclavian. Now to answer the question. That would be the left carotid. Again, let the answers be a guide as to the correct answer.

Author's Note: Some would argue that the Lt. and Rt. main coronary arteries are the 1st branches off aorta, and they would absolutely be correct. Here is a case where you need to see the answers that are given to make your choice. In everyday scanning, unless you are doing cardiac imaging, are you really concerned with the coronaries?

## Mnemonics

#2. *Cranial nerves: OOOTTAFAGVAH*

**O**lfactory, **O**ptic, **O**cular Motor, **T**rochlear, **T**rigeminal, **A**bducens, **F**acial, **A**coustic, **G**lossal-Pharyngeal, **V**agal, **A**ccessory, **H**ypoglossal.

**O**n **O**ld **O**lympus's **T**owering **T**ops, **A** **F**in **and** **G**erman **V**iew **A**ncient **H**opps. *OR:*

**O**H, **O**H, **O**H, **T**o **T**ouch **and** **F**eel **A** **G**ood **V**elvet **A**h, **H**eaven

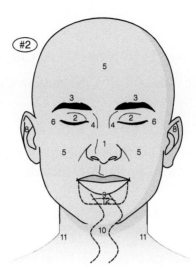

#2: Artists' numerical depiction of cranial nerve coverage on the face.

## Mnemonics

**#3.** *Carpal bones:* **S**he **L**ooks **T**oo **P**retty, **T**ry **t**o **C**atch **H**er OR:

Some Lovers Try Positions That They Can't Handle

*Prox. Row: Thumb to Pinky:* **S**caphoid, **L**unate, **T**riquetrum, **P**isiform

*Distal Row: Thumb to Pinky:* **T**rapezium, **T**rapezoid, **C**apitate, **H**amate

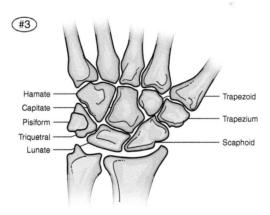

#3: Artist depiction of the carpal bones, here is a PA view of left wrist.

## Mnemonics

**#4.** *Tarsal bones:* **O**liver **T**wist **N**ever **C**ould **C**ha, **C**ha, **C**ha.

**O**s-Calcis (Calcaneus), **T**alus, **N**avicular, **C**uboid, **1st, 2nd, and 3rd** Cuneiforms

OR:

**T**iger **C**ubs **N**eed **MILC**: **T**alus **C**uboid, **N**avicular, **M**edial, **I**ntermediate **L**ateral **C**uneiforms. *Remember to include the Calcaneus (Heel) which is excluded in this saying.*

#4: Artist depiction of the tarsal bones. Here is a A/P view of the right foot.

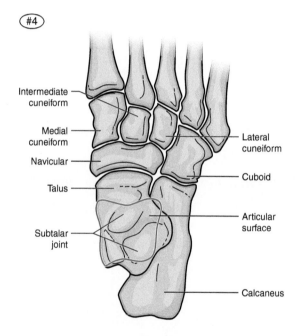

## Mnemonics

**#5.** *Rotator cuff:* **S**upraspinatus, **I**nfraspinatus, **T**eres Minor, **S**ubscapularis. Remember: **S.I.T.S**

#5-1: Axial GRE of Lt. shoulder at the level of the supraspinatus tendon.

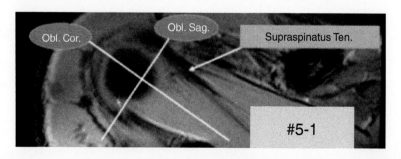

#5-2 + 3: Artist renditions of A/P and P/A anatomy of the shoulder.

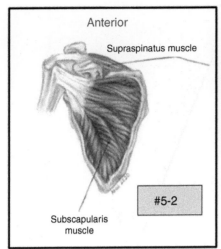
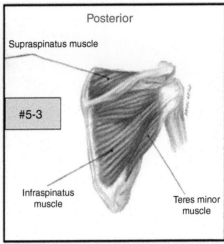

## Mnemonics

**#6.** To remember the order of the gradient applications in any sequence, it is **S.P.F.** Think: Sunscreen Protection Factor: **S**LICE, **P**HASE, **F**REQUENCY

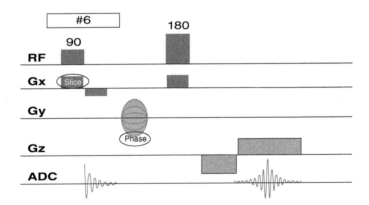

**#7.** 3 tissues that are bright on T1 weighted images are FAT, GAD, and PROTEINS: **FGP**

#8. *There are 3 different boney "OID's" in the body.*

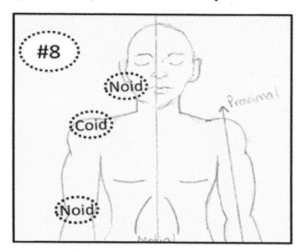

CORO**NOID**: MANDIBLE. CORO**COID**: SHOULDER. CORO**NOID**: ELBOW. Here is how to remember them: point to your JAW: **NOID**, point to your Shoulder: **COID**, point to your Elbow: **NOID**.

Use the saying:

#9. Wrist: The **Tri**angular Fibro Cartilage Complex attaches to the **Trique**trum Bone. So, think: "TRI to TRI."

Why point this out? You should, be able to find the TFCC on a wrist. When asked to name a particular carpal bone, you may forget (due to stress) which is the proximal row? Is the ulna medial or lateral? Use the TFCC as a landmark, or, remember that the radius is on the thumb side (RT). The TFCC attaches to the triquetrum and is medial in the proximal row.

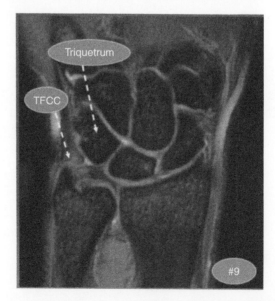

#10. There are different spellings of Ileum: Ileum and Ilium. Ilium is in the pelvis while Ileum is the terminal portion of the small bowel. The parts of the S.B are the **Duodenum, Jejunum, and Ileum**. Easy way to remember: An MR Enterography is done to evaluate the bowel. It has an E. The "E" in Ileum is the bowel while the "Ilium" is the pelvis. If you can remember one of them, then the other is true.

#11. The **Cap**itate in the elbow (distal humerus) is the biggest and in the middle (medial). "The **Cap**itol" as it were.

#12. Medial malleolus is on the tibia. Tibia is medial, the Fibula is lateral. Easy way to remember is: The FibuLa has an **L** in it so think: Lateral. The tibia is also the weight-bearing bone in the lower leg, and is why somebody can walk fairly easily with a broken fibula.

## Helpful Anatomy: The Basil Ganglia

The brain stem and basil ganglia anatomy are two anatomical regions that you should be familiar with.

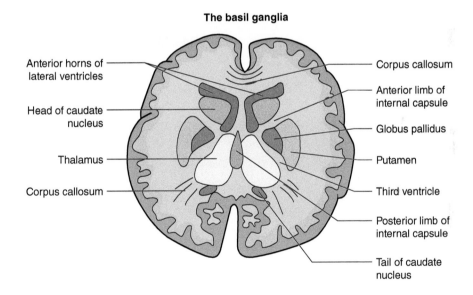

The basil ganglia

Anterior horns of lateral ventricles

Head of caudate nucleus

Thalamus

Corpus callosum

Corpus callosum

Anterior limb of internal capsule

Globus pallidus

Putamen

Third ventricle

Posterior limb of internal capsule

Tail of caudate nucleus

## Helpful Anatomy: T2 Axials of Basil Ganglia

What about the Foramen of Monroe? Bottom right image. It is pointed out by the scanner cursor. Now you know where it is.

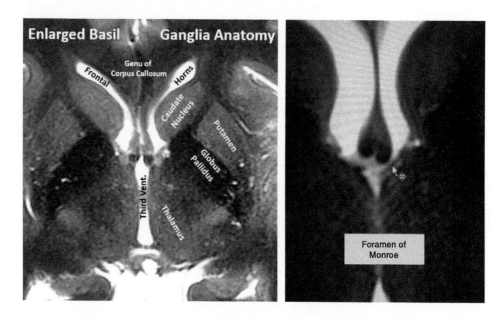

## Helpful Anatomy: T1 Sagittal of Brain Stem

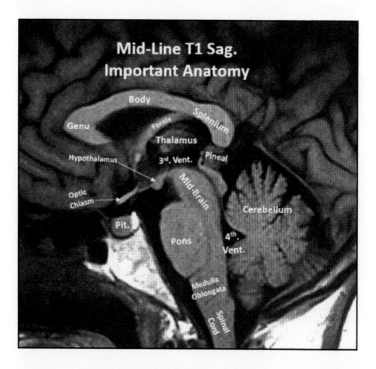

## Other Helpful Anatomy: The Brachial Plexus

The brachial plexus is an anatomical "entity" that can be difficult to visualize in your mind. I offer it here in order to give you a visual concept of where it is located along with its general pat or course out of the spine and into the arm.

*Please note* that it actually runs behind the clavicle meeting up with subclavian artery and Vein at the level of the clavicle to form what is called a "Neuro-Vascular Bundle."

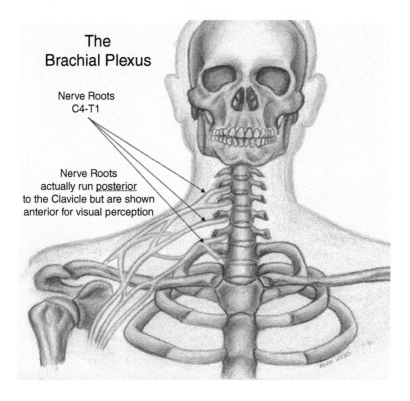

First what is a "Plexus"? It's a group or collection of nerves or vessels. These two are often grouped together. The difference is simply location of or the origins of the nerve roots. The lumbar plexus (in orange) originates from the lumbar spine: T12 and L1–L4. It courses down anterior to the hip and is contained in the psoas major muscle. It supplies enervation for the anterior thigh. The sacral plexus (purple) actually provides much of the enervation of the leg. It originates from out of L4–S4 levels. The sacral plexus is the major nerve supply to the posterior thigh, lower leg, and also the foot. An artist rendition is shown below of both. I have had them drawn on opposite sides of the body and in different colors to give you a better idea of what and where they are anatomically. Imaging of either the brachial or L/S plexus is usually part of a metastatic or infection work-up.

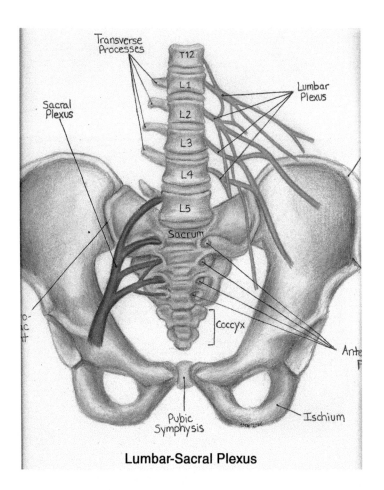

**Lumbar-Sacral Plexus**

# The Boney Pelvis

There are multiple different anatomical structures you need to know in the pelvis. The **Iliac Crest** is probably the most important. It serves as a very common landmark in both X-ray and MRI for positioning of the lumbar spine. It falls at the **L3/4** level and only slightly above the **S/I Joint.** The **Anterior Superior Iliac Spine** (ASIS) can be used for finding the level of the sacrum. The ischium is further inferior and is the bone upon which we sit. The symphysis pubis is in between the ischium. Recall that the very large foramen of the ischium is called the obturator foramen. Through the obturator foramen passes the obturator nerve, artery, and vein. The obturator nerve is part of the lumbar plexus.

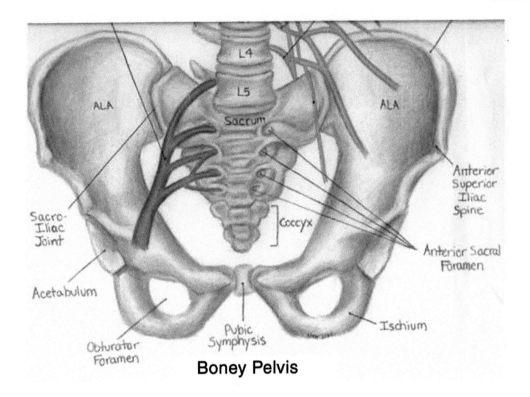

**Boney Pelvis**

# The Cranial Nerves: O O O T T A F A G V A H

There are many ways to remember the names for the cranial nerves. Pick one and stay with it. The more you try to use the more confused it will be come. Also included, is by color are they sensory, motor, or a combination of the two.

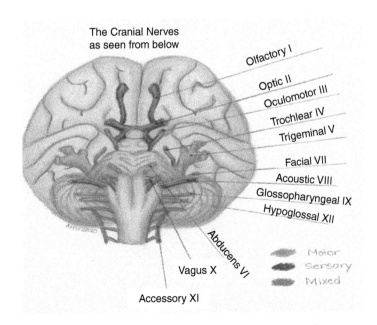

The Cranial Nerves as seen from below

Olfactory I
Optic II
Oculomotor III
Trochlear IV
Trigeminal V
Facial VII
Acoustic VIII
Glossopharyngeal IX
Hypoglossal XII
Abducens VI
Vagus X
Accessory XI

Motor
Sensory
Mixed

# Cranial Nerve: Study

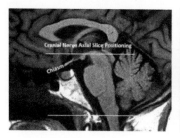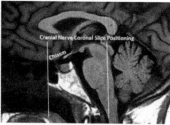

Positioning the slices for a cranial nerve study may be challenging for the newer technologists. It really is easy. Off of a mid-line sagittal of the brain all you really have to go by is the optic chiasm. It is the nerve that crosses the mid-line so use that fact. The rest of the pairs of nerves come off laterally and you cannot see them on a sagittal. I use the optic chiasm as my landmark and place my top slice a couple of mm's higher to include the olfactory nerve and cover down to just below the inferior tip of the clivus portion of the sphenoid bone. The coronal coverage should be from the center of the brain stem and forward to just inside the sphenoid sinus. There is a lot of anatomy in a very small area. See the drawing of the cranial nerves as seen from below on the previous page.

# T1 and T2 Contrast Differences in the Brain

In brain imaging, the gray matter/white matter differentiation is often spoken of, and is of great importance. Below are two enlarged images of the same slice in the same patient. On the T1 image, white matter is bright due to its higher fat content from (myelin) (it is doing what fat is supposed to do) and gray matter is dark (gray) due to its high water content. It is doing what water is supposed to be doing on a T1. Compare it to the CSF.

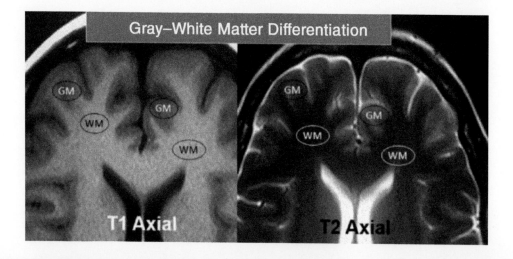

On the T2 weighted image, white matter is now darker because again it is mostly fat and is doing what fat does on a T2, it drops in signal. Grey matter is bright now on the T2 because it is doing what water does on a T2, it is bright because of its long T2 relaxation time. Compare it to the CSF.

## Answers

1. **B.**

2. **B.** The T wave can elevate during scanning mimicking an M.I.

3. **C.** Avascular.

4. **A.** Femoral head.

5. **C.**

6. **B.**

7. **C.** T2 FLAIR (scanning with Fat Sat is rather common).

8. **A.** Aortic arch. The great vessels off the aorta: A, B, C, S. Question 71 Section 1. Number 1 in Mnemonics.

9. **B.**

10. **A.** There are two plexus's: The lumbar includes nerve roots from L1–L4, and the sacral L5–S4.

11. **B.**

12. **C.** The Mnemonic here is S.I.T.S. See number 5 in Mnemonics.

13. **D.**

14. **A.** Median nerve.

15. **B.**

16. **C.**

17. **A.**

18. True.

19. **B.** The three parts of the corpus collosum: Anterior: The genu, body and posteriorly the splenium.

**20. B.**

**21. A.**

**22. D.**

**23. B.**

**24. A.**

**25. D.** The adrenal is a.k.a. the supra-renal.

**26. B.**

**27. D.**

**28. D.**

**29. B.** Crus (Crura is the pleural) or Crux of the diaphragm. Refers to one of two tendinous structures extending below the diaphragm to attach to the vertebral column. Together they form an attachment/tether for muscular contraction for respirations.

**30. B.**

**31. A.** The psoas muscle(s) attach at the lumbar verts. (L2–L4), extend down through the pelvis and connects to the femur at the lesser trochanter. This muscle flexes the hip and helps lift the leg toward the body. Movement created from the psoas is key to walking.

**32. A.** The adrenal gland a.k.a. the suprarenal gland, supra meaning "Above the Kidney."

**33. D.**

**34. B.** This is the first/upper most part of the biliary tree, intra-hepatic.

**35. C.** The duct coming from the GB is the cystic duct. Here truncated from surgery.

**36. A.** The hepatic bile duct and the cystic duct join to form the common bile duct (CBD).

**37. D.** The pancreatic(s) are duct part of the biliary tree. It joins the CBD making the ampulla of Vater. The ampulla dumbs bile into the duodenum through the sphincter of Oddi. The sphincter of Oddi is a one-way valve that keeps stomach contents out to the ampulla/biliary tree.

**38. C.** The celiac is the 1st branch off the abdominal aorta. There are three branches off the celiac axis: Hepatic, Splenic, and Left Gastric. The 2nd branch off the AA is the superior mesenteric artery or SMA the next major branch is the IMA or inferior mesenteric. Remember, If there is a "Superior Something, there will most likely be an Inferior Something."

**39. B.**

**40. D.** There are two mesenteric arteries. If there is an inferior, then logically there is a superior.

**41. A.**

**42. A.** (Review Figure 4-29)

**43. A.** The symphysis is where the pubic bones meet.

**44. C.**

**45. C.** Junctional zone. The uterus has three zones or layers. The outer most is the **Myometrium** (Myo) muscle, a **Junctional zone** which is the muscle turning/transforming into **Endometrium**. Endo meaning the interior.

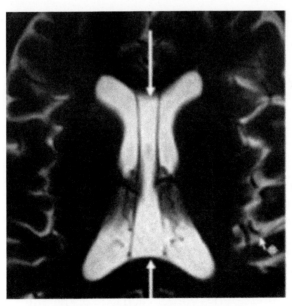

**Question number 53 Shown is a
"Cavum Septum Pellucidum"
or Accessory Ventricle**

**46. C.**

**47. B.**

**48. B.**

**49. D.**

**50. C.**

**51. D.**

**52. A.** The position of the uterus can change as the bladder fills over time.

**53. C.** The division between the lateral ventricles is a midline, double layer of tissue called the septum pellucidum. The septum pellucidum separates the left from right ventricles. There is a potential space between the septum which is usually empty but can fill with CSF. This condition is called "Cavum Septum Pellucidum." Cavum meaning "open." This condition is commonly referred to as an accessory ventricle.

**54. D.** Also called the lateral sulcus. It separates the frontal and parietal lobes from the temporal lobe.

**55. D.** The stalk of the pituitary is also known as the infundibulum. Infundibulum means a funnel-shaped tube or cavity. The infundibulum connects the posterior pituitary gland to the hypothalamus. Some cells in the infundibulum are neurons that also have endocrine-type properties. It is not just a "Cherry Stem" attaching the pituitary gland to the brain.

**56. C.**

**57. B.**

**58. B.** It is a dural venous sinus bordered by the temporal bone and the sphenoid bone. It is lateral to the sella turcica. It enhances vividly with IV Contrast on both CT and MRI.

**59. C.** The optic chiasm is well seen in this coronal view. Chiasm means "A crossing."

**60. B.** The carotid arteries border each side of the pituitary gland. Here, due to flowing blood, there is a "Flow Void" more correctly expressed/termed a high-velocity signal loss, HVSL.

**61. A.** In this axial view, the optic chiasm is well seen "crossing." This slice is just *above* the pituitary.

**62. C.**

**63. A.** Cerebral peduncle.

**64. C.** This structure that looks like "Mickey Mouse" is the PONS. The ears are called the peduncles.

**65. B.** Mammary bodies. The mammary bodies are part of the limbic system. They aid in memory and help send impulses to the thalamus. These are often seen on T2 axials.

**66. A.** All ventricles have choroid plexus. Choroid plexus makes CSF. It will enhance with IV Contrast.

**67. C.**

**68. A.**

**69. C.** All ventricles contain choroid plexus to make CSF. It will enhance with IV contrast.

**70. C.** The arachnoid space filled with CSF between the temporal lobe and the brain is the "Sylvian Fissure." This fissure is an important anatomical land-mark you need to be able to identify in the coronal and axial planes. This fissure separates the frontal and parietal lobes from then temporal lobe.

**71. A.**

**72. C.** (and Question 205) Interhemispheric fissure or falx cerebri is a double layer of dura mater which will enhance with IV contrast. This is especially true in a patient with meningitis. It is very common to see calcifications in the interhemispheric fissure especially in older patients.

**73. B.**

**74. C.**

**75. D.**

**76. A.**

**77. C.**

**78. C.** Carotid siphons. The "Siphon" portion is part of the internal carotid, and runs through the sphenoid bone.

**79. B.**

**80. D.**

**81. A.**

**82. A.**

**83. D.** The 2nd cervical vertebrae has two names: obviously C-2 the other is the "Axis." The boney projection sticking up through C-1 is called the odontoid or dens.

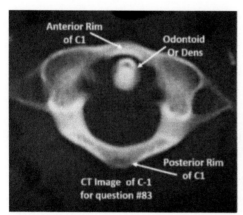

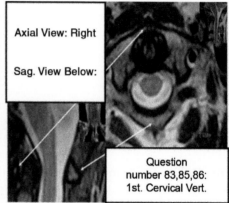

**84. B.** Cerebral tonsils. The tonsils can protrude downward or through the foramen magnum, a condition called a "Chiari Malformation." It can happen when part of the skull is abnormally small/misshapen, which presses the brain downward toward the foramen. During Chiari malformation surgery, a small section of occipital bone is removed to make room for the cerebellum to relieve pressure off the brainstem, cerebellum, and spinal cord.

**85. A.** Anterior rim of C-1. C-1 is a.k.a. the Atlas, articulates with the occipital bone. It is an atypical vertebra, ring-like vertebra with no body. Number 3 points to the anterior arch while number 5 points to the posterior arch.

**86. A.** Posterior rim of C-1.

**87. B.** An Arnold Chiari malformation is when the cerebella tonsils project down to or through the foramen magnum. This can put pressure on the spinal cord and even cause hydrocephalus.

**88. B.** T1 FLAIR. Many sites do T1 FLAIRs instead of T1's, especially at 3T. In FLAIR's, the CSF is very dark (darker than expected on SE T1) as CSF is targeted by the TI to be nulled or suppressed.

89. **C.** The conus medullaris. Conus medullaris syndrome often comes from trauma and has symptoms of: Severe back pain, jarring sensations in the back, described as a buzzing, tingling, or numbness, bowel and bladder dysfunction. Usually a stack of T2 weighted axials are performed covering the conus.

90. **D.** Cauda equina or horses' tail. It is a long bundle of spinal nerves originating from the conus.

91. **B.** Disc.

92. **D.**

93. **A.**

94. **A.**

95. **D.** LABRUM.

96. **D.**

97. **D.**

98. **D.** ARTHROGRAM.

99. **B.**

100. **C.**

101. **B.**

102. **D.** Bicipital groove. The biceps tendon is located within the bicipital groove.

103. **B.**

104. **D.**

105. **C.** The PCL is a solid single tendon which is less often torn vs. the ACL which is a series of almost feather-like smaller tendons. The ACL/PCL cross from front to back. Cruciate means "Cross shaped."

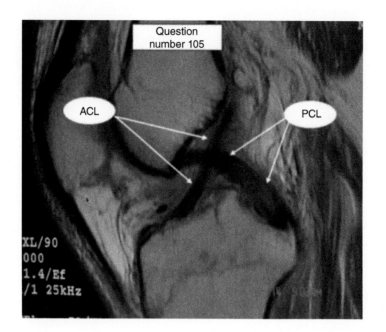

106. A.

107. A.

108. B.

109. D.

110. B.

111. A.

112. A.

113. D.

114. B.

115. B.

116. C.

117. D.

118. A.

119. D.

120. C.

121. **A.**

122. **B.**

123. **C.**

124. **B.**

125. **A.** The obturator muscle. The obturator muscles are a pair of muscles, one on each side of the obturator foramen: Internus and Externus. Internus is the one inside the pelvis, so logically, the Externus is outside the pelvis.

126. **A.** Ischium. This is the bone you actually sit upon.

127. **C.**

128. **D.** Coronoid (Process) Time out here. Another coronoid? Yes. But there are easy to remember. Think "NOID, COID, NOID." *Coronoid* in the Mandible, *Coracoid* in the Shoulder finally *Coronoid* in the Elbow. Also think: High to Low. Mandible, Shoulder, Elbow. *See the Mnemonics sections for more.*

129. **D.**

130. **D.** The brachialis muscle is the other muscle that helps flex the elbow besides the biceps. Biceps attaches to the radius (lateral aspect of elbow), brachialis attaches medially on the coronoid process.

131. **D.**

132. **A.** Radial head.

133. **A.** Capitulum.

134. **D.** The distal condyles of the humerus are the capitulum and the trochlea. Which is which? An easy way to remember, if looking at a coronal or sag, if it is near the Radial **Head** it is the **Cap**itulum. REMEMBER this: You put a **CAP** on your **HEAD**.

135. **C.**

136. **B.**

137. **D.**

138. **D.**

139. **B.** In the anatomical position, the radius is lateral to the ulna. An easy way to remember it is *after* you pass this test you are an **R.T.**, so think **R**adius is on the **T**humb side.

140. **C.**

141. **A.** The ulna bone has a distinct "Pointy Thing" in the ulna styloid process, the radius does not.

142. **D.**

143. **B.**

144. **C.**

145. **C.** The **H**amate has, if imaged in the axial plane, a distinct "**H**ook" shaped projection. Think H-H.

146. **B.**

147. **D.** The median nerve in "Carpal Tunnel" is being compressed by the transverse carpal ligament (flexor retinaculum). So, "How am I supposed to see that?" Right, it is a small structure mixed in with all those tendons. And I do not know the names of all those tendons! They would not be asking you some lesser important nerve or tendon's name so its got to be the median nerve. A Rad will know them of course. Again, let the answers answer the question. What is a very common reason to scan a wrist? Carpal Tunnel, right? So, its got to be the medial nerve. Simple logic.

148. **B.**

149. **D.**

150. **C.**

151. **D.**

152. **D.**

153. **A.** Sinus tarsi. The tarsal sinus contains a neuro-vascular bundle (nerves, arteries, and veins grouped together is a NV bundle) as well as a fat and ligaments. It is a tube or tunnel between the talus and the calcaneus bones. Sinus tarsi syndrome is pain or injury to this area. Trauma to the ankle/foot (multiple ankle sprains) and overuse are the main causes of this sinus tarsi syndrome.

154. **B.**

**155. C.**

**156. D.**

**157. A.**

**158. B.**

**159. A.**

**160. B.**

**161. A.**

**162. C.**

**163. B.** Infraspinatus muscle. Well if there is a supraspinatus, there must logically be an infraspinatus. These two muscles live above (Supra) and below (Infra) to the "Spine" of the scapula.

**164. C.** Teres minor (**Minor** not major). The Teres major is obviously larger but lower down in the shoulder away from the rotator cuff complex. Number 5 in Mnemonics.

**165. D.** Subscapularis meaning it is under the scapular.

**166. A.** Number 1 is an oblique sagittal, Number 2 is an oblique coronal. An oblique sagittal shows the rotator cuff better end on. The angle of the oblique sagittal view should be orthogonal (90°) to the oblique coronal which is angled to the supraspinatus tendon found in the axial views. *See the Mnemonics section for more info on shoulder anatomy.*

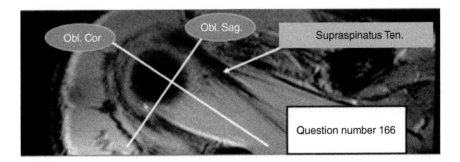

**167. C.**

**168. B.**

**169. A.**

170. C.

171. C.

172. B.

173. C.

174. C.

175. B.

176. D.

177. B.

178. A.

179. **C.** The portal vein. This is a delayed post gado coronal image.

180. B.

181. **C.** The is a small meniscus or "DISC" within the temporal mandibular joint.

182. **B.** Behind the TMJ's are the mastoid air cells.

183. C.

184. D.

185. C.

186. C.

187. A.

188. A.

189. C.

190. D.

191. B.

192. A.

193. C.

194. D.

195. **C.** "Dys" means difficulty whereas, **A** means not or none as in **A**pnea, not breathing.

196. **A.**

197. **C.**

198. **C.**

199. **C.** SEPTUM. Septum means a division or dividing membrane.

200. **D.**

201. **C.**

202. **D.**

203. **C.**

204. **A.**

205. **B.**

206. **D.**

207. **C.**

208. **A.**

209. **C.**

210. **A.**

211. **D.**

212. **C.**

213. **B.**

214. **A.** The 7TH. Cranial nerve is anterior to the 8th in the axial plane. An easy way to remember it is remember the soft drink: "7-Up." Number 2 in Mnemonics.

215. **C.**

216. **B.**

217. **C.**

218. **D.**

**219. B.**

**220. B.**

**221. B.** The 5th cranial nerve or trigeminal is affected by Bell's palsy. Number 2 in Mnemonics.

**222. C.**

**223. A.**

**224. D.**

**225. D.**

**226. D.**

**227. D.**

**228. A.**

**229. C.**

**230. D.**

**231. B.**

**232. A.**

**233. D.**

**234. B.**

**235. A.**

**236. C.**

**237. A.**

**238. C.**

**239.** True.

**240. B.**

**241. D.** All ventricles have choroid plexus. Choroid plexus makes CSF. It enhances with IV Contrast.

**242. A.**

243. C.

244. C.

245. B.

246. B.

247. D.

248. B.

249. A.

250. B.

251. D.

252. C.

253. C.

254. D.

255. A.

256. A.

257. A.

258. A.

259. D.

260. D.

261. C.

262. A.

263. C.

264. A.

265. B.

266. A.

267. D.

**268. D.**

**269. A.** The S/I joints.

**270. B.** Gluteus muscle. There are three pairs of gluteal muscles: Maximus, Medius, and Minimus. The larger is of course the maximus with minimus being the smallest. Hopefully they would not get that nit-picky that you need to know the difference. General knowledge is the key here. A radiologist needs to know the difference between the 3.

**271. B.**

**272. A.**

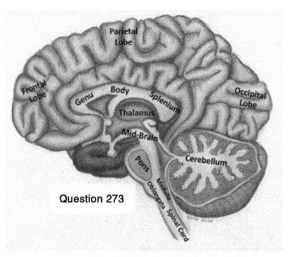

Question 273

**273. B.** Pons. The pons is the middle portion of the brain stem. The upper most is the mid-brain, pons is the middle and is the fattest/thickest, and narrowing down into the medulla oblongata the uppermost portion of the spinal cord.

**274. A.**

**275. C.**

**276. D.**

**277. D.**

**278. A.**

**279. D.** Dose is 0.2 ml/kg OR 0.1 mmol/kg.

**280. C.**

**281. C.**

**282. C.**

**283. C.**

**284. A.**

**285. B.**

**286. D.**

**287. C.** C is the best answer. A has T1 factors so fat would be bright but it is dark, B maybe with T2 factors, and D has conflicting contrasts: Short TR for more T1 and a long TE for more T2. Which is it?

**288. C.**

**289. A.**

**290. C.**

**291. B.**

**292. C.**

**293. B.**

**294. D.** Medial malleolus. The tibia is medial, bigger, and the weight-bearing bone in the lower leg. The fibula is lateral. Easy way to remember: The FibuLa has an **L** in it so think: Lateral.

**295. A.**

**296. C.** The articular surface of the talar bone is curved and sometimes referred to as the talar dome.

**297. B.**

**298. C.** A STIR sequence works very well for detecting bone marrow edema.

**299. C.** STIR. T1 weighting shows it well, T2 will show it a bit better, but STIR is usually the go-to sequence for marrow edema. T2 Fat Sat will also show edema very well.

**300. B.** AC JOINT.

**301. A.** SUPRASPINATOUS number 5 in the Mnemonics section.

**302. B.**

**303. C.** Subscapularis: Sub means under, so it is under the Scapula: SUBSCAPU-LARIS.

**304. B.** Coracoid: (MNENOMIC: NOID, COID, NOID). Number 8 in Mnemonics.

**305. D.**

**306. C.**

**307. C.** Sigmoid or "S" shaped like the sigmoid colon.

**308. D.**

**309. A.** Superior Sag. Sinus.

**310. B.** If there is a "superior" something, there will more than likely be an "inferior" something.

**311. B.**

**312. A.**

**313. D.**

**314. B.**

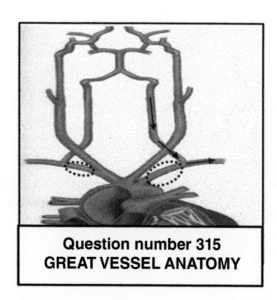

**Question number 315**
**GREAT VESSEL ANATOMY**

**315. B.** In a subclavian steal, due to possible pathology (circled) in *either* of the subclavian arteries, blood flows the wrong way (Retrograde) in the vertebral artery to supply blood to the arm.

**316. C.**

**317. A.**

**318. A.**

**319. C.**

**320. A.**

**321. C.**

**322. A.**

**323. A.**

**324. A.**

**325. A.**

**326. D.**

**327. D.**

**328. D.**

**329. A.**

**330. C.** Also known as the intraventricular septum.

**331. B.**

**332. A.** Fovea capitis. The fovea capitis ovoid depression in the head of the femur that serves as an attachment for the ligamentum teres or teres ligament. *** Here is one of those questions where you need to let the answers answer the question for you. *** You may want to answer with fovea capitis, but what if that is not one of the choices. Teres ligament is the next best answer. Pick that one. Tell them what they want to here.

**333. D.**

**334. B.**

**335. B.**

**336. A.**

**337. D.**

**338. A.**

**339. D.**

**340. B.**

**341. A.** The A/C-P/C line (above) is used by some facilities. These two anatomical landmarks give a more consistent angle for positioning axial slices. This is important for the patient who is having serial exams during treatment.

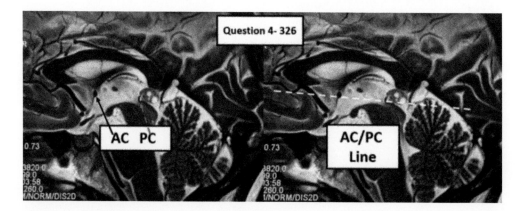

Question 4- 326

AC PC

AC/PC Line

**342. C.** Angle coronal slices perpendicular to the temporal lobe as shown below. Visualization of the temporal lobes is a staple in the work up for seizures. Typically, Hi-Res. T2 and T2 FLAIR coronals are performed to evaluate for sclerosis of medial aspect of the temporal lobes a.k.a. mesial temporal sclerosis. Mesial is another term "Medial."

**343. C.**

**344. B.**

**345. A.**

**346. D.**

**347. B.**

**348. B.**

**349. C.**

**350. B.** External rotation puts tension on the subscapularis, so it is easier to distinguish.

**351. C.**

**352. C.**

**353. C.** The 5th C.N.

**354. B.**

**355. C.**

**356. C.**

**357. D.**

**358. A.**

**359. D.**

**360. D.** Shortening the scan time will almost always affect I.Q. ↓ the TR can change the image contrast or if shortened enough cause tissue saturation (Chapter 3), ↓ the Phase: loss resolution and cause truncation (Chapter 12), ↓ nex/acq and lose SNR (Chapter 11).

**361. B.** When motion, (Breathing/Cardiac/Pulsatile) all of which are both repetitive and periotic, the artifact is seen as/at regular intervals in the phase encoding direction. This is especially well demonstrated on long TR/TE sequences.

**362. D.**

**363. D.**

**364. B.**

**365. B.**

**366. D.**

**367. B.** True. If the artifact consistently in the image, then simply repeating the sequence with a swap in phase and frequency will place the artifact in a different direction and location.

**368. D.**

**369. C.** Aliasing, Wrap, and Fold-over are all interchangeable terms for the same thing.

370. **C.** A superiorly placed Sat. band will not help in this case where wrap is left/right. An increase in phase only lengthens scan time and lowers the SNR. Increasing the FOV will lessen or eliminate the artifact but will lower the image resolution.

371. **C.** Anterior/Posterior.

372. **A.**

373. **B.** See Chapter 12 specifically about Wrap and the Nyquist theorem.

374. **C.**

375. **D.** While scanning perpendicular to flow in the vessel is of prime importance in an MRA, of the given choices/answer C is the best choice.

376. **C.**

377. **B.**

378. **A.** Small and SQUARE pixels are always your friend. They lessen the Gibbs/Truncation artifact.

379. **A.**

380. **D.**

381. **C.**

382. **B.**

383. **B.**

384. D

385. **A.**

386. **A.**

387. **C.**

388. **C.**

389. **D.** The chemical shift artifact can be rather subtle just like here in this image.

390. **D.**

**391. C.** Fat Sat will eliminate the artifact but changes the image contrast. A swap of phase and frequency only places the artifact in a different direction but does not reduce or eliminate the artifact.

**392. C.**

**393. C.**

**394. B.**

**395. A.**

**396. D.**

**397. B.** Entry slice phenomenon. Due to the very short TR/TE, you are seeing a time of flight effect before the blood saturates.

**398. B.**

**399. D.** The artifact is called either di-electric effect or standing wave.

**400. B.**

**401. D.**

**402. D.**

**403. C.** You would not see an OOP TE effect **(EVER)** on a SE or FSE sequence because of the effects of the 180°. The 180(s) ALWAYS put the Transverse NMV in phase at TE. Even if you select an "OOP" ms TE in a SE, you still would not see/get the OOP or Opposed TE effect. The lack of a 180 in GREs allows the NMV to be OOP at TE, so you will see that OOP effect.

**404. B.** False.

**405. B.** False.

**406. A.**

**407. C.**

**408. C.**

**409. D.**

**410. C.**

**411. D.**

**412. A.**

**413. A.**

**414. A.**

**415. D.**

**416. C.**

**417. C.**

**418. C.**

**419. B.**

**420. C.**

**421. C.**

**422. C.**

**423. B.**

**424. A.** A, C, D, G. Annifact is signal from outside the FOV that gets mis-mapped to inside the FOV. **A: Less Coils** to acquire less signal from outside the FOV. **C: Sat pulses** causes tissue outside the FOV to give little to no signal. **D: Swapping** Phase/Freq places the artifact in another place or direction. **G: Over-sampling** will correctly/fully sample and place the signal in the correct location.

**425. C.**

**426. B.** When the pixels are large and there is also a sharp contrast between two tissues you can get Gibbs/Truncation artifact. By making increasing the scan matrix (go from 192 × 320 to say 256$^2$) this will lessen the artifact. Making the pixels smaller and squarer will lessen the Gibbs/Truncation artifact.

**427. C.** The conus medullaris is the lower/lowest portion of the spinal cord. In the vast majority of patients, it is at the level of L1/2. During fetal development, the cord is actually attached down in the sacrum. At some point that attachment releases and as we further develop the cord (conus) ends up at the L1/2 level. In a tethered cord, that attachment does not release and as the child grows the cord never retracts up to its normal/common position.

**428. C.** Scar tissue has a richer blood supply than an intervertebral disc, therefore it will enhance 1st with the disc enhancing about five minutes later.

**429. A.** Flow types include: Laminar, Turbulent, Vortex, and Stagnant.

**430. B.** Coronal

**431. C.** The vertebral arteries join to form the basilar artery. It enters the skull via the foramen magnum anterior to the brain stem feeding the cerebellum. The major vessels off the basilar are the posterior cerebral arteries.

**432. B.**

**433. C.**

**434. B.**

**435. C.**

**436. C.**

**437. C.**

**438. B.** This is a common question. This pair of openings (two of them) are called The Foramen of Monroe. The lateral ventricles each have one foramen draining into the 3rd ventricle.

**439. A.** They also love to ask this one. The aqueduct runs in the midline from the 3rd to 4th ventricle.

**440. C.** You see this all the time; you just do not know its name. Commonly seen on STIR sagittals.

**441. C.** When the pixels are large and there is a sharp contrast between two tissues, you can get Gibbs/Truncation artifact. By making increasing the scan matrix (go from 192 × 320 to say $256^2$) this will lessen the artifact. Making the pixels smaller helps.

**442. C.** The conus medullaris is the lower/lowest portion of the spinal cord. In the vast majority of patients, it is at the level of L1/2. During fetal development, the cord is actually attached down in the sacrum. At some point that attachment releases and as we further develop the cord (conus) ends up at the L1/2 level. In a tethered cord, that attachment does not release and as the child grows the cord never retracts up to its normal position.

**443. C.** Scar tissue has a richer blood supply than an intervertebral disc, therefore it enhanced 1st and the disc about five minutes later.

**444. A.** Flow types include: Laminar, Turbulent, Vortex, and Stagnant.

**445. B.**

**446. A.** Bone to Bone. Tendons attach Muscle to Bone.

**447. B.** The common iliac arteries. Femoral arteries come from the bifurcation of the iliac arteries.

**448. B.** The carotids and the basilar arteries feed the C.O.W.

**449. C.** The pituitary part of the endocrine system and is sometimes referred to as the "Master Gland" as it controls a rather long list of the body's endocrine functions. It regulates hormonal activity in multiple other endocrine organs and glands. The anterior portion or **Adeno Hypophysis** is key in producing ACHT the "Stress hormone" and prolactin affects your mammary glands and helps women make breast milk. Then, there is the posterior portion a.k.a. the neuro hypophysis which produced ADH to regulate the water balance in the body. The other big hormone from the **Neuro Hypophysis** is oxytocin used for lactation and child birth and human behavior. If you go back to the Mnemonics section and look at the mid-Line T1 Sag. image of the brain stem, and notice the pituitary gland. The word "Pit" is in the adeno hypophysis while the bright white tissue directly behind it is the neuro hypophysis. The neuro hypophysis is bright on a T1 as it has a high protein content from different hormones so has a short T1 relaxation time. The third portion the **Intermediate portion**, is seldom talked about. It controls skin pigmentation.

**450. D.** The supra-renal or adrenal glands.

**451. B.**

**452. B.**

**453. B.**

**454. D.** An alternative name for the manubrium is the gladiolus.

**455. C.** The name "Ala" is an older name but still valid. Ala actually means a flat or wing-like process especially that of a bone.

# MRI Math

Figuring out math equations is not something we do on a routine basis while scanning, but you should have a basic understanding of it. This is a base knowledge you will need when you sit for the MR Advanced Registry. Demonstrated will be:

- Larmor Equation
- SNR from nex
- Scan time formulas
- Pixel size and Voxel Volume
- Bandwidths Conversion
- In and Out of Phase TE's
- Dixon Math
- SNR and 3D Sequence
- Match the scan time formula
- Let's do some Math

## The Larmor Equation

The most important number you need to know in MRI is the gyromagnetic ratio of hydrogen. It is 42.57 MHz at 1 T. **It is a constant, it never ever changes.** Some texts round it number up to 42.60. This number is the precessional frequency of hydrogen at 1 T.

Larmor equation:

$$\text{Gyromagnetic Ratio}(\gamma) \times \text{field strength}(B_0) = W_0$$

$$W_0 = \gamma B_0$$

*MRI Registry Review: Tech to Tech Questions and Answers*, First Edition. Stephen J. Powers.
© 2021 John Wiley & Sons Ltd. Published 2021 by John Wiley & Sons Ltd.

# The Larmor Equation Examples

$$\gamma \times B_0 = W_0$$

at 0.5 T: $42.57 \times 0.5 = 21.28$ MHz
at 0.7 T: $42.57 \times 0.7 = 29.79$ MHz
at 1.5 T: $42.57 \times 1.5 = 63.87$ MHz
at 3 T: $42.57 \times 3 = 127.71$ MHz

There is also a couple of more ways the Larmor equation can be displayed: These are a bit obscure but still valid.

$$F = \gamma B_0$$

$$W_0 = \gamma / 2\pi B_0$$

# SNR from Acquisitions or NEX or NSA

The SNR increases with the square root of the number of nex. What's a nex or average? A NEX or NSA is how many times you fill the k-Space with *concurrent* TRs. 1 nex, fills each line once (1 line for each TR), 2 nex: fill line 1 with TRs number 1 and 2, line 2 with TRs number 3 and 4, line 3 with TRs number 5 and 6. See the pattern developing?

If you say "I doubled my nex from 1 to 2, my scan time doubled but not my SNR." Why? As I stated in Chapter 11 of Tech to Tech Explanations, signal is thought to be a "constant" which means we generate a certain amount of signal with each acquisition while noise is at a **random** or inconsistent level in the background of any electronic system. Noise may be lower on one acq, and higher the next and maybe even higher still on a third. If you average out the SNR of all the nex, it comes out to the square root of the number of nex.

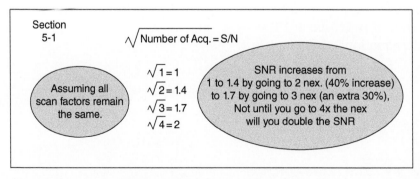

Figure 5.1 Signal to noise changes with the square root of the number of acquisitions.

**There are only three scan time formulas to know:**

2D, 3D, and FSE / TSE

A lot of people stress about this topic. **First, get the basic spin-echo scan time formula down. Practice it.**

Memorize the Basic Scan Time formula

**TR × phase steps × nex = scan time in ms. Then ÷ 60 000.**

The math will give you a big number which is the *scan time in ms*. Now you need to convert the scan time in ms to minutes.

Take that big number of ms and divide it by 60 000. **What is 60 000?** It is the number of ms in 1 minute. You need to break the scan time into minutes. 1 second is 1000 ms. This step is needed to convert ms into minutes. Now you have a scan time in minutes. Something like 3.65 minutes or 4.7 minutes.

Next, keep the minutes (3:), and multiple the 0.65 by 60, this will equal the scan time seconds. The final answer for a scan time of 3.65 minutes is 3 : 39. (3 minutes and 39 seconds.)

## Scan Time Equations

**Example: Conventional 2D SE Sequence**

- 500 ms TR × 192 Phase steps × 2 nex = 192 000 ms
- 192 000 ÷ 60 000 = 3.2 minutes
- 3.2 minutes = 3 minutes and 2/10ths of a minutes.
- 0.2 × 60 seconds = 12 seconds.
- The answer is a 3 : 12 seconds scan time

## Now for Turbo or Fast Spin Echo

FSE has an Echo train so that needs to be factored into the 2D SE equation.

- **TR × phase × nex = scan time in ms, divide by the ETL.**
- Example: 5000 TR, 192 Phase, 2 nex, and an ETL of 7.
- 5000 × 192 × 2 = 1 920 000 ms
- 1 920 000 ÷ 7 = 274 285 ms
- 274 285 ÷ 60 000 = 4.57 minutes

- 60 seconds × 0.57 = 34 seconds.
- Answer: 4.57 minutes = 4 : 34 minutes.

Convert 10ths into seconds. You will need to practice!!

The last equation is for **3D**. (A **2D sequential** equation uses the same math as the 3D.)

## 3D Sequence or a 2D Sequential Scan Time Formula

Uses the basic scan time formula **but you need to factor in the number of partitions or Locs (locations).**

Example: Conventional 3D Sequence

- TR × Phase × nex × **partitions** (or locations) = scan time.
- 36 × 192 × 1 × **64** = 442 368 ms.
- 442 368 ÷ 60 000 = 7.37 minutes
- 60 seconds × 0.37 = 22 seconds
- Answer: 7 : 22 seconds of scan time

How about a 2D sequential? **Sequential** is the key word here. A 2D TOF MRA of the Carotids is a sequential sequence so use the 3D equation.

- TR × Phase × nex × number of slices = scan time in ms.
- Yes, that is right, **it is exactly the same as the 3D.**
- 45 × 224 × 1 × 75 = 756 000 ms
- 756 000 ÷ 60 000 = 12.6 minutes
- 60 × 0.6 = 36 seconds.
- Answer is 12 : 36 minutes.

What about an inversion recovery sequence?

**If asked an IR sequence, do not use the TI. It is not in the basic scan time formula.**

If you are studying for the registry, I highly suggest that you practice these formulas. The scanner figures it out for you, so do the math for yourself and see if it matches.

Here are a couple of what ifs or FYI's on scan time questions.

1) You could be asked what is the scan time in ms (milliseconds). In this case, just figure out the time and do not break it down to minutes and seconds. Look at the FSE math on the preceding page, your answer for a question like this would be 274 285 ms.

2) Sometimes they do not want you to break it down into minutes and seconds, just minutes. So again, for the FSE sequence previously shown, the answer would be 4.57 minutes. Not 4 minutes and 57 seconds, but 4.57 minutes.
3) Careful, they could put in both answers: 4.57 and 4 : 57. Slow down and be sure of your answer you choose.

## Resolution: Pixel Size

To figure out pixel size, divide the FOV by the scan matrix. The equation is: **FOV ÷ Matrix = Pixel size**. This math will give you pixel dimensions of width and height.
Example:

- A FOV of 250 or 25, and a matrix of 256×256 ($256^2$).
- 250 ÷ 256 = 0.97 mm in each direction, 0.97×0.97 mm. Which is a square or **Isotropic** pixel.

**What about a not square matrix?**

- 250 FOV with a 192×256 matrix.
- 250 ÷ 192 = 1.3 mm.
- 250 ÷ 256 = 0.97 mm.
- The pixel size is 1.3×0.97 mm. This is an **Anisotropic** pixel.
- Newer scanners calculate pixel size for you, but *I still suggest you practice this math.*

Fig 14-2

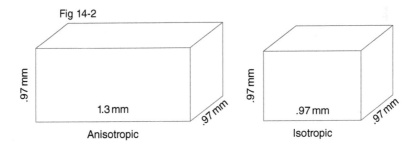

.97 mm    1.3 mm    .97 mm
Anisotropic

.97 mm    .97 mm    .97 mm
Isotropic

## Voxel Volume

There is a pretty good chance you will be asked to calculate the volume of a voxel. Recall that a Voxel is a Pixel with a Slice Thickness, as the third dimension. To find voxel volume: multiply Height by Width by Thickness. Here is the math for an **Isotropic** 0.97 voxel:

- 0.97 mm × 0.97 mm × 0.97 mm = a 0.91 mm³ voxel volume.

## Anisotropic Voxel Volume

- $1.3 \times 0.97 \times 0.97 = 1.22$ voxel volume.
- **Isotropic Voxels are ideal for 3D reformatting.**

## In-plane Resolution

A tricky kind of question is to ask "the in-plane resolution" of a sequence. You may be given all the scan factors, TR, TE FOV, Matrix Flip Angle, etc. The slice thickness is mixed into the scan factors. The "In-Plane Resolution" is the slice thickness. Nothing more, nothing less.

## How to Convert Hz/Px to MHz

If you work on multiple vendor systems like many of us, going back and forth is difficult enough terminology wise. A common difficulty is Hertz per Pixel (Hz/Px) and Megahertz. Hz per Pixel is just that: the number of Hz (frequencies) in each pixel while the MHz is the number of Hz (frequencies) across the FOV. They are basically the same. Know that increasing Hz/Px is the same as increasing the MHz, both widen the bandwidth which results in a: lower SNR, shortens the minimum TE, and decreases the Chemical Shift artifact.

If you really want to do the math:

- Take the Hz/Px and multiply by the Frequency Matrix.
- Then divide by 2.
- Move the decimal point over to the left three places.

For example:

- $172\,\text{Hz/Px}$ times 256 (frequency matrix) $= 44\,800$.
- $44\,800 \div 2 = 22\,400$.
- Move decimal point over three places $= 22.40\,\text{kHz}$.
- $172 \times 320 = 55\,040$.
- $55\,040 \div 2 = 27\,520. = 27.520\,\text{kHz}$.

## In and Out of Phase TE's

Where do those numbers come from? The IP and OOP TE's that we use vary by field strength. If you have been scanning for a while, you have them memorized as 2.2, 4.4, and 6.6 ms at 1.5T and 1.1, 2.2, and 3.3 ms at 3T. They are probably saved into the scan protocol, all is well.

In truth, those TE's are defined by an equation. This equation is seldom if ever mentioned but here it is.

**The 1st In phase TE is : $1/(3.5\,\text{ppm} \times PF) \times 1000$.**

## In and Out of Phase TE's

What's this 3.5 ppm? In the Artifact Chapter, I explained Chemical Shift. 3.5 ppm is the numerical difference or shift in PF's between fat and water. It means that for every 1 million rotations, 1 000 000 that water does, fat does 3.5 less or 999 996.5 rotations.

Example:

- $1/3.5 \times 63.86 \times 1000 =$ **1st In-phase TE in ms.**
- First step is: multiply $3.5 \times 63.68$, this equals 223.51, next, divide 1 by 223.51.
- $1/223.51 = 0.004\,46$, now, multiply by 1000 or just move the decimal point over three places, your choice.
- $0.004\,46 \times 1000 =$ **4.46 ms is the first in phase TE.**
- **To find the first Out of Phase TE:** (Standard method.)
- Take the 1st IP TE and divide by 2, add the 1st IP TE.
- $4.46/2$ which $= 2.23$, then add that to the first IP TE. $4.46 + 2.23 = 6.69$ ms is the OOP TE.

It is not really that hard, try it a few times, you will get it.

Now for the non-standard method:

**To find the first Out of Phase TE: non-standard.**

At 1.5 T we now use the 1st OOP TE of 2.2–2.3 ms, this is because years back, gradients were not as fast as they are now so the 1st OOP TE obtainable was 6.6 ms. A 2.2 ms TE was not possible back then. **A general rule on OOP TE's:** is when acquiring a dual echo seq. like in the Adrenals, always acquire the OOP first and the IP second. That is because of a signal loss as the TE gets longer. As a quick reminder: At 1.5 T, the protons are in Phase at 0 ms (we cannot image there), dephase to out of phase by 2.2 ms, become in phase again at 4.4 ms, out of phase at 6.6, and in phase again at 8.8 ms. Do you see a pattern developing there?

## Dixon Math

The Dixon technique is a way to get Fat Sat-like images at low fields. It is not a true Fat Sat, just fat sat-like images. This is done mathematically by adding or subtracting the In and OOP echoes.

You would not be doing this math while sitting at the console, but I want you to see the basic math done behind the scenes by the scanner.

As a reminder, the Dixon technique evolved from not being able to get good fat-Sat at magnetic fields at 0.7 or lower.

The sequence acquires two echoes, an **In** and an **Out** of phase then does some math with them to give you four different contrasts:

(i) An **In-Phase**, (ii) An **Out of Phase**, (iii) a **Water-only** image which shows signal from tissues with a lot of water, and (iv) a **Fat-only** image which shows high signal from tissues that contain a lot of Fat.

## Dixon Math

1) $IP = (water + fat)$
2) $OOP = (water - fat)$
3) $Fat\ only = IP - OOP = (water + fat) - (water - fat)$
4) $Water\ only = IP + OOP = (water + fat) + (water - fat)$

## SNR and the 3D Sequence

A 3D sequence, with all factors being the same, has a higher SNR than a 2D sequence. It also has a better resolution owing to its thinner slices or locations. There are a number of ways to describe the "slices" in a 3D. First, think of a 3D slab as a very big thick slice divided into lots of little slices. These little slices are referred to as: Partitions, Locations, Loc's, or slices. Now the math.

SNR in a 3D increases with the number of locations or partitions. You may have noticed that the SNR in a 3D goes up as you add slices? Either another slab or slices. Scan time goes up as well but so does the SNR increases with more slices. The SNR gain/loss is the square root of the number of partitions. Figure 5.2 depicts an axial slab and the effects of changing the partition or slab thickness.

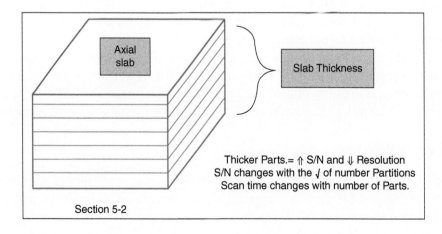

Axial slab

Slab Thickness

Thicker Parts.= ⇑ S/N and ⇓ Resolution
S/N changes with the √ of number Partitions
Scan time changes with number of Parts.

Section 5-2

Figure 5.2 Think of a 3D slab as a big thick slice. That slice is divided into "Partitions" or "LOCS" by an additional Slice Select Gradient. 3D sequences inherently have higher SNR and Resolution compared to a 2D sequence.

## SNR and the 3D Sequence

SNR of a 3D: The $\sqrt{}$ of 36 = 6. The number 6 really means nothing **YET.** Let us think of the "6" as a baseline or 100%. If you need more coverage and increase your partitions to 64, then the $\sqrt{}$ of 64 = 8. That is about a 35% **increase** in SNR. Obviously 8 is more than 6.

The number "6" we got from the math does not really mean much until you compare it to the "8," we got from adding partitions to the 3D. That math I just did is just shows you how the number of slices or partitions in a 3D will affect the SNR of the sequence. The SNR goes up in a 3D with the addition of partitions because you are making the slab thicker. Just like a 2D sequence, when you make the slices thicker, you increase the SNR because you are making the pixels bigger and there are more protons in a thicker slice.

Adding slices to a sequential 2D sequence **DOES NOT increase SNR.** It only makes the sequence longer. More slices, more work for the scanner, more work means a longer scan time.

Making the slices thicker in a 2D will _____ the SNR and _____ the Resolution. (Just had to ask one last question)

## Match the Scan Time Formula to the Sequence

TR×phase×nex = scan time, ÷ ETL, ÷ 60000 _____
TR×phase×nex = scan time, ÷ 60000 _____
TR×phase×nex×number of slices = scan time, ÷ 60000 _____
TR×phase×nex×number of partitions = scan time, ÷ 60000 _____
   A) Spin-echo
   B) Fast-spin
   C) Inversion recovery
   D) 3D
   E) 2D sequential

Answers at the end of this section

**Let us practice some math on the sequence below.**
Number 1: TR 4521, TE 102, Flip angle=90°, FOV 235 mm, 224×256 matrix, Head coil, ETL = 17, 25 5 mm thick slices, 3 nex or acq =, with no gap between slices.

1) What is the scan time in ms? _____
2) What is the scan time in minutes? _____
3) What is the scan time in minutes + seconds? ___
4) What is the pixel size? _____
5) What is the voxel volume? _____
6) What is the in-plane resolution? _____
7) Is the TE an in-phase or out of phase TE? _____
8) Explain your answer for Question 7.
9) Is the above sequence a 2D or a 3D sequence?
10) How many millimeters of coverage will this sequence give you?
11) What weighting is the sequence?

# Answers for Sequence Number1

1) 178 712 ms
2) 2.97 minutes
3) 2 : 58
4) 1.04×0.97 mm
5) 5.04 mm³
6) 5 mm
7) It is neither in or out
8) The sequence is an FSE (the Echo train), you do not/ cannot get an IN or OOP echo. You only get IN or OOP echoes with Gradient echo. This is a tricky question.
9) 2D. A 3D would list the number of "Locs or Partitions." While some vendors do have 3D FSE sequences, they are fairly new (a few years) to MRI. When "Slices" are stated, it usually means a 2D sequence.
10) 125 mm's: 25 slices × 5 mm = 125 mm's
11) T2

**Let us do some math on sequence number 2 below.**
Number 2: TR 35, TE 6.6, Flip angle = 75°, FOV 275 mm, 256×256 matrix, Head coil, 45 3 mm thick sequential locations with a 20% overlap, 1 nex or acq=, 1.5 T scanner, MRV in the pelvis.

12) What is the scan time in ms? _____
13) What is the scan time in minutes? _____
14) What is the scan time in minutes + seconds? ___
15) What is the pixel size? _____
16) What is the voxel volume? _____
17) What is the in-plane resolution? _____
18) Is the TE an in-phase or out of phase TE? _____
19) Explain your answer for Question 7.

20) Is the above sequence a 2D or a 3D sequence?
21) How many millimeters of coverage will this sequence give you?
22) Where should the saturation pulse be placed?
23) Are the pixels isotropic?

## Answers for Sequence Number 2

1) 403 200 ms
2) 6.72 minutes
3) 6 : 43
4) $1.07 \times 1.07$ mm
5) 3.68 mm³
6) 3 mm
7) Out-phase
8) The sequence is an GRE, at 1.5T the first out-phase TE is 2.2 ms, the 1st in-phase TE is at 4.4 ms, the next OOP is at 6.6 TE.
9) 2D. The overlap of the slices gives it away. 2D MRA sequences have overlap of the slices where as a 3D would overlap the slabs if there were more than one.
10) 108 mm's: 45 slices × 3 mm = 135 mm's. Then take 135 and subtract 20% for the overlap = 108 mm.
11) The saturation pulse should be placed superiorly (above the slices) to saturate the arterial blood flowing down the aorta and iliac arteries.
12) Yes, isotropic pixels have the same dimensions in both directions. The voxel is not however isotropic. It does not have the same dimensions in all three directions. The dimensions from sequence number 2 are 1.07 × 1.07 × 3 mm.

## Sequence/Scan Time Matching Answers

TR × phase × nex = scan time, ÷ ETL, ÷ 60 000 **B: FSE or TSE**
TR × phase × nex = scan time, ÷ 60 000 **A: Spin-echo**
TR × phase × nex × number of slices = scan time, ÷ 60 000 **E: 2D Seq**
TR × phase × nex × number of partitions = scan time, ÷ 60 000 **D: 3D**
** The IR option was meant to trick you. An IR sequence has a TI, **but TI is not part of any of the scan time formulas** so do not use it. Do not try to force it into one. Your math will be very wrong.

# Glossary

**2D sequence** When Fourier transform is applied in two directions – phase and frequency – for image production.

**3D sequence** Fourier transform is applied in three directions – slice, phase, and frequency. The third dimension in 3D comes from the slice select gradient, which is applied in a varying amplitude just like the PEG. This requires a third calculation for image processing, hence the name 3D.

**Acceleration factor** Relates to using a "parallel imaging" technique in order to scan faster. As the acceleration factor is made higher and higher, scan times are made shorter and shorter. Faster scan times come at the expense of signal to noise and resolution.

**Acquisition/nex/NSA** All three mean the same thing. They are vendor-specific terms for how many times the k-spaces are to be filled: 1, 2, or 3 times.

**Active shim** An electronic adjustment to the main magnetic field.

**ADC map** An extra set of images produced that shows an acute cerebrovascular accident (CVA) as dark. A corresponding area on the b-1000 should be bright.

**Adiabatic** In thermodynamics, an adiabatic process is one in which no heat is lost or gained by a system. In MR, adiabatic RF pulses in an inversion recovery sequence more precisely excite or invert (180°) tissues with less heating so SAR is less of a concern.

**Aliasing (also known as Wrap or Fold-over)** Happens when there is tissue outside of the field of view in the phase direction. Tissue outside the field of view is not sampled enough to satisfy the Nyquist theorem and is misplaced on the opposite side of the image.

**Analog** In MRI, the echo that forms at TE is considered an "analog" signal. It is displayed or pictured as a continuously varying and physically decreasing sine wave. The array processor cannot work on a sine wave so the echo (a sine wave) is converted into numbers for conversion to the image.

**Analog to digital converter (ADC)** The signal received in the coil

*MRI Registry Review: Tech to Tech Questions and Answers*, First Edition. Stephen J. Powers.
© 2021 John Wiley & Sons Ltd. Published 2021 by John Wiley & Sons Ltd.

is analog. It is converted into numbers by the ADC.

**Angiogenesis** A physiological process in which new blood vessels form/develop from pre-existing vessels, much like the root system of a plant that continues to develop. Angiogenesis is common in pathological tissues (tumors).

**Anisotropic** When referring to a pixel, if the pixel is not square (e.g. 1 mm × 1 mm), then the pixel is anisotropic.

**Annifact artifact** Artifact caused by signal from outside of the field of view due to having too many coils turned on.

**Arterial spin labeling (ASL)** A proton density weighted sequence that can give perfusion-like information without an injection of IV gadolinium-based contrast. It gives the relative cerebral blood flow (rCBV) for an area of interest.

**Artifact** An area or point in the image(s) that contains false information or data. There are many causes of image artifacts, as outlined in Chapter 12. FYI: All images have artifact(s) of some sort from some cause or reason. Artifacts cannot be eliminated; they can only be minimized/lessened.

**Axial plane (also known as the "Z" plane)** Assuming the patient is head first and supine, axial slices transect the patient from head to toe.

**b-Value or b-Factor** In diffusion weighted imaging, the "b" value is relative to the **strength and/or duration** of the diffusion gradients being applied for the sequence. The higher or greater the b-value, the more sensitive the sequence is to decrease cellular diffusion. For example, a 500 b-value is less sensitive to a stroke in the brain than is a 1000 b-value.

**$B_0$** The main magnetic field. It is also known as the longitudinal field, and sometimes termed "B-naught" (naught = zero). It is also called the Z axis.

**$B_0$ (image)** In DWI, image acquired without DW gradients applied. Basically, low-resolution T2 weighted images.

**$B_1$** The RF field applied for slice selection and refocusing. The RF flips the protons into the transverse plane.

**Bandwidth (B/W)** In MRI, bandwidth is a range of frequencies. There are two different bandwidths: Receiver B/W, which is taken while sampling the echo; and Transmitter B/W, which is a range of frequencies that excites a slice.

**Big three (The)** Local and main magnetic field inhomogeneities, and magnetic susceptibility.

**Bird cage coil** A coil type similar to a saddle coil where the anatomy is placed inside of the coil for imaging. It may slide over the anatomy or close over the top.

**Black blood** An SE sequence with an RF pulse specifically used to make blood appear black on the images. A similar effect is often seen on CSE sequences where the blood has moved out of the slice and been replaced by "unexcited" blood. Unexcited tissue cannot give signal. This effect is often referred to as a "flow void."

**Blood brain barrier (BBB)** A semipermeable matrix of tissues and fibers that only lets certain molecules and drugs into the brain. Gadolinium is one such molecule that **will not cross** an intact BBB. Pathology such as tumors and infection will make the BBB a less effective barrier and will allow gadolinium to cross and be taken up by the abnormality.

**Body coil** Typically refers to the large "inherent" or internal transmit/receive RF transmitting coil located inside the bore of the scanner.

**Bound protons** A group or pool of protons that are tightly bound/attached to another molecule and are not able to be "flipped" by an RF pulse. They will not give any signal at TE. Hydrogen protons in cortical bone, tendons, or ligaments are bound.

**Brownian movement or motion** An erratic/random movement of microscopic particles that results in collisions with other molecules in a surrounding medium. In other words, water and other intracellular chemicals are moving within, into, and out of the cell. Equate this to "bumper cars" at an amusement park. If the cells are perfused, there is energy to move around; if they are not perfused, the energy is shut off and the bumper cars stop moving.

**Cartesian coordinates** The X, Y, Z coordinate system of localization. It is used to locate a point relative to a fixed reference. In MR, that fixed reference is isocenter, whose coordinates are 0, 0, and 0. The coordinates specify each point along a plane as set by numerical coordinates, which are assigned distances along the three fixed perpendicular planes.

**Cellular respiration** A process in which cells combine oxygen and nutrient molecules and use the chemical energy from these substances to perform activities such as discarding waste products, carbon dioxide, and water.

**Center frequency (CF)** The precessional frequency of the center slice of a stack or slab.

**Center lines (of $k$-space)** Those lines in the middle or center portion of $k$-space. The center 25% of lines in k-space contribute close to 90% of an image's contrast.

**Centric k-space filling** A filling scheme that fills the center lines first for maximum image contrast. The outer lines are filled last. This scheme is often used in contrast MRA or dynamic imaging studies.

**Cerebral spinal fluid (CSF)** Fluid surrounding the brain and spinal cord. It has the highest PD of all human tissue as it is mostly water. Urine is a close second.

**Chemical saturation or "Chem Sat"** When a specific chemical (tissue) like fat or water is targeted with RF pulses to not give signal at TE. A fancy name for fat-sat.

**Chemical shift** The frequency difference between fat and water.

**Chemical shift artifact** An artifact seen in the frequency direction. A black border is seen on one side of a structure, a white border on the other. It is caused by narrow receiver B/Ws. There are really two kinds of chemical shift artifact. The first is chemical shift as described above. The second kind is also known as the OOP echo, where there is a black line around all tissues in both the phase and frequency directions.

**Cine loop** A series of MR images acquired rapidly and repeatedly like an MR movie. Also known as "real-time."

**Circle of Willis (COW)** The major "cross roads" of connections for all the major arteries supplying blood to the brain. It is comprised of the anterior, middle, and posterior cerebral arteries.

**Coil(s)** A generic term in MR for a loop or loops of wires that collect the signal produced at the TE. Some coils are designed for very specific purposes or more general imaging.

**Collapsed images** All scanners produce these. When an MRA sequence has finished running, a set of images, usually an anterior/posterior (A/P), superior/inferior (S/I), and right/left (R/L), are processed by the scanner. Collapsed means that all the slices or locations are projected as one image. You might say that they are stacked up onto one another as if you were looking at all the data at once. It is a quick way to check image quality in the form motion and coverage. These images are truly the "MIPs" (MIP stands for maximum intensity projection). Basically, it is showing you all the bright pixels (maximum intensity) in one projection. See "Maximum intensity projection" for more information.

**Concatenations (Acquisitions)** A number that is input to allow you to use a lower TR to maintain image contrast. It can let you halve the TR. It can also be used to shorten a breath-hold

in chest/abdomen/pelvis studies. Example: 30 slices needs 1000 ms to acquire at 1 concat, but 2 concats lets you use a 500 TR. Fifteen slices are acquired in 500 TR, the other 15 slices in another 500 TR. In another example, a 42 second breath-hold at 1 acquisition becomes two 21 second breath-holds with 2 acquisitions.

**Conjugate symmetry of k-Space** There is symmetry or redundancy in $k$-space which is a fundamental property for Fourier transformation. Basically, one only needs half the data to characterize any place in k-space. This means that if there is a +2X3Y data point, then because of the symmetry in k-space there will be a −2X3Y data point. This symmetry can be taken advantage of to fill lines of $k$-space without actually scanning them.

**Contrast** A difference in signal intensities between tissues.

**Contrast-enhanced MRA (CE-MRA)** IV contrast is injected, and data acquisition is timed to contrast reaching the target vessel(s).

**Contrast to noise ratio (CNR)** Amount of contrast over the level of noise.

**Contrast triangle** A visual depiction of the three different topics or concerns to that contribute to image quality: contrast, signal to noise, and resolution.

**Conventional spin echo (CSE)** 90°, 180°, followed by an echo.

**Corduroy artifact** Artifact resulting from a single or multiple "spike" (abnormally high signal amplitudes) in the data causing the classic "corduroy" look to the image. There are several causes of these "spikes."

**Coronal plane** Assuming the patient is head first and supine, the coronal plane transects the patient A/P. The "Y" direction.

**Cross-excitation** Often used synonymously with cross-talk. Cross-excitation happens when two or more slices cross each other. The common tissue of the slices is seen as dark as the common tissue has not had time to T1 relax and is actually saturated to a point. This artifact is commonly seen posterior to the cord in lumbar spine images.

**Cross-talk** This artifact was more common many years ago. Basically, the RF profile of one slice had some RF in common with the slice next to it. Slice A would excite a little bit of slice B, signal in slice B was a little bit less. Slice B excited a little bit of slice C and so on. Putting a gap between slices is the most common way to eliminate this artifact.

**Cryogen** A substance capable of producing very low temperature(s).

**dB/dT** Rate of change (d) of a magnetic field (B) over change (d) in time (t). This indicates how fast the gradient field changes over time.

**Decay curve** A T2 curve. A graph depicting a number or volume of protons that have left (de-phased) the X/Y plane over a given time. Typically, two curves are shown in order to compare a fast-decaying tissue against a lower decaying tissue. Protons will stay together (be in phase) in the X/Y for only a short period of time. Signal quickly begins to decay. See also "Relaxation curve."

**De-phasing** The act of protons getting out of sync with each other.

The direction of de-phasing is a function of the main magnetic field. De-phasing can be recovered by two methods: a 180° refocusing RF pulse or a magnetic gradient application.

**Diamagnetic** A substance with no permanent magnetic dipole such as water, nickel, or bismuth, that, in the presence of an external magnetic field, sets up an opposite magnetic field to that of the external field. This means it is mildly repulsed by a magnetic field. Diamagnetic substances have unpaired electrons, which is the opposite of "paramagnetic" substances that have unpaired electrons. Gadolinium is a paramagnetic material.

**Dielectric effect or Standing wave artifact** This is often seen at 3 T but it can happen at any field strength. It is related to the wavelength of the RF at 3 T having a propensity to "bounce back" or echo out. One RF is bouncing back out while a second is coming into the anatomy. They cancel each other out, causing the classic area of signal loss. Two waves exist at the same time, hence the name "standing wave."

**Diethylenetriamine pentaacetate (DTPA)** A chelating agent with multiple uses in metal-containing diagnostic agents such as MRI contrast agents, and nuclear medicine scanning. It is a synthetic compound that can sequester (bind to) metal ions and form highly stable DTPA–metal ion complexes. Bonding to the gadolinium molecule makes it too large to get through an intact BBB, but big enough to be taken out of the blood stream by glomerular filtration.

**Diffusion** At the cellular level, the act of a cell moving nutrients, waste, and water in and/or out through its membrane. Diffusion requires energy in the form of a blood supply to the tissue.

**Diffusion weighted imaging (DWI)** An echo planar type of sequence where the image contrast comes from differences in tissue diffusion. DW imaging is a staple sequence in brain imaging for stroke.

**Digital to analog converter (DAC)** The RF pulse instruction from the computer to the radio frequency power amplifier (RFPA) is numeric. The DAC converts numbers to analog so the RFPA can transmit the RF. This works opposite to the way the ADC works. They do not oppose each other; they just have two separate and different jobs.

**Dixon method or technique** A method of producing fat-sat images at low field strengths. It has recently become popular at high fields. An IP and OOP echo are acquired and mathematically manipulated to produce four different contrasts: IP, OOP, fat, and water images.

**Driven equilibrium (DE, also known as DRIVE)** This uses an extra +180° then a −90° set of RF pulses at the end of the echo train to force, drive, or accelerate T1 relaxation.

**Duty cycle** A statement on gradient performance that is sequence dependent. It is a percentage of time that the gradients are able to work at their maximum strength. A 95–100% duty cycle is to be expected in most of the modern high-field scanners.

**Dynamic susceptibility of contrast (DSC, also known as Perfusion)** DSC is often performed in the brain to aid in the planning of treatment for a stroke or CVA. It requires a rapid injection of IV contrast with repeated rapid sets of images of the brain. That is the **"dynamic"** part. The **susceptibility** part is taking advantage of the "metallic" properties of the contrast as it reaches the brain. As the gadolinium reaches and "perfuses" the brain, signal in the brain will decrease. Portions that are not perfused will not decrease in signal. Tissues that are not being perfused very well will take longer to decrease in signal. DCS studies show which tissues are either perfused, not perfused, or poorly perfused. See also "Perfusion weighted imaging." **Terms associated with DSC or perfusion studies include:**

  ▪ **Mean transit time (MTT):** The **average** (mean) time it takes for the contrast to reach (wash in) and exit (wash out) the region of interest (ROI). Basically: How long does the gadolinium hang around in the tissue?

  ▪ **Time to peak (TTP):** The time it takes for the gadolinium bolus to reach its highest concentration, causing maximum signal loss in the ROI.

  ▪ **Relative cerebral blood flow (rCBF):** A red, yellow, and blue colored map showing red as high flow, yellow less, and blue even less flow. Important in stroke evaluation, it is a qualitative representation of the amount of blood flow in the tissue.

- **Relative cerebral blood volume (rCBV):** A similar color map as in rCBF and used most often in tumor evaluation/characterization. It is a qualitative representation of the amount of blood in the tissue.

**Echo (also known as the TE)** Where a signal is induced in the coil by the effects of a refocusing mechanism.

**Echo planar imaging** An imaging technique where a complete "planar" image (slice) is obtained with one selective excitation pulse.

**Echo spacing (ES)** The time in ms (milliseconds) in between echo formation. Typically, the first TE (the minimum TE) is also the echo spacing. Echo spacing in spin echo sequences is about 10 ms or lower. A low ES is desirable to decrease blurring. Factors affecting ES are: FOV, receiver B/W, and frequency matrix.

**Echo train balancing** The ideal of "echo train balancing" is to have the effective TE be the center or middle echo of the echo train. This will place the effective TEs in the center of k-space for the best image contrast.

**Echo train length (ETL)** In turbo or fast spin echo imaging, multiple echoes are produced during the sequence. The number of echoes can vary from as low as two to 24 or even more. The number of echoes produced is called the ETL. The ETL has an effect on image contrast. Short ETLs are used for T1 weighted imaging with an ETL of 2–4, while T2 weighted contrast images often have an ETL of 18–24 or more. The more echoes, the more T2 contrast is placed into the k-space. RF exposure (SAR) increases with longer ETLs.

**Effective TE (ETE)** In fast or turbo spin echo sequences, multiple echoes are produced per TR. The echo chosen for the image contrast is said to be the "effective TE." The effective TEs will be placed in the center lines of k-space during the run of the sequence.

**Elliptical centric k-space filling** In MRA sequences, the center lines are filled in an outwardly spiraling direction starting from the center and moving outward.

**Equilibrium** A state or condition of a "system" in which all parts have the same temperature. Equilibrium occurs in MR, when, over a sufficient amount of time (ms), the tissues have released all of their RF energy into the lattice.

**Ernst angle** A flip angle that produces the maximum signal in a tissue for a particular TR. At a constant TR (e.g. 500 ms), SNR increases with higher and higher flip angles, but only to a point. At a certain flip angle, the Ernst angle, tissue starts to saturate (not enough time to T1 relax) and signal begins to decrease. Ernst angle sequences are more often used at 3 T than at 1.5 T. This is because SAR is a concern at 3 T and getting good T1 contrast can also be a challenge at 3 T. Ernst angle sequences can give better T1 contrast than conventional SE sequences.

**Estimated glomerular filtration rate (eGFR)** See "Glomerular filtration rate" for additional information.

**Excitation pulse** The initial application of RF to push the longitudinal NMV to a certain angle into the transverse, e.g. 90° for a SE, or 20° for a GRE. **Note:** The RF pulse does not have a "flip angle" in it; the amount of "flip" or "tip" is a function of the amount of time the RF is applied. **A 180° pulse means the RF is applied for twice as long as it was for a 90°.** Excitation is sometimes symbolized as α.

**Exponential ADC map (eADC map)** In DWI imaging, a calculated image set used to further exclude T2 shine through. The calculation is the $B_0$ divided by (÷) the DWI image.

**Faraday cage** Copper lining in the ceiling, walls, and floor of the scan room to keep external RF out and the RF transmitted during a sequence in the scan room.

**Faraday's law of induction** A law of physics where a magnetic field moving through or past a conductor will induce current in that conductor.

**Fast Fourier transform (FFT)** A numerical algorithm to compute a discrete Fourier transform for a sequence. Fourier transform converts signals from their original form into a representation in the frequency domain. It breaks down a group of frequencies into the individual frequencies.

**Fast spin echo (FSE) or Turbo spin echo (TSE)** A variation on the spin echo pulse sequence where multiple echoes (more than one), called an echo train, are produced per TR in order to decrease scan time. Scan time decreases as a function of the ELT.

**Fast spoiled gradient recalled (FSPGR)** The FSPGR sequence uses an RF pulse to "spoil" residual transverse net magnetization vectors. Hear SPGR, think T1 weighted GRE.

**Fast recovery, Drive, or Driven equilibrium** In spin echo and FSE imaging, there will be some residual transverse net magnetization (long T2 tissue vectors). Given enough time, these vectors will relax equilibrium on their own. This, though, takes time. Fast recovery or DRIVE uses negative polarity RF pulses to force or drive the vectors back to longitudinal.

**Fat saturation** (fat-sat, F/S) There are several methods to decrease signal from fat-containing tissue. Fat-sat uses RF pulses **specifically tuned to the precessional frequency of fat** which are applied at the beginning of the pulse sequence. Consequently, fat has received multiple RF pulses and is rendered unable to give much signal at TE. Often abbreviated as F/S or FS.

**Fat suppression** As in a STIR sequence, signal from fat is suppressed by the application of an inversion pulse, waiting an appropriate amount of time in ms (the TI) before beginning the pulse sequence. The affect is that fat (and other short T1 relaxing tissues) is able to give very little signal at TE.

**Ferrous** Containing a percentage of iron and so forcibly attracted to a magnet (**nonferrous** means having little to no iron content and not attracted by a magnet). Common ferrous materials are hair pins (bobby pins and paper clips). These common objects can and will be pulled into the scanner. MR-safe wheelchairs are made of "nonferrous" material such as aluminum which is not attracted to a magnet.

**Field of view (FOV)** Analogous to the film size in X-ray, this is the area to be scanned in the slice select direction. It is assumed to be square (200 mm× 200 mm or 20 cm× 20 cm) unless otherwise stated as in a rectangular FOV. The FOV is a function of or comes from the FEG. A smaller FOV can cause the minimum TE to increase slightly. A small FOV needs a strong application of the FEG.

**Flip angle (F/A)** The angle or degrees away from longitudinal the NMV achieves from an RF pulse. This is a function of time that the RF is turned on. See "Excitation pulse." F/A can also be a function of the strength or amplitude of the RF application. A stronger pulse flips the protons over faster, which may allow a shortening of the TR and or the TE.

**Flow compensation (Flow comp, also known as gradient motion refocusing (GMR) or gradient motion nulling (GMN))** A series of gradient applications applied before TE to compensate for loss of signal from flow, or to reduce pulsatile artifacts.

**Flow-related enhancement** A newer term used interchangeably with TOF MRA. Think of it this way: the vessel's **enhancement** is **related** to its **flow**.

**Flow types** Flowing blood can be categorized or described by four basic types: laminar = normal; vortex = jet like; turbulent = tumbling; and finally, stagnant = very slow to not flowing at all.

**Flow void**
A very commonly used description of a lack of signal in a blood vessel(s). This is meant to state/indicate that the lack of signal in a vessel is due to flowing blood. This is synonymous with high-velocity signal loss (HVSL). Both of these terms indicate that excited blood has moved out of the slice before the TE.

For example: On CSE and FSE sequences where blood has moved out of the slice, it is replaced by "unexcited" blood at the TE. Unexcited tissue cannot give signal. This effect is often referred to as a "flow void."

**Fluid attention inversion recovery (FLAIR)** A variation on a spin echo sequence used in the brain and spine to suppress signal from CSF.

**Fold-over** Another name or term for the artifact wrap.

**Fourier transform** An algorithm used to divide or separate the frequency components of an echo from its various amplitudes as a function over time. Fourier transform is vital to all modalities, and especially in MRI. Signals received by coils in MRI are a complex of periodic signals made up of a large number of different frequencies (the bandwidth). Fourier transform represents/breaks down data over its frequency axis. An MR spectroscopy image is a simple example in which different molecules are at different frequencies along an axis.

**Fractional echo or Partial echo** When only part of or a fraction of the echo is sampled at TE. Most often this is done when acquiring a CE-MRA sequence in order to save time (shorten the TR).

**Free induction decay (FID)** A signal generated by the excitation RF pulse.

**Free protons** Protons that are not tightly affixed to another structure or molecule. They are "free" to be flipped by an excitation pulse and can therefore contribute to the signal at TE. Almost all protons in the body are "free," examples are those in muscle, liver, brain, and bone marrow. See also "Bound protons."

**Frequency** This has more than one meaning in MRI. Frequency as related to RF is the number of times something repeats or occurs in a given period of time. It can also be referred to as "temporal frequency." Temporal is an adjective relating to "time." Radiofrequency (RF) is measured by units of Hertz (Hz). This is equal to one occurrence, oscillation, or repetition per second. Megahertz (MHz) means Million Hertz or million repeats. 63 MHz is 63 million oscillations per second.

**Frequency direction** One of the three cardinal directions in MRI. The other two are phase and slice.

**Frequency encoding** This happens after the refocusing event. As the protons rephase, the FEG is applied while the echo is sampled.

**Frequency encoding gradient (FEG)** Gradient applied during the TE. Sometimes symbolized by $\nu$ (nu).

**Frequency matrix** The number of pixels in the scan matrix in the frequency direction. This is also the number of times the echo is sampled. A higher frequency matrix may cause the TE to lengthen. Remember that the more work is asked of the scanner (more frequency encodes), the more time it will take. In this case, asking for more samples of the echo, the FEG has to be left on for a longer period of time.

**Fringe field** In MR, a weaker surrounding magnetic field that gets stronger as one gets closer to the scanner/bore. The equivalent to "scatter radiation" in X-ray.

**Gadolinium** A rare earth metal with seven unpaired electrons that help protons lose energy (T1 relax) that was acquired from the RF pulses. Gadolinium is considered "paramagnetic" because of the unpaired electrons.

**Gamma** Term for the gyromagnetic ratio of hydrogen. Symbol: $\gamma$.

**Gauss** A unit of magnetic strength where $10\,000\,G = 1\,Tesla\,(T)$.

**Generalized auto calibrating partially parallel acquisition (GRAPPA)** A parallel imaging method in which the center lines of $k$-space are fully sampled while the outer lines are "under-sampled," thus saving time. There is a slight loss in resolution with this method.

**Ghosting artifact** A vague repeated duplication of a structure in the phase direction. It is caused by repetitive motion from the heart, or respirations. It is a motion artifact but should not be confused with gross patient motion.

**Gibbs artifact** Commonly substituted with truncation, Gibbs artifact commonly comes from extremely anisotropic pixels. If the phase matrix is less than half the frequency matrix, Gibbs artifact will occur. See also "Ringing artifact."

**Glomerular filtration rate (GFR)** A number that indicates how well a patient's kidneys are working (or if they are failing). The estimated (eGFR) calculation that is performed uses the factors of age, gender, race, and a current serum creatinine. The "e" means it is an estimate, which also means there can be a significant margin for error.

**Glutamate/Glutamine (Peaks)** Glutamate and glutamine are two brain metabolites and indicate neuronal transmitters.

**Gradient** A gradient is a hill. In MRI it indicates an "magnetic hill" that is high (strong) on one side, and weak on the other.

**Gradient echo or Gradient recalled echo (GRE)** One of the two pulse sequences in MRI. It is characterized by an excitation pulse without a refocusing pulse. It uses a gradient pulse to refocus the protons.

**Gradient magnetic fields** These are time-varying magnetic fields applied to the static magnetic field. They temporarily and selectively change the strength of the main magnetic field.

**Gradient warp** When imaging at the edge of a gradient uniformity, the image is seen as warping or bending. Gradients need to be linear, constant, and reproducible. Imaging out near the end of a gradient's limit for linearity is where the IQ starts to suffer.

**Grey matter (GM)** The more superficial layer of brain tissue that contains mostly nerve cell bodies and few myelinated fibers and therefore appears grey on dissection. Compare with "White matter."

**Gyromagnetic ratio (GMR)** A mathematical constant in the Larmor equation. Its value is 42.57 MHz for hydrogen at 1 T. See "Larmor equation."

**Half Fourier** Uses $k$-space symmetry to interpolate data points and fill $k$-space faster. Is also called complex conjugate symmetry.

**Half Fourier acquired single shot turbo spin echo (HASTE)** Half of the data is acquired with one excitation pulse, the other half with a second RF excitation pulse. Basically, the two single shots are then interleaved or combined.

**Hard shim** Shimming is used to make something level. In MRI, to shim is make the magnetic field uniform. A hard shim is a permanent adjustment to the field via small pieces of aluminum attached inside the bore.

**Helium (He** An inert (not flammable) naturally occurring gaseous element.

**Helmholtz coil** A pair of coils designed to generate a uniform signal from the tissue in between them.

**High-velocity signal loss (HVSL)** Lack of signal in a vessel due to moving (flowing) blood. Excited blood has moved out of the slice before the 180° and gives no signal at TE. Synonymous with, or used instead of, "Flow void."

**Hunter's angle** A term used when speaking about spectroscopy. Dr. Hunter, a neurologist, would look at a spectroscopy, and if a line drawn from the *N*-acetyl aspartate (NAA) peak to the creatine-choline peaks was about 45°, that spectroscopy was likely normal.

**Image quality (IQ)** An image with good tissue contrast, SNR, and resolution is said to have good "image quality or IQ." Other aspects of good image quality can include being free of artifacts and well positioned to demonstrate the desired anatomy.

**In phase (IP)** There are two definitions: (i) In a GRE sequence when the **TE** is at a time in ms when the fat and water vectors point in the same direction, thus adding up to make the overall SNR higher. This is opposed by the out of phase (OOP) TE when vectors point in opposite directions. Signal will drop. (ii) When protons of all tissues are all pointing in the same direction they are said to be "in phase."

**In-phase echo** An "in-phase" echo is when both fat and water vectors are pointing in the same direction within a pixel. They combine their signal and the pixel(s) becomes brighter.

**In-plane saturation** In an MRA sequence, this refers to the loss of signal from blood due to the blood flowing in the slice or slab (the plane) for too long. That blood has received many RF pulses and begins to "saturate" just like the background tissue. Contrast between the vessel and the background is lost.

**Internal auditory canal/Internal auditory meatus (IACs/IAMs)** The foramen in the petrous portion of the sphenoid bone from which the seventh and eighth cranial nerves exit.

**Inversion** When a set of vectors is flipped or inverted from its original position (e.g. 0° flipped to 180°) by an RF pulse.

**Inversion pulse** Usually a 180° RF pulse that flips the NMV halfway around. Vector ↑ gets hit with a 180° and becomes vector ↓ as a STIR or FLAIR sequence.

**Inversion recovery (IR)** A pulse sequence that allows suppression of tissues by varying the TI in the sequence. See "Inversion time." An inversion recovery sequence contains three RF pulses: 180°, 90°, and 180°. TIs or inversion times, measured in milliseconds (ms), can be changed from short to long depending on which tissue is to be suppressed.

**IR prep** An 180° (inversion) RF pulse (or pulses) is applied in order to "prep" tissue(s) to either enhance or suppress signals from certain tissues by varied TIs. If you think about it, STIR and FLAIR can be considered IR-prepped sequences. If the base sequence is a 3D spoiled gradient echo (SPGR), the TI can be varied to enhance grey/white matter (GM/WM) differentiation or actually suppress WM to increase tissue conspicuity between WM and multiple sclerosis (MS) plaques.

**Isotropic** When referring to a pixel, if the pixel or voxel is square (e.g. $1 \times 1 \times 1$ mm), then the pixel/voxel is isotropic.

**J-coupling** A quantum mechanics interaction between nuclear spins within the same molecule. A full explanation is beyond the scope of this book. In short, J-coupling is responsible for the modulation (multiplication) of the signal of fat during a fast spin echo sequence.

**k-Space** A temporary storage area for image data (raw data) prior to image processing. **k** is an arithmetic symbol that denotes frequency. A k-space is an imaginary entity that you cannot touch or see. It is a space to store k's or frequencies. There is one k-space per slice for that slice's raw data. There are multiple ways or methods to fill k-space.

**Lactate** A metabolite found in the brain. It is displayed on a spectroscopy image and is a marker of cellular death.

**Laminar flow** In a blood vessel, normal undisturbed or unobstructed flow of blood.

**Larmor equation** The equation used to find the precessional frequency of hydrogen at any field strength: Wo = $\gamma B_0$ where Wobble (Wo) or frequency, $\gamma$ is the gyromagnetic ratio of hydrogen at 1 T. This number is a constant. $B_0$ is the field strength of the magnet for which you are trying to find the precessional frequency. Example: Wo = $42.57 \times B_0$; Wo = $42.57 \times 0.75$ T; Wo = $31.91$ MHz.

**Larmor frequency** The precessional frequency (PF) of hydrogen at 1 T = 42.57 MHz.

**Lattice** The local environment to which protons give off or exchange energy in longitudinal relaxation. See "T1" relaxation.

**Linear filling of *k*-space** A k-space filling method that fills one line at a time. It is less efficient time-wise than the method used in fast/turbo spin echo.

**Logical gradients** The X, Y, and Z gradients do the three jobs of spatial encoding. Each one can do any job, but which one will do which job? This is the thinking or logical portion.

**Longitudinal magnetization** The net magnetization vector (NMV) that runs along the static magnetic field or Z direction. Its counterpart is the transverse NMV.

**Longitudinal plane** The north/south direction of the magnet. The $B_0$ or Z plane.

**Magic angle artifact** An artifact sometimes seen on T1 and PD weighted images. If a tendon is positioned at approximately 55° to $B_0$ and with a short TE, then high signal can be seen on the tendon mimicking pathology.

**Magnetic resonance spectroscopy (MRS)** A sequence that allows a determination of the concentration of different metabolites in a specific region of interest. Different disease processes have different concentrations of metabolites.

**Magnetic susceptibility** A measure of a tissue' or substance's ability to be magnetized. Air cannot be magnetized whereas soft tissues can be magnetized.

**Magnetization prepared (MP, or Mag prepped)** The use of an RF pulse before the start of a sequence in order to either null signal from a tissue or to enhance a tissue's contrast.

**Magnetization transfer (MT)** A technique with an off-center RF pulse used to decrease the signal from a tissue, thus increasing conspicuity of another. Very commonly used in brain MRAs to decrease signal from the background white matter, thus brightening blood vessels.

**Main magnetic field (MMF)** Also known as $B_0$.

**Matrix** A term to describe the resolution of an image. The matrix is an array of rows and columns, each having a direction: phase and frequency. A scan matrix of $256 \times 256$ $(256^2)$ means that there are 256 pixels in both the phase and frequency directions. Pixel size is determined by the FOV and the scan matrix.

**Maximum intensity projection (MIP, also known as collapsed images)** We all call the "cut-outs" we do of the vessels from an MRA data set an "MIP." They are not. That is a misnomer. "Cut-outs" is a bit more accurate, but "MIPs" is and what has been used for a long time so that is what we call them. Scanners have post-processing programs that allow us to "cut out" or remove background/low-signal intensity structures from MRA data sets to better see blood vessels. You want to see just the "maximum intensity" (bright pixels) structures (i.e. the blood vessels. See "Collapsed images" for more information.

**Metabolites** Chemicals that are produced in the brain as a result of cellular activity. Normal brain tissue has a certain amount/level of the various metabolites. Metabolite levels will change (raise/lower) in the presence of different disease processes or conditions.

**Metal artifact** Metal inside the FOV causes the precessional frequencies to drift off the center frequency determined by the scanner during pre-scan. This, in turn, causes an area to be unable to be imaged.

**Metal artifact reduction series or sequence (MARS)** A generic non-vendor-specific term for adjusting a sequence's scan parameters to lessen the metal artifact in the images. Any scanner can be adjusted to scan with this series of parameter adjustments. Factors adjusted are: echo train length, receiver B/W, and TE.

**Minimum intensity projection (Min. IP)** A post-processing program used to display or project pixels with the **least** or **minimum signal intensity**, usually blood vessels. It is used in reformatting 3D susceptibility weighted images or sequences. These sequences are specifically done looking for the presence of blood or petechial hemorrhage post trauma or post operatively.

**Minimum TE (Min. TE)** The shortest possible TE obtainable after excitation and refocusing. There are several scan factors that can affect the Min. TE such as the FOV, frequency matrix, slice thickness, and receiver B/W.

**Moiré fringe artifact** Artifact caused by several things on a steady-state GRE sequence, usually from wrap combining with magnetic field inhomogeneities, especially at the edge of the FOV.

**Motion artifact** Artifact always seen in the phase direction because the phase direction is encoded many times during the course of the sequence, causing the associated "smearing" in the phase direction.

**Multiple overlapping thin section angiography (MOTSA)** In MRAs, having blood in the slice or slab for as short a time as possible in order to minimize in-plane saturation. To lessen the effects of in-plane saturation, several thin slabs or sections are positioned so that they overlap. Overlap is vital. You do not want to miss any of the vessel.

**Multi-shot** When multiple TRs are required to fill a $k$-space for a slice. This is what is being done for the vast majority of imaging in MR. See also "Single shot."

**Nephrogenic systemic fibrosis (NSF)** A possible consequence of the breakdown of the bonds between the gadolinium molecule and its chelating agent, leading to free gadolinium radicals being released into the body. Fibrous tissue can form in multiple locations in the body related to the reaction to the presence of gadolinium.

**Net magnetization vector (NMV)** The sum of many small vectors adding up into a larger vector.

**Nex/NSA/Acq** Vendor-specific terms or acronyms stating the number of times each k-space will be filled (e.g. 2 "nex" means that each line is filled twice before filling the next line, example: line 1 is filled twice, then line 2 gets filled twice, followed by line 3 being filled twice).

**Noise** Something that is present in all electronic equipment. It is low-level meaningless random signal that detracts from image quality. It is the second factor in the signal to noise ratio equation. Ideally there is more signal received by the coils than there is noise.

**Non-Cartesian** Describes k-space filling. Cartesian filling is "line by line"

and has been the most common method for filling $k$-space since MRI began 30 or more years ago. In the last 10–15 years, other methods of filling k-space have evolved and are in wide use. Some of these other non-Cartesian methods include elliptical centric (spiral), radial (blade like), and rectilinear, common in EPI sequences.

**Nonferrous** A quality of a metal meaning that it contains little to no iron and thus is not attracted toward a magnetic field.

**No phase wrap (GE), Phase oversampling (Siemens), Fold-over suppression (Philips)** Sequence options to eliminate or minimize the artifact called wrap, aliasing, or fold-over.

**Null point** A term referenced when describing IR sequences. The null point is determined by multiplying a tissue's T1 relaxation time by 0.69. This math determines what TI to use to suppress signal from a tissue. For example, the T1 relaxation of fat is approximately 230 ms at 1.5 T, so $230 \times 0.69 = 158$ ms. If the TI is set to 158 ms, signal from fat will be nulled. If you know the T1 time of a tissue, do the math, set the TI and suppress signal from that tissue. In Chapter 6, I referred to the null point as the transverse plane. My description showed the NMV of fat and water T1 relaxing during the sequence. Here, whatever tissues were in the X/Y or transverse plane (null point) at the end of the TI would be suppressed.

**Nyquist theorem** An important principle in digital signal processing (sampling) stating that a sine wave or signal needs to be sampled at twice its frequency to be accurate or "faithful."

**Orthogonal** At 90° to another plane. Analogous to a P/A and lateral view chest X-ray. The lateral view is orthogonal to P/A.

**Outer lines** In *k*-space, these edge lines contribute mostly to an image's resolution or edge detail and only a small percentage to image contrast.

**Out of phase (OOP) TE** In a GRE sequence, if the TE is such that fat and water vectors within a pixel are pointing in opposite directions, signal in that pixel will be decreased. At 1.5 T, the vectors are out of phase every 2.2 ms, so OOP at 2.2 ms, in-phase (IP) at 4.4 ms, OOP at 6.6 ms, and IP at 8.8 ms.

**Parallel imaging (PI)** The prime objective in parallel imaging is to image faster. The way to accomplish this is to sample fewer lines of phase. Sampling fewer phase lines comes at a price, which is SNR and resolution. There are several methods to perform parallel imaging, two of which are GRAPPA and SENSE. See "Acceleration factor" for additional information.

**Paramagnetic** If a substance has a small and positive amount of magnetic susceptibility (like gadolinium), it is considered "paramagnetic" and is weakly attracted to an external magnetic field. This quality can and will shorten the longitudinal (T1) relaxation time of a tissue. A property of paramagnetism is having unpaired electrons, which is the opposite of a diamagnetic material.

**Partial echo (also called Fractional echo)** This option is usually employed during a CE-MRA sequence. Here, only about three quarters of the echo is sampled. The reason for truncating (cutting) the echo is purely to save scan time.

**Partial Fourier** Related to symmetry of *k*-space. Slightly more than half the *k*-space is filled so a pattern in *k*-space is recognizable. The unfilled lines are filled with data discerned from the pattern in the filled lines.

**Partial volume effect** When a tissue appears less bright or less dark than it actually should be. When large pixels contain both bright and dark tissues, the resulting pixels will display as grey. A pixel's signal intensity is the average of all tissues inside of it. Fix: smaller pixels and/or thinner slices.

**Passive shim** See "Hard shim."

**Perfusion** When a tissue has a blood supply, you could say that it is perfused. Perfusion sequences are commonly performed in the brain during the workup process for a stroke.

**Perfusion study** See "Dynamic susceptibility of contrast."

**Perfusion weighted imaging (PWI)** Another name for DSC. Basically, like any other sequence or set of images, its contrast is based on or "weighted with" the perfusion of the tissues as IV gadolinium arrives and enters the tissues.

**Peripheral nerve stimulation (PNS)** A consequence of very rapid and intense magnetic field gradient applications. It actually comes from the rapid switching or alternating polarity of the magnetic fields. This rapid switching causes small amounts of current to form and flow in the nerves of the hands and feet while the sequence is running. PNS stops when the sequence stops.

**Permanent magnet** A type of magnet made up of many magnetic bricks so that, when aligned in the right orientation, their collective magnetic fields will add up to a strength great enough to be used for imaging.

**Phase** Describes the state or quality of an NMV. When all vectors/protons are pointing in the same direction, they are thought to be in phase. As they spread or fan out, they are thought to be de-phasing and signal drops.

**Phase conjugate synthesis** A mathematical premise that a number (scanned data in k-space) has an equal and opposite number value. Basically k-space is a mirror image of itself. This is the half or partial Fourier option to save time.

**Phase contrast (PC)** A GRE-based sequence used in MRA, MRV, CSF flow studies, and some cardiac exams.

**Phase encoding** In a pulse sequence, phase encoding happens in between excitation and refocusing. It puts each echo just a little bit more out of "phase" with the preceding echo.

**Phase encoding gradient (PEG)** A gradient applied between the 90° and the 180° RF pulses as part of spatial localization. The PEG and/or phase is sometimes symbolized as "$\varphi$."

**Phase over-sampling** An option used to decrease or eliminate the wrap artifact or aliasing. Aliasing is seen in the phase direction. The "over-sampling" means that extra lines of phase are sampled so that the tissue that is outside the FOV in the phase direction is "sampled" enough to satisfy the Nyquist theorem. Those extra lines are then discarded by the scanner and not displayed in the final images.

**Physical gradients** The X, Y, and Z gradients that make the classic noise during an MR sequence.

**Pixel** Is a two-dimensional picture element. A pixel's dimensions result when the FOV is divided by the scan matrix. A pixel's dimensions are width × height. Pixels are the smallest visible part of a digital image.

**Poor man's Fat-Sat** A way to lower signal from fat and other background tissue simply by increasing the flip angle (F/A) in a 2D TOF MRA sequence. Increasing the F/A while using a very short TR increases the contrast between the bright vessels and a dark background, which is a desirable effect in MRA studies. Note the key term here is "in a 2D TOF MRA." The same effect in a 3D TOF comes from using a ramped pulse.

**Post labeling delay (PLD) in arterial spin labeling (ASL)** This is the time from "labeling" the spins (actually exciting the arterial blood flow) with an RF pulse to the TE. "Labeled" spins entering tissues will cause a small amount of signal loss whereas tissue that is not perfused will be slightly brighter, a non-contrast perfusion study as it were. The PLD is a user-selectable value. A typical adult PLD is in the 1500–2000 ms range. As blood flow slows (i.e. in the elderly), the PLD should be increased to about 2500–3000 ms; with fast flow the PLD should be decreased to say 1000–1500 ms. These are general numbers/guidelines and are empirical. There are several factors that influence what PLD to use. These include of course age, cardiac output, the patient's hematocrit, and sickle cell anemia.

**Precession** Rhythmic gyrations or spins of a body (proton) around its axis like a spinning top. The angle off of its axis is a function of a torque or pulling from an external force, that force being the magnet.

**Precessional frequency (PF)** Sometimes symbolized as ω (omega). PF does not exist with the presence of $B_0$.

**Pre-scan** At the beginning of a sequence, the scanner will adjust or tune several critical things: the center frequency of the center slice, the transmitter gain (strength), and the receiver gain.

**Proton density (PD, also termed Hydrogen density or Spin density)** A tissue characteristic related to the number of protons in a $mm^3$ (cubic mm) for a given tissue (e.g. CSF vs. muscle). CSF has many more protons in a $mm^3$ than does muscle.

**Proton electron dipole interaction (PEDI)** Water protons attach to the free electrons in a gadolinium molecule, letting the water release its extra energy from the RF quicker than it normally would. The T1 time of water is shortened.

**Pulse sequence design or Line diagram (PSD)** A group of lines with symbols depicting RF and gradient applications over a time line.

**Quantum mechanics** A branch of physics centered on very small objects. The body of scientific laws describing the behavior of protons, electrons, and other subatomic particles.

**Quench** A sudden loss of the super-conductivity of the current in the magnet's coil. Loss of the cryogen causes resistance in the coil and magnetism is lost rapidly.

**Radial imaging** Often used when imaging the bile duct and gall bladder during an MRCP exam. Multiple thick slices are imaged at increasing (or decreasing angles), all having a common "pivot" point. These slices fan out like a wagon wheel.

**Radiofrequency (RF)** An oscillation rate of alternating electric current/voltage or electromagnetic field. The frequency range is from approximately 20 kHz (kilohertz or thousand hertz) to around 300 GHz (gigahertz or billion hertz).

**Ramped pulse** In a 3D MRA sequence, to lessen the effects of in-plane saturation, the RF pulse applied to the 3D slab has an increasing flip angle. This special kind of RF pulse increases the flip angle related to its position in the imaging slab. The idea of this higher flip angle is not to make the blood brighter, but to increase the saturation of the background tissue even further, which will increase the contrast between vessels and the background.

**Rapid acquisition with rapid excitation (RARE)** The original term that eventually became FSE/TSE.

**Raw data** This term for the MR tech typically refers to the images generated from the TOF MRA sequence.

**Real time** See "Cine loop."

**Rectangular FOV (Rec. FOV, sometimes called Phase FOV)** The FOV is square (e.g. 200 × 200 mm) unless otherwise stated, as in Rec. FOV (e.g. 150×200 mm). In order to save time, Rec. FOV does not scan all the lines in the phase direction as dictated by the scan matrix. Resolution is **not** affected as the scan matrix is not changed; it is just that fewer lines in the phase direction are scanned. For example, if phase is left to right in the brain, and the FOV in the phase direction includes some area without anatomy, this area (likely to be air) will not be scanned. SNR does/will decrease when using the Rec. FOV option.

**Refocusing pulse** The 180° pulse applied at half the TE and used to correct for magnetic field inhomogeneities and susceptibilities. The 180° pulse is placed "symmetrically" (halfway) between the 90° and TE.

**Region of interest (ROI)** When scanning an area of suspected pathology such as a soft tissue mass within a larger area, this is called the region of interest.

**Relaxation** In MRI, the act of the protons returning to a lower energy state (releasing energy) from the effects of an RF pulse. See also "T1" and "T2" relaxation.

**Relaxation curve** A graph depicting a number or volume of protons that have returned (regrown) to $B_0$ over time. Typically, two curves are shown in order to compare a fast-relaxing tissue to a slower-relaxing tissue. See also "Decay curve."

**Re-ordered k-space filling** In FSE or TSE where lines of k-space are not filled sequentially but in an order where ETE goes into center lines of k-space for best image contrast.

**Re-phasing gradients** These magnetic field gradients are used to refocus or re-phase a set of vectors much like the 180° RF pulse does in a spin echo pulse sequence. These gradients are applied in an equal and opposite polarity to the previous gradient to counter its effects. They are often used in "steady-state" GRE sequences. See "Rewinding gradients."

**Resistive magnet** A type of magnet that is a large coil of wire with current flowing through. The flowing current produces a magnetic field strong enough to be used for imaging. This type of magnet also produces heat as a result of resistance in the conductor.

**Restricted diffusion** Usually used to describe an area in the brain that is involved in or an evolving CVA. When brain cells have a good blood supply, they will diffuse in a normal fashion or rate. When the blood supply is interrupted, cells begin to run out of fuel and diffusion begins to slow down/stop. This is called restricted diffusion.

**Rewinding gradients** Another name for re-phasing gradients. These magnetic field gradients are used to refocus or re-phase a set of vectors much like the 180° RF pulse does in a spin echo pulse sequence. They are often used in "steady-state" GRE sequences.

**Ringing artifact** Sometimes exchanged with the term truncation. This is an "edge" or ringing artifact that looks like alternating black and white stripes. It is caused by sharp edges of high and low signal intensities as in the bright CSF and the dark cord in the spine. It can never be completely eliminated, only lessened. The fix is to increase the scan matrix.

**Rise time** How fast a gradient can get up to a required strength. It is stated in ms and can be anywhere from 0.4 ms down to a fast 0.1 ms. Overall, rise time is useless unless coupled with slew rate.

**Rupture view** View used when performing a breast study looking for a "ruptured" implant. The image contrast desired to see a ruptured implant changes with the type of implant. A saline rupture is easily seen with either a T2 fat-sat or STIR (sequence of choice is a radiologist preference). A silicone rupture view may require a STIR sequence to suppress fat, and a "water suppression" pulse which will leave only silicone to be bright on the resulting images. These two techniques are only stated as descriptions. Your department protocol should be followed.

**Saddle coil** A coil configuration in which one coil is placed on top of another surrounding the anatomy to be imaged.

**Sagittal plane** Assuming the patient is head first and supine, sagittals transect the patient from left to right. The "X" direction.

**Saturation** When a tissue receives too many RF pulses over a short period of time, that tissue loses its ability to generate signal because it has little time to T1 relax. Saturation usually means that a specific tissue such as fat was targeted with RF to give little signal.

**Saturation pulse (Sat Pulse, Sat Band)** An RF pulse applied either inside or outside the FOV, either for artifact control or to saturate one side of the vascular tree to null signal in blood vessels entering the slab or slice during an MRA/MRV.

**Sensitivity encoding (SENSE)** A parallel imaging method where individual coils are assigned to gather specific lines of $k$-space. Scan time decreases in relation to the number of elements in the coil. Wrap artifact can be an issue with this method.

**Sequential** In increasing (e.g. 1, 2, 3, 4) or decreasing (4, 3, 2, 1) order. Acquiring slices in said order.

**Short time (Tau) inversion recovery (STIR)** Variation on a spin echo sequence to suppress signal from short T1 relaxing tissues, usually fat.

**Signal to noise ratio (SNR, S/R)** Simply put, the amount of signal generated in the coils over an amount of background noise. Ideally there is more signal generated by the sequence than there is background noise in the system.

**Single shot** When imaging rapidly and all the lines of phase are filled in one (1) TR period from a single 90° RF excitation pulse.

**Slew rate** A statement of gradient performance which is a combination of rise time and maximum gradient strength. It is stated as Tesla/meter/second (T/m/s). Maximum gradient strength ÷ rise time = slew rate. A good slew rate is 150–200 T/m/s; average 100–120; low fields come in at around 50–60. Slew rate affects TR, TE, and echo spacing.

**Slice excitation** An RF pulse that excites a particular region of tissue into the X/Y plane, whether it be an axial, sagittal, coronal, or somewhere in between as an oblique. It is either a 90° RF pulse in a spin echo or a partial F/A in the case of a GRE sequence.

**Slice gap** An area in between slices that is not imaged. It is usually a small percentage of the slice thickness, about 10–20%.

**Slice refocusing** An RF pulse that refocuses or re-phases a slice's X/Y plane NMV.

**Slice select gradient (SSG)** Is the gradient applied during the RF excitation to produce either an axial, sagittal, or coronal slice.

**Smart prep/Fluoro trigger** Vendor-specific options/sequences to inject a bolus of IV contrast and initiate data acquisition when the bolus reaches the target vessel.

**Sodium pump** In cellular respiration, a living cell pumps or diffuses various chemicals and waste products in and out of itself to maintain homeostasis. The sodium pump requires a blood supply to perform this task.

**Spatial resolution** The ability to see or image a structure in "space." A fancy way of saying resolution.

**Specific absorption rate (SAR)** The amount of RF energy absorbed by the patient. It is measured in watts of energy per kilogram of body weight.

**Spectral attenuation (or adiabatic) inversion recovery (SPAIR)** Basically, a STIR sequence with the exception being that the 180° RF pulse is tuned to the PF of fat whereas in STIR it is not. The 180° RF pulse is also repeated several times during the TR to suppress fat better. In STIR, the 180° is a wide bandwidth RF pulse that excites the entire slice. The 180° in SPAIR excites only fat.

**Spectral inversion recovery (SPIR)** A STIR sequence in which the 180° is tuned to the PF of fat and is applied only once. SPAIR and SPIR are a bit more forgiving when doing fat-sat than a true fat-sat sequence when the FOV is large and/or off-center.

**Spin angular momentum** Protons spin on their axis like wobbling tops. Spin angular momentum comes from the proton's spin being pulled on by the magnet. The proton wants to spin upright; the magnet is trying to pull it down. The proton's "momentum" is altered.

**Spin echo** One of the two pulse sequences in MRI, the other being the GRE. Spin echo is characterized by a 90–180° RF pulse which then leads to an echo. The 90° RF pulse knocks the protons down into the X/Y plane; the 180° flips or spins them around. The resulting echo is called a "spin echo."

**Spoiled gradient echo (SPGR)** A T1 weighted GRE sequence. Vendor-specific names include BRAVO, MP-RAGE, LAVA, VIBE, VIBRANT, TRIVE, TIGRE, T1-FFE, SARGE, 3D-Fast FE, etc.

**Spoiling/Spoiled** Spoiling is a method to remove residual magnetization in the transverse plane. It is done with either an RF or gradient pulse.

**Spectroscopy** A sequence that is able to give a quantitative value for the concentration of metabolites. Spectroscopy is most often used in the brain to characterize brain lesions. See also "Metabolites."

**Spin-lattice** Protons heat slightly from the energy of an RF pulse. They give off this heat/energy to the surrounding tissues, known as the "lattice," in order to reach thermal equilibrium. Another name for T1 relaxation.

**Spin-spin relaxation** When a group of protons are spinning and interacting with each other and affecting the magnetic field between them, they will de-phase. This de-phasing from bumping into each other is called spin-spin relaxation, also known as T2.

**Stagnant flow** In a blood vessel, this is blood flowing at a very slow rate.

**Static magnetic field** The stationary (not time-varying) main magnetic field which is the heart of the MR scanner. It is sometimes referred to as $B_0$. Varying magnetic fields are the gradients.

**Steady state** Refers to the state of the NMV when the TR is shorter than both the T1 and T2 of a tissue. The transverse NMV stays at the F/A imparted by the RF so it neither increases nor decreases. It stays "steady."

**Subtraction** A post-processing function done either manually or automatically by the scanner where a "pre contrast" data set is subtracted from a "post contrast" set. The resulting set of images should be a representation of gadolinium-filled structures or tissue.

**Superconducting magnet** The most common type of magnet. It is a resistive magnet with the conductor bathed in a liquid cryogen that all but eliminates resistance in the conductor, allowing for much more current to flow and produce a stronger static magnetic field.

**Suppression** A tissue or tissues are purposely made to give less signal at TE. Usually done in an IR-type sequence through a combination of RF pulses and timing to allow more or less T1 relaxation. See also "Saturation."

**Surface coil** A flat RF receiver placed over or under an ROI.

**Susceptibility** The idea that something can be influenced by another and to what degree. Some human tissue (e.g. fat or CSF) is susceptible to a magnetic field whereas air is not.

**Susceptibility weighting imaging (SWI)** Obtaining image contrast based on susceptibility differences between tissues. There are some vendor-specific sequences that obtain these kinds of images. These sequences are EPI and are higher resolution than most EPI sequences. If you think of it, your basic GRE (T2*) sequence, run routinely in the brain, is susceptibility weighted. You are looking for blood/hemorrhage which causes a susceptibility artifact.

**Swap phase and frequency** There are three directions in an MR image: slice, phase, and frequency. In swapping phase and frequency, you change their directions by 90°. This is done to "move" an artifact, make motion go in a different direction, or take advantage of a rectangular FOV and decrease scan time.

**T1** Related to a relaxation rate. It is a logarithmic time constant for when 63% of a tissue has returned to (regrowing into) the longitudinal or $B_0$ (37% remains in the X/Y).

**T2** Also related to a relaxation rate. A logarithmic time constant for when 37% of a tissue's NMV are still in the transverse or X/Y plane after the excitation pulse has been turned off (think: 63% went back to $B_0$).

**Note T1 and T2 are completely independent of each other but occur simultaneously. Tissues T2 and T1 at the same time.**

**T2*** Always associated with a GRE sequence, T2* contrast comes from inhomogeneities in the main and local magnetic field. Basically, it is the contrast you get as a result of not having a 180° pulse cleaning up for the Big three. GRE axials in the brain are T2* and are used to look for blood.

**T2 shine through** In DWI imaging, tissues with a very long T2 relaxation time are bright (shine through) and do not represent areas of restricted diffusion. The long T2 times can mimic stroke. The eADC is sometimes used by the radiologist as a "tie-breaker" to differentiate between a CVA or some other pathology. The eADC map removes T2 shine through from a DWI image.

**Tau** Greek letter (T or τ) symbolizing time. 1 Tau = ½ the TE.

**Temporal resolution** The ability to image quickly over time. A dynamic CE-MRA is said to have high "temporal resolution."

**The Big three** Local and main magnetic field inhomogeneities, and magnetic susceptibility.

**Time of flight (TOF)** An MRA concept that images with very short TRs and TEs. The TR/TE times are shorter than the T1 relaxation time of the background tissue. Background tissues quickly saturate because of the short TR/TE and with fresh **unsaturated** spins entering the slice/slab, they give off more signal than background tissue. An alternative term for time of flight is flow-related enhancement.

**Time of inversion (TI)** The TI is stated in ms. Long TIs suppress long T1 relaxing tissue, short TIs suppress short T1 relaxing tissue.

**Time of repetition (TR)** The time from the 90° RF pulse that excites slice 1 to the next 90° that excites the same slice again.

**Time to echo (TE, also known as 2 Tau)** The time from the 90° to the 180° is 1 Tau, and from 180° to the echo is 1 Tau. 1 Tau + 1 Tau = 2 Tau. Time to echo is the time when the protons come into phase and generate signal in the coil.

**Timing bolus** In CE-MRA, filling the center lines of $k$-space at the same time the gadolinium bolus arrives at the target vessel is vitally important. A timing bolus sequence tells you how much time it takes for the gadolinium to get to the target vessel. See also "Smart prep/Fluoro trigger."

**Tissue saturation** When a tissue or tissues are exposed to RF pulses, they will want to "relax" after the RF to release the energy. If they are re-exposed to another RF pulse before sufficient relaxation has occurred, they will not be able to give off much signal at TE and are considered to be "saturated."

**Torso coil** A large receive-only surface coil used for imaging larger body parts such as the abdomen, pelvis, or long bones.

**Transmit/Receive (T/R)** A coil that can transmit an RF pulse as well as receive one. This kind of coil is different from coils that can only receive RF, not transmit RF.

**Transmitter bandwidth** Used in describing an RF pulse. A wide transmitter B/W contains many frequencies and will excite or refocus a wide or thick slice vs a narrow B/W which excites a thinner slice as it has fewer frequencies.

**Transverse net magnetization vector** The sum of vectors in the transverse plane or X/Y plane. It is at 90° to $B_0$. Sometimes the word "residual" is added to the beginning. This refers to how much transverse NMV is still in or left over in the X/Y plane after the TE. Its opposite or counterpart is the longitudinal NMV. This is what exists prior to excitation.

**Transverse plane (also known as the X/Y plane)** It is at 90° to the longitudinal or $B_0$.

**Truncation artifact** Often substituted or exchanged with Gibbs artifact. It is commonly seen where there is a high degree of signal intensity differences between tissues, as on sagittal views of the cervical spine. It looks like a zebra stripe. It is caused by the signal being sampled too slowly. If we could sample the signal continuously an infinite number of times, we would not get truncation artifact.

**Turbo spin echo (TSE)** A sequence where multiple echoes are acquired per slice per TR. Synonymous with "Fast spin echo."

**Tuning** The scanner is adjusting resonant frequency of the system components' receivers and transmitters to the Larmor frequency for the optimum signal return.

**Turbulent flow** In a blood vessel, this is a flow pattern that is starting to get/go back to normal. Vectors are "pointing" all over the place. Signal from this blood is less than that from laminar flow.

**Vector** A quantity of having both magnitude (amount) and a direction (Z or X/Y). Often represented by an arrow with its length proportional to its magnitude and pointing in a direction.

**Velocity encoding (Venc)** A user-selectable parameter in PC imaging referring to the speed of the tissue you want to image. The venc is the maximum velocity that will be encoded into the image. Venc is increased for fast-flowing blood and decreased for slow.

**Vortex flow** In a blood vessel, a tumbling, swirling pattern of flow. It results from the blood jetting through a stenosis. Signal from blood is rather low from this flow pattern when compared to that of laminar flow.

**Voxel** A three-dimensional picture element (pixel) that has height, width, and depth or thickness: $H \times W \times D$.

**Water excitation** A sequence that has excitation and/or refocusing pulses tuned to the PF of water. Fat is not excited, so gives no signal.

**Water saturation** A sequence that starts out with RFs tuned to the PF of water for saturation. See also "Fat saturation."

**Water suppression** Usually talked about when performing spectroscopy. The precessional frequencies of the metabolites being imaged during a spectroscopy are between those of fat and water. There is more water in the brain than fat so, for a better spectroscopy, the sequence contains a "water suppression" pulse.

**Weighted or Weighting** A concept of having more of one thing over another. When an image is described as T1 weighted, it means that the contrast seen is mostly due to the T1 relaxation characteristics of tissues. There is always a mixture of all three contrasts present in any image. You cannot eliminate any one contrast, just minimize it. See the weighting triangle in Chapter 3.

**White matter (WM)** Is the inner layer of brain tissue made up mostly of myelinated axons. Myelin is a fatty (lipid-rich) substance surrounding nerve cells (the nervous system's "wires"). Myelin insulates the "wires" from each other.

**White matter tractography diffusion tensor imaging (DTI)** A DWI sequence capable of imaging the white matter tracts in the brain. It is akin to or has a similar imaging theory to that of TOF MRA. Diffusion of white matter cells or tracts runs mostly within the cells, similar to blood flowing in a vessel. It diffuses little through the cell membrane. White matter tractography shows the location of the tracts and can be useful in surgical planning in the brain.

**Wobble (Wo, or Frequency)** Also symbolized as "gamma," symbol $\gamma$.

**Wrap (also known as Aliasing or Fold-over)** An artifact caused by tissue being outside of the FOV in the phase direction. The Nyquist theorem was not satisfied.

**X/Y plane** Another term for the transverse plane.

**Z plane or axis** Longitudinal or $B_0$.

# Index

## A

Abdominal aorta, 12, 36, 194, 315
Aberrant, 28, 41
Achilles tendon, 11, 193
ACL, 14, 319, 320
Acquisition/Nex/NSA, 99, 101, 340–341
Aliasing, 87, 333
Allergic reaction, signs and
     symptoms of, 7
Analog to digital converter (ADC), 129
Anaphylactic reaction, signs or
     symptoms of, 23
Anisotropic, 132, 181, 343, 344
Annifact artifact, 294, 336
Anosmia, 16, 38, 231
Anterior, 26
Anti-aliasing options, 59
Aortic arch, 13, 35, 195, 301, 302, 313
Arnold Chiari, suspected, 14
Artifact, 92, 109, 127, 137, 152, 157,
     180, 181, 245, 275–296, 299,
     333–337, 344, 345
Aseptic technique, 25
Atrophy, 28
Avascular necrosis, 11, 35, 76, 193
Axial plane (aka Z plane), 160, 174, 176,
     182, 190, 197, 205, 208, 215, 220,
     225, 231, 232, 241, 252, 257, 268,
     272, 304, 308, 316, 317, 319, 322,
     323, 325, 332, 346

## B

$B_0$, 46, 47, 51, 55, 60, 94–97
$B_1$, 34, 48, 51, 56, 95, 182
Background noise, 53
Background suppression of MRA
     sequences, 91
Bandwidth (B/W), 80, 82, 94, 100, 105,
     109, 130, 152, 164, 180, 181, 344
Basic scan time formula, 125
BBB. See Blood brain barrier (BBB)
Bell's palsy, 16
Beneficence/benefactor, 22
Blood brain barrier (BBB), 8, 33, 34, 41
     non-contact, gadolinium
          administration and, 5, 27
     normal enhancing structures outside, 8
Blood pressure
     instrument, 4
     systolic, 3, 32
Blood supply to bone, decreased, 11
Blood vessels
     pressure in, 12
     tangled collection of, 16
Blurring, 64
Body coil, 58
Body temperature, 8
Bolus, 27
Bound protons, 51
Bowel and bladder dysfunction, 10, 16
Bradycardia, 23

*MRI Registry Review: Tech to Tech Questions and Answers*, First Edition. Stephen J. Powers.
© 2021 John Wiley & Sons Ltd. Published 2021 by John Wiley & Sons Ltd.

Brain hemorrhage, 17
B-Value or b-Factor, 161

C

Cardiac arrest, 2, 27
Carpal tunnel syndrome, 13
Cellular diffusion, 149
CE-MRA. *See* Contrast-enhanced
MRA (CE-MRA)
Center frequency (CF), 150, 293
Center lines (of *k*-space), 103, 119
Centric *k*-space filling, 138, 141, 150
Cerebral spinal fluid (CSF), 12, 36, 37, 84,
181, 190, 195, 248, 312, 313, 316,
317, 318, 326
Chemical shift, 67, 106, 150, 183, 345
Chemical shift artifact, 109, 127, 180,
181, 334, 344
Circle of Willis (COW), 208, 209, 300
Coarctation, 30
Coil(s), 9, 35, 39, 45, 49, 58, 59, 61–63, 72,
73, 93, 94, 96–98, 253, 336, 347, 348
angle orientation, 58
inherent body, 58
long row, 58
quadrature, 58
signal in, 59
size of, 62
surface, 62
Collapsed images, 141
Concatenations (acquisitions),
101, 340–341
Contrast, 34, 39, 41, 53, 54, 64, 67, 75, 83,
89–91, 94, 97–99, 101, 103, 105–
107, 120, 122, 138–140, 145–147,
151, 158, 161, 162, 165, 183, 187,
189, 190, 286, 299, 312–313, 316,
317, 326, 329, 333, 335–337, 346
Contrast-enhanced MRA (CE-MRA),
105, 139, 301
Conventional bore scanner, 54
Conventional spin echo (CSE),
138, 156, 176
COPD, 19
Copper lining, in scan room, 10
Corduroy artifact, 290
Coronal plane, 37, 201

COW. *See* Circle of Willis (COW)
Cranial nerves, largest diameter, 16, 26
Cryogen, 9, 33–35
CSE. *See* Conventional spin echo (CSE)
CSF. *See* Cerebral spinal fluid (CSF)

D

dB/dT, 7, 33–34
De-oxygenated blood in arteries, 18
De-phasing, 49, 180
Desiccate, 28
Diamagnetic, 54, 56, 96, 97
Diethylenetriamine
pentaacetate (DTPA), 8
Difficulty swallowing, 15
Diffusion, 89, 149, 185
Diffusion weighted imaging (DWI), 40,
89, 149, 161, 185
Dipole–dipole interaction, 72
Dixon method or technique, 182,
183, 345–346
DTPA. *See* Diethylenetriamine
pentaacetate (DTPA)
DWI. *See* Diffusion weighted
imaging (DWI)
Dyspnea, 15

E

Echo, 77
partial, 114
spacing, 88, 98
train, 119–121, 135, 143, 176,
182, 341, 348
Ectomy, 27
Eddy currents, 72, 85
Effective TE (ETE), 84m, 122, 138
Elliptical centric *k*-space filling, 138, 141
Emesis, 4
Equilibrium, 46, 47, 63, 72, 94, 95, 98
Ernst angle, 104
Erythrocyte, 18
Estimated glomerular filtration rate
(eGFR), 21, 39, 256
ETE. *See* Effective TE (ETE)
Excitation pulse, 47, 50, 59, 60, 77,
78, 95, 96, 98, 101, 103,
104, 176, 181

## F

Faraday cage, 10, 35
Faraday's law of induction, 49, 94, 96
Fast spin echo (FSE), 33, 57, 64, 73, 84, 97,
    101, 105, 121, 127, 135, 138, 148,
    156, 161, 174, 176, 178, 180, 335,
    341–343, 348
Fat
  brightest, 92
  saturation (fat-sat, F/S), 64, 101, 127,
      137, 180, 189, 346
  and water
    chemical shift between, 67
    processional frequency difference
        between, 45, 92
FDA
  limit for clinical scanning, 21
  limits for heating due to RF, 6
  safe Gauss line limit, 2
Febrile, 24
Ferrous, 6, 56, 96, 97
Ferrous object, 6
FID. See Free induction decay (FID)
Field of view (FOV), 69, 70, 73, 76, 82,
    100, 102, 105, 106, 117, 122–124,
    125, 132, 133, 142, 152, 154, 159,
    163, 164, 174, 178, 179, 181, 187,
    334, 336, 343, 344, 347, 348
FLAIR. See Fluid attention inversion
    recovery (FLAIR)
Flip angle (F/A), 21, 34, 39, 71, 80, 81, 86,
    91, 100, 104–106, 129–131, 134,
    159, 181, 182, 187, 347, 348
Flow compensation (flow comp, gradient
    motion refocusing (GMR),
    gradient motion nulling (GMN)),
    134, 136, 157, 182, 186
Flow-related enhancement, 70, 188
Flow types, 337, 338
Flow void, 71, 100, 316
Fluid attention inversion recovery
    (FLAIR), 35, 73, 90, 190,
    313, 318, 332
Fold-over, 333
Fourier transform, 59, 162, 163, 180, 184
FOV. See Field of view (FOV)
Fractional or partial echo, 114

Free induction decay (FID), 48, 55, 94,
    97, 98, 177
Free protons, 56
Frequency, 54, 92, 99, 102, 103, 106, 141,
    159, 163, 174–176, 179, 277–279,
    333, 335, 339, 344
  direction, 84, 130, 135, 180–182, 185,
      282
  Larmor, 46, 100
  matrix, 129, 159, 344
  processional, 45, 56, 78, 79, 87, 94,
      109, 152, 166
  radiofrequency, 54
Frequency encoding gradient (FEG), 83,
    100, 103, 115
Fringe field, 6
Fringe magnetic fields, controlling/
    limiting, 12
FSE. See Fast spin echo (FSE)

## G

Gadolinium, 34, 84, 133, 139, 146,
    160, 254, 257
  and allergic reactions, 29
  caution for, 8
  contraindications for, 3, 32
  ions, 75
  and non-intact BBB, 5, 27
  for normal intracranial tissues
      enhancement, 27
  to nursing mother, 3
  short tau inversion recovery
      sequence, 83
Gauss, 2, 6, 31–33, 35, 52, 53, 95, 108
Gibbs artifact, 299
GMR. See Gyromagnetic ratio (GMR)
GM. See Grey matter (GM)
Gradient, 40, 62, 83, 94, 103–105, 114,
    119, 128, 134, 138, 146, 164, 168,
    169, 190, 305
  echo, 50, 54, 74, 81, 101, 116, 117, 121,
      174, 176, 348
  during echo formation, 114
  field, 33, 34
  frequency encoding, 115
  phase, 115
  warp, 284, 286, 290, 296

Gradient recalled echo (GRE), 33, 74, 77, 82, 88, 101, 105, 106, 113, 115, 129, 130, 135, 144, 150, 151, 160, 174, 176, 177, 180–183, 185, 187, 191, 286, 288, 304, 335, 349
GRE. *See* Gradient recalled echo (GRE)
Grey matter (GM), 313
Gyromagnetic ratio (GMR), 52, 53, 55, 56, 94, 339

**H**

Half Fourier, 142, 162
Heart chamber
    most anterior, 14
    most posterior, 14
Heat, factors influencing patient's ability to dissipate, 5
Heavy blood loss, 25
Helium, 33, 34, 59, 97
Hematocrit, 10, 15
High-resolution imaging, 76
High-velocity signal loss (HVSL), 100, 316
Hives, 18
HVSL. *See* High-velocity signa loss (HVSL)
Hydrogen
    gyromagnetic ratio of, 52, 53, 55
    in MR medical imaging, 55, 57
    precessional frequency of, 79
    proton, magnetic moment of, 55
    spins, distribution or concentration of, 60
Hydrogen density, 54, 62
    weighted image, 68
Hypertrophy, 28
Hypo, 29
Hypoglycemia, 21

**I**

Image contrast, 67
Image quality, 126, 139
Imaging coils, inspection of, 9
Imaging procedure, 22
Implants status, 20
Inability to speak, 15
Indwelling urinary foley catheters, 23
Infectious process, 15

Inferior, 26
Informed consent, 1, 7, 31
In phase, 98, 138, 333–335, 345, 346
In-plane saturation, 101
Insulin administration, excessive, 22
Intraocular metallic foreign body, standard of care, 20
Inversion pulse, 81
Inversion recovery, 81, 83, 100, 101, 105, 159, 342
IR (STIR or FLAIR) sequence, 73
Islet cells, 11
Isocenter
    magnetic strength in, 9
    objects away from, 7
    objects closest to, 6
Isotropic, 68, 69, 125, 126, 179, 343, 344, 349
Itis, 29
I.V. bag, 4

**K**

*k*-space, 74, 84, 86, 97, 103, 105, 119, 121, 135, 138, 139, 141–143, 150, 161, 162, 176, 177, 184, 340

**L**

Lack of oxygen to brain, condition of, 23
Laminectomy, 29
Larmor equation, 49, 56, 94, 95, 339, 340
Larmor frequency, 46, 100
Lateral, 25
Leukocyte, 19
Libel, 2, 32
Ligamentum teres, 13
Liquid helium, 59
Localization
    light, and eye damage, 4
    spatial signal, 46
LOCS, in 3D sequence, 78
Longitudinal NMV, 82
Longitudinal relaxation, 62
Lumbar plexus, nerve roots of, 15

**M**

Magnetic dipole, 52
Magnetic dipole moment, 48
Magnetic field inhomogeneity, 88

Magnetic states of material, 56
Magnetic susceptibility, 49, 56, 88,
    90, 105, 148
Magnetism, 61
Main magnetic field, 48
Mask, conditions for wearing, 3
Matrix, 68–70, 74, 101, 106, 117,
    122–125, 129, 132, 133, 142,
    159, 163, 182, 336, 337, 343,
    344, 347, 348
Maximum intensity projection, 183
Medial, 25
Medical emergency, in scan room, 23
Meninges
    inner and outer most, 17
    layers of, 17
Minimum TE (Min. TE), 80, 89, 344
Monitoring, 5
    verbal, 3
    visual, 5
MR conditional, 20
MRCP, 24, 76
MR safe, 20
MR unsafe, 20
M.S. plaques, sequence of, 11
Multiple slices, imaging of, 92
Multi-shot, 188

N

Nephrectomy, 28
Net magnetization vector (NMV), 46, 47,
    49, 50, 55, 58, 63, 72, 73, 78, 82, 94,
    95, 98, 104, 181, 335
Nex/NSA/Acq, 83, 99
NMV. *See* Net magnetization
    vector (NMV)
Noise, 7, 33–34, 53, 56, 58, 62, 97, 340
Nonmaleficence, 22
Nosocomial infection, 22
N.P.O., 7
Nyquist theorem, 334

O

One T1 time, 47, 55, 73
One T2 time, 47, 55
Oophorectomy, 28
Orthogonal, 95, 323
Ostomy, 27

Outer lines, 138, 141
Out of phase (OOP) TE, 136–138, 183,
    288, 289, 344–346
Oxygenated blood, 21

P

Pacemakers, fringe field line for, 6
Parallel imaging, 86, 87, 158, 160, 163
Paramagnetic, 96
Partial Fourier, 184
Partial volume effect, 103, 108
Patent airway, 18
Pathogens, 25
Patient interactions and
    management, 1–44
Pediatric brain, gray/white matter
    differentiation in, 14
Perfusion, 40, 64, 158, 185, 273
Peripheral nerve stimulation (PNS), 24,
    34, 40, 185
Permanent magnet, 65
Phase contrast, 105, 145, 146
Phase encoding, 77, 333
Phase encoding gradient, 115, 117, 119
Photo phosphenes, 7, 62
Pituitary stalk, 13
Pixels, 68–70, 92, 100, 101, 105, 109,
    122, 132, 179–181, 334, 336, 337,
    343, 344, 347
Popliteal, 29
Posterior, 26
Precession, 73
Precessioninal frequency, 45, 56, 78, 79,
    87, 94, 109, 152, 166
Prefixes, 30
Pre-scan, 87
Prostate and bladder, relation between, 11
Protons
    bound, 51
    density, 35, 50, 58, 85, 96
    equilibrium state of, 63
    free, 56
    in magnetic field, 63
    parallel aligned, 63
    realigned with $B_0$, 60
    spin, 79
    states of, 51
Pulse measurement, typical sites for, 10

## Q

Quench, 4, 6, 7, 33–35

## R

Radiofrequencies, transmitted range of, 54
Radiofrequency, 54
Radiologists
    order or protocol revision, 26
Raw data, 97, 162
Readout gradient, length of time of, 83
Receiver bandwidth, 82
Refocusing pulse, 91, 182
Relaxation, 67, 99, 126
    definition of, 50
    longitudinal, 62
    magnetic susceptibilities and, 49
    shortest time, 66
    spin–spin, 97, 182
    T1, 50, 57, 72, 103, 107, 181, 258, 338
    T2, 49–51, 57, 72, 107, 176, 182, 313
Relaxation curve, 99, 107
Rephasing, 49
Residual transverse NMV, 82
Res Ipsa Loquitur, 2
Resistive magnets, 6, 33
Resolution, 60
Revolving/alternating magnetic field, 45
RF application to patient, higher, 6
RF deposits in the body, 8
RF pulses, in MR imaging, 80
Right lateral recumbent position, 29
Right to the patient's medical history, 19
Rise time, 169, 190
R/O metallic foreign body, 3

## S

Safety zones in MRI suite, 19
Sagittal plane, 37, 273
SAR. *See* Specific absorption rate (SAR)
Saturated tissue, 81
Saturation, 101, 133, 137, 181, 333
Saturation pulse, 75, 77, 80, 133, 152, 160, 163, 349
Scan time, 117
Sciatic nerve, 12

Scoliosis in spine, visualization of, 14
Sequence identification, 114
Sequential, 348
Serum creatinine, 13
Shimming, 90
Shortest relaxation time, 66
Short time (Tau) inversion recovery (STIR), 105, 179
Signal intensity between tissues, 48, 65, 66
Signal to noise ratio (SNR, S/R), 58, 62, 63, 68, 69, 72, 76, 80, 82–86, 97, 99, 100, 102–105, 121, 125, 130, 131, 133–135, 154, 163, 165, 181, 182, 333, 334, 340–341, 344, 346–347
Sims/Recovery position, 19
Single shot, 148, 150, 161
Slew rate, 169, 190
Slice location, 68
Slice select gradient (SSG), 169, 174, 347
Slice thickness, 70, 71, 86
Small pixels, 68
Spatial localization, 79
Spatial resolution, 51, 96, 139
Spatial signal localization, 46
Specific absorption rate (SAR), 33, 34, 39, 80, 84, 104, 116, 119, 123, 124, 148, 178, 187
    definition of, 5
    limits of, 9, 105
Spin echo, 50, 55, 74, 75, 80, 101, 105, 115, 116, 121, 135, 138, 150, 165, 174, 176, 177, 181, 341
Spin-lattice, 97, 101
Spin–spin relaxation, 97, 182
"SPOILED" GRE sequence, 77
Spoiling/Spoiled, 77, 82, 83
SSG. *See* Slice select gradient (SSG)
Static magnetic field, 193
Steady state, 144, 180
Stenosis, 30
STIR. *See* Short time (Tau) inversion recovery (STIR)
Stricture, 30
Subtraction, 105
Superconductor, 61
Superior, 26

Suppression, 91, 105, 165, 181, 185, 187
Supraspinatus muscle, 25
Surface coil, 62
Swap phase and frequency, 285, 295
Syncope, 17, 18
Systolic blood pressure, 2, 32

## T

Tau, 102
TE. *See* Time to echo (TE)
Technologists to wear
   contact precautions for, 3
   respiratory precautions for, 4
Temporal resolution, 56, 139
Tesla, 78
3D sequence, 70, 78, 84, 101, 105, 107,
   126, 131–133, 135, 140, 154–157,
   160, 164, 181, 182, 188, 246
Time, 82
Time of flight (TOF), 70, 75, 77, 100,
   133, 140, 141, 155–157, 160–162,
   298, 335, 342
Time to echo (TE), 49, 67, 68, 74, 80, 81,
   84, 86, 89, 94, 101–103, 105, 106,
   115–117, 122–125, 129, 130, 132–
   134, 136–138, 141, 144, 154, 158,
   159, 163, 178, 179, 181, 182, 187,
   226, 329, 333, 335
Time-varying magnetic fields, 5, 61
Tissue contrast, 64
Tissue saturation, 333
TOF. *See* Time of flight (TOF)
T1 relaxation, 72, 103, 107, 181, 258, 338
   long, 73
   and proton density, 50, 57
Tortuosity, 30
Transmission of infection, 22
Transmitted range of frequencies, 46
Transmitter bandwidth, 164
Transverse magnetization, at
   equilibrium, 46
Transverse net magnetization, 61
Transverse plane, 78, 94, 107
Truncated, 30

Truncation artifact, 334, 336, 337
TSE/FSE sequence, 64
TSE. *See* Turbo spin echo (TSE)
T2 relaxation, 49, 57, 72, 107, 176, 182, 313
   long, 73
   and proton density, 50
   timing of, 51
Turbo spin echo (TSE), 33, 64, 105, 118,
   138, 165, 341, 349
T wave elevation, during an MRI, 12
2D sequence, 70, 101, 105, 129, 132, 133,
   140, 155–157, 160, 161, 180, 181,
   298, 341, 342, 346, 347
Tympanoplasty, 9

## U

Unresponsive/unconscious patient, 23

## V

Vascular necrosis, femur issues and, 11
Vasovagal/syncopal episode, 17
Vectors
   accumulation, with external static
      external magnetic field, 78
   attributes of, 48
   properties of, 61
Venous drainage of the liver, 13
Verbal monitoring, 3
Vertebral arteries, 16
Vertebral bodies, identification of, 76
Visual monitoring, 3
Voxel(s), 105, 109, 156
   isotropic, 125, 126, 179, 343
   size, 69, 90, 100, 187
   volume, 69, 100, 122, 132, 343–344

## W

White matter, 14, 37, 102, 106,
   273, 312, 313
Wilms tumor, 7
Wobble, 48

## Z

Zone 1, for general public, 19